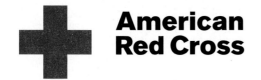

American
Red Cross

P9-CLR-763

American Red Cross
First Aid/CPR/AED

PARTICIPANT'S MANUAL

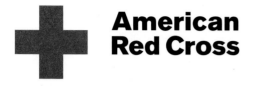
American Red Cross

This participant's manual is part of the American Red Cross First Aid/CPR/AED program. By itself, it does not constitute complete and comprehensive training. Visit redcross.org to learn more about this program.

The emergency care procedures outlined in this book reflect the standard of knowledge and accepted emergency practices in the United States at the time this book was published. It is the reader's responsibility to stay informed of changes in emergency care procedures.

Published by StayWell Health & Safety Solutions

Printed in the United States of America

ISBN: 978-1-58480-479-6

Acknowledgments

This is the fourth edition of the *American Red Cross First Aid/CPR/AED Participant's Manual*. This is a revised version of the text that was previously published under the title, *First Aid/CPR/AED for Schools and the Community*.

This manual is dedicated to the thousands of employees and volunteers of the American Red Cross who contribute their time and talent to supporting and teaching life-saving skills worldwide and to the thousands of course participants and other readers who have decided to be prepared to take action when an emergency strikes.

This manual reflects the 2010 Consensus on Science for CPR and Emergency Cardiovascular Care (ECC) and the Guidelines 2010 for First Aid. These treatment recommendations and related training guidelines have been reviewed by the American Red Cross Scientific Advisory Council, a panel of nationally recognized experts in fields that include emergency medicine, occupational health, sports medicine, school and public health, emergency medical services (EMS), aquatics, emergency preparedness and disaster mobilization.

The *American Red Cross First Aid/CPR/AED Participant's Manual* was developed through the dedication of both employees and volunteers. Their commitment to excellence made this manual possible.

Table of Contents

About This Manual

This manual has been designed to help you acquire the knowledge and skills you will need to effectively respond to emergency situations. The following pages point out some of the manual's special features.

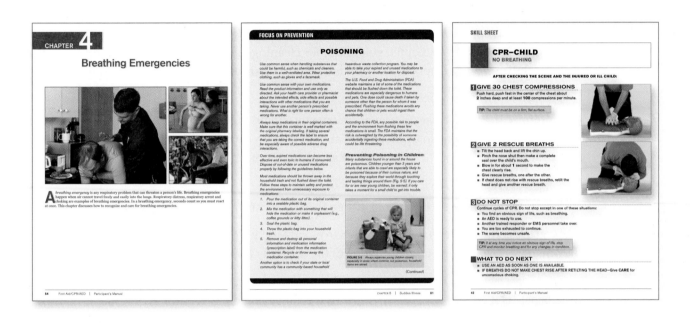

Chapter Openers
Each chapter concentrates on an essential component of the American Red Cross First Aid/CPR/AED course. Material is presented in a clear and concise manner, complete with color imagery.

Prevention and Preparedness Boxes
These sidebars expand on the essential prevention and preparedness information covered in the course. They appear in most chapters.

Skill Sheets
At the end of certain chapters, skill sheets give step-by-step directions for performing specific skills. Photographs enhance each skill sheet. Learning specific skills that you will need to give appropriate care for victims of sudden illness or injury is an important part of this course.

Health Precautions and Guidelines During First Aid Training

The American Red Cross has trained millions of people in first aid and cardiopulmonary resuscitation (CPR) using manikins as training aids. The Red Cross follows widely accepted guidelines for cleaning and decontaminating training manikins. **If these guidelines are adhered to, the risk of any kind of disease transmission during training is extremely low.**

To help minimize the risk of disease transmission, you should follow some basic health precautions and guidelines while participating in training. You should take precautions if you have a condition that would increase your risk or other participants' risk of exposure to infections. Request a separate training manikin if you—

- Have an acute condition, such as a cold, a sore throat, or cuts or sores on the hands or around your mouth.

- Know you are seropositive (have had a positive blood test) for hepatitis B surface antigen (HBsAg), indicating that you are currently infected with the hepatitis B virus.*

- Know you have a chronic infection indicated by long-term seropositivity (long-term positive blood tests) for the hepatitis B surface antigen (HBsAg)* or a positive blood test for anti-HIV (that is, a positive test for antibodies to HIV, the virus that causes many severe infections including AIDS).

- Have had a positive blood test for hepatitis C (HCV).

- Have a type of condition that makes you unusually likely to get an infection.

To obtain information about testing for individual health status, visit the CDC Web site at: **www.cdc.gov/ncidod/diseases/hepatitis/c/faq.htm**

After a person has had an acute hepatitis B infection, he or she will no longer test positive for the surface antigen but will test positive for the hepatitis B antibody (anti-HBs). Persons who have been vaccinated for hepatitis B will also test positive for the hepatitis antibody. A positive test for the hepatitis B antibody (antiHBs) should not be confused with a positive test for the hepatitis B surface antigen (HBsAG).

If you decide you should have your own manikin, ask your instructor if he or she can provide one for you to use. You will *not* be asked to explain why in your request. The manikin will not be used by anyone else until it has been cleaned according to the recommended end-of-class decontamination procedures. Because the number of manikins available for class use is limited, the more advance notice you give, the more likely it is that you can be provided a separate manikin.

*A person with hepatitis B infection will test positive for the hepatitis B surface antigen (HBsAg). Most persons infected with hepatitis B will get better within a period of time. However, some hepatitis B infections will become chronic and will linger for much longer. These persons will continue to test positive for HBsAg. Their decision to participate in CPR training should be guided by their physician.

Some people are sensitive to certain allergens and may have an allergic reaction. If you start experiencing skin redness, rash, hives, itching, runny nose, sneezing, itchy eyes, scratchy throat or signs of asthma, wash your hands immediately. If conditions persist or you experience a severe reaction, stop training and seek medical attention right away.

GUIDELINES

In addition to taking the precautions regarding manikins, you can further protect yourself and other participants from infection by following these guidelines:

- Wash your hands thoroughly before participating in class activities.

- Do not eat, drink, use tobacco products or chew gum during class when manikins are used.

- Clean the manikin properly before use.

- For some manikins, this means vigorously wiping the manikin's face and the inside of its mouth with a clean gauze pad soaked with either a fresh solution of liquid chlorine bleach and water ($\frac{1}{4}$ cup sodium hypochlorite per gallon of tap water) or rubbing alcohol. The surfaces should remain wet for at least 1 minute before they are wiped dry with a second piece of clean, absorbent material.

- For other manikins, it means changing the manikin's face. Your instructor will provide you with instructions for cleaning the type of manikin used in your class.

- Follow the guidelines provided by your instructor when practicing skills such as clearing a blocked airway with your finger.

PHYSICAL STRESS AND INJURY

Successful course completion requires full participation in classroom and skill sessions, as well as successful performance in skill and knowledge evaluations. Due to the nature of the skills in this course, you will be participating in strenuous activities, such as performing CPR on the floor. If you have a medical condition or disability that will prevent you from taking part in the skills practice sessions, please let your instructor know so that accommodations can be made. If you are unable to participate fully in the course, participate as much as you can or desire. Be aware that you will *not* be eligible to receive a course completion certificate unless you participate fully and meet all course objectives and prerequisites.

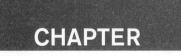

CHAPTER 1

Before Giving Care and Checking an Injured or Ill Person

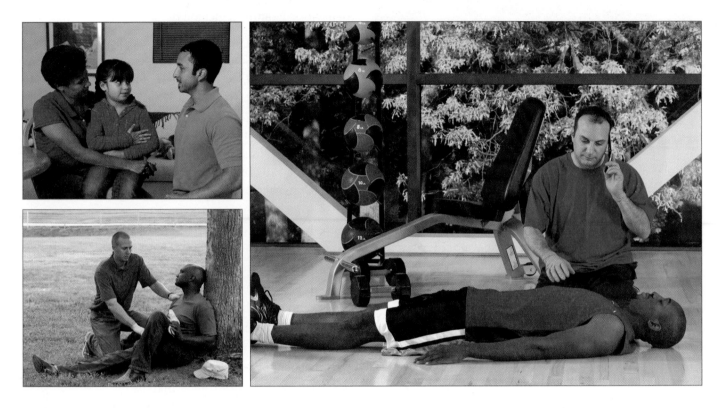

Medical emergencies can happen every day, in any setting. People are injured in situations like falls or motor-vehicle accidents, or they develop sudden illnesses, such as heart attack or stroke.

The statistics are sobering. For example, about 900,000 people in the United States die each year from some form of heart disease. More than 300,000 of these deaths are caused by sudden cardiac arrest. Heart disease is the number one cause of death in this country.

Another leading cause of death is unintentional injury. In 2008, approximately 118,000 Americans died from an unintentional injury and another 25.7 million were disabled.

Given the large number of injuries and sudden illnesses that occur in the United States each year, it is possible that you might have to deal with an emergency situation someday. If you do, you should know who and when to call, what care to give and how to give that care until emergency medical help takes over.

This chapter discusses your role in the emergency medical services (EMS) system, the purpose of Good Samaritan laws, how to gain consent from an injured or ill person and how to reduce your risk of disease transmission while giving care.

In addition, you will read about the emergency action steps, **CHECK—CALL—CARE**, which guide you on how to check and give emergency care for an injured or suddenly ill person. You also will read about the effects of incident stress and how to identify the signals of shock and minimize its effects.

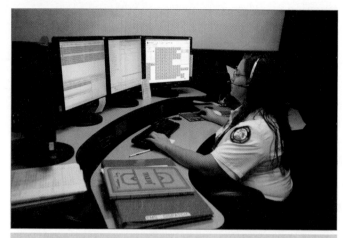

FIGURE 1-1 *EMS call taker or dispatcher*

YOUR ROLE IN THE EMS SYSTEM

You play a major role in making the EMS system work effectively. The EMS system is a network of community resources, including police, fire and medical personnel—and you.

The system begins when someone like you recognizes that an emergency exists and decides to take action, such as calling 9-1-1 or the local emergency number for help. The EMS dispatcher or call taker answers the call and uses the information that you give to determine what help is needed (Fig. 1-1). Emergency personnel are dispatched to the scene based on the information given. These personnel then give care at the scene and transport the injured or ill person to the hospital where emergency department staff and other professionals take over.

Early arrival of emergency personnel increases a person's chance of surviving a life-threatening emergency. Calling 9-1-1 or the local emergency number is the most important action that you can take.

Your role in the EMS system includes four basic steps:

Step 1: Recognize that an emergency exists.

Step 2: Decide to act.

Step 3: Activate the EMS system.

Step 4: Give care until help takes over.

Step 1: Recognize that an Emergency Exists

Emergencies can happen to anyone, anywhere. Before you can give help, however, you must be able to recognize an emergency. You may realize that an emergency has occurred only if you become aware of unusual noises, sights, odors and appearances or behaviors. Examples include the following:

- Unusual noises
  - Screaming, moaning, yelling or calls for help
  - Breaking glass, crashing metal or screeching tires
  - A change in the sound made by machinery or equipment
  - Sudden, loud noises, such as the sound of collapsing buildings or falling ladders
  - Unusual silence
- Unusual sights
  - A stopped vehicle on the roadside or a car that has run off of the road
  - Downed electrical wires
  - A person lying motionless
  - Spilled medication or empty container
  - An overturned pot in the kitchen
  - Sparks, smoke or fire (Fig. 1-2, A)
- Unusual odors
  - Odors that are stronger than usual
  - Unrecognizable odors
  - Inappropriate odors
- Unusual appearances or behaviors
  - Unconsciousness (Fig. 1-2, B)
  - Confusion, drowsiness or unusual behavior (Fig. 1-2, C)
  - Trouble breathing
  - Sudden collapse, slip or fall

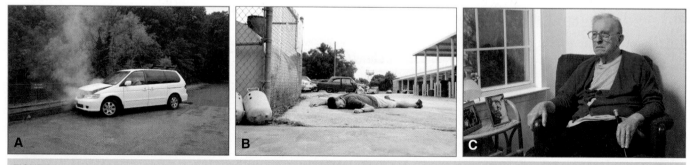

FIGURE 1-2, A–C *Unusual sights or behavior may indicate an emergency.*

- Clutching the chest or throat
- A person doubled over in pain
- Slurred, confused or hesitant speech
- Sweating for no apparent reason
- Uncharacteristic skin color
- Inability to move a body part

Step 2: Decide to Act

Once you recognize that an emergency has occurred, you must decide how to help and what to do. There are many ways you can help in an emergency, but in order to help, you must act.

Overcoming Barriers to Act

Being faced with an emergency may bring out mixed feelings. While wanting to help, you also may feel hesitant or may want to back away from the situation. These feelings are personal and real.

Sometimes, even though people recognize that an emergency has occurred, they fail to act. The most common factors that keep people from responding are:

- Panic or fear of doing something wrong
- Being unsure of the person's condition and what to do
- Assuming someone else will take action
- Type of injury or illness
- Fear of catching a disease (see the Disease Transmission and Prevention section in this chapter)
- Fear of being sued (see discussion of Good Samaritan laws in this chapter)
- Being unsure of when to call 9-1-1 or the local emergency number

Panic or Fear of Doing Something Wrong

People react differently in emergencies. Some people are afraid of doing the wrong thing and making matters worse. Sometimes people simply panic. Knowing what to do in an emergency can instill confidence that can help you to avoid panic and be able to provide the right care. If you are not sure what to do, call 9-1-1 or the local emergency number and follow the instructions of the EMS dispatcher or call taker. The worst thing to do is nothing.

Being Unsure of the Person's Condition and What to Do

Because most emergencies happen in or near the home, you are more likely to find yourself giving care to a family member or a friend than to someone you do not know. However, you may be faced with an emergency situation involving a stranger, and you might feel uneasy about helping someone whom you do not know. For example, the person may be much older or much younger than you, be of a different gender or race, have a disabling condition, be of a different status at work or be the victim of a crime.

Sometimes, people who have been injured or become suddenly ill may act strangely or be uncooperative. The injury or illness; stress; or other factors, such as the effects of drugs, alcohol or medications, may make people unpleasant or angry. Do not take this behavior personally. If you feel at all threatened by the person's behavior, leave the immediate area and call 9-1-1 or the local emergency number for help.

Assuming Someone Else Will Take Action

If several people are standing around, it might not be easy to tell if anyone is giving care. Always ask if you can help. Just because there is a crowd does not mean someone is caring for the injured or ill person. In fact, you may be the only one on the scene who knows first aid.

Although you may feel embarrassed about coming forward in front of other people, this should not stop you from offering help. Someone has to take action in an emergency, and it may have to be you.

If others already are giving care, ask if you can help. If bystanders do not appear to be helping, tell them how to help. You can ask them to call 9-1-1 or the local emergency number, meet the ambulance and direct it to your location, keep the area free of onlookers and traffic, send them for blankets or other supplies such as a first aid kit or an automated external defibrillator (AED), or help to give care.

The Type of Injury or Illness

An injury or illness sometimes may be very unpleasant. Blood, vomit, bad odors, deformed body parts, or torn or burned skin can be very upsetting. You may have to turn away for a moment and take a few deep breaths to get control of your feelings before you can give care. If you still are unable to give care, you can help in other ways, such as volunteering to call 9-1-1 or the local emergency number.

Fear of Catching a Disease

Many people worry about the possibility of being infected with a disease while giving care. Although it is possible for diseases to be transmitted in a first aid situation, it is extremely unlikely that you will catch a disease this way. (For more information on disease transmission, see the Disease Transmission section in this chapter.)

Fear of Being Sued

Sometimes people worry that they might be sued for giving care. In fact, lawsuits against people who give emergency care at a scene of an accident are highly unusual and rarely successful.

Good Samaritan Laws

The vast majority of states and the District of Columbia have Good Samaritan laws that protect people against claims of negligence when they give emergency care in good faith without accepting anything in return. Good Samaritan laws usually protect citizens who act the same way that a "reasonable and prudent person" would if that person were in the same situation. For example, a reasonable and prudent person would:

- Move a person only if the person's life were in danger.
- Ask a conscious person for permission, also called consent, before giving care.
- Check the person for life-threatening conditions before giving further care.
- Call 9-1-1 or the local emergency number.
- Continue to give care until more highly trained personnel take over.

Good Samaritan laws were developed to encourage people to help others in emergency situations. They require the "Good Samaritan" to use common sense and a reasonable level of skill and to give only the type of emergency care for which he or she is trained. They assume each person would do his or her best to save a life or prevent further injury.

Non-professionals who respond to emergencies, also called "lay responders," rarely are sued for helping in an emergency. Good Samaritan laws protect the responder from financial responsibility. In cases in which a lay responder's actions were deliberately negligent or reckless or when the responder abandoned the person after starting care, the courts have ruled Good Samaritan laws do not protect the responder.

For more information about your state's Good Samaritan laws, contact a legal professional or check with your local library.

Being Unsure When to Call 9-1-1

People sometimes are afraid to call 9-1-1 or the local emergency number because they are not sure that the situation is a real emergency and do not want to waste the time of the EMS personnel.

Your decision to act in an emergency should be guided by your own values and by your knowledge of the risks that may be present. However, even if you decide not to give care, you should at least call 9-1-1 or the local emergency number to get emergency medical help to the scene.

Step 3: Activate the EMS System

Activating the EMS system by calling 9-1-1 or the local emergency number is the most important step you can take in an emergency. Remember, some facilities, such as hotels, office and university buildings, and some stores, require you to dial a 9 or some other number to get an outside line before you dial 9-1-1.

Also, a few areas still are without access to a 9-1-1 system and use a local emergency number instead. Becoming familiar with your local system is important because the rapid arrival of emergency medical help greatly increases a person's chance of surviving a life-threatening emergency.

When your call is answered, an emergency call taker (or dispatcher) will ask for your phone number, address, location of the emergency and questions to determine whether you need police, fire or medical assistance.

You should not hang up before the call taker does so. Once EMS personnel are on the way, the call taker may stay on the line and continue to talk with you. Many call takers also are trained to give first aid instructions so they can assist you with life-saving techniques until EMS personnel take over.

Step 4: Give Care Until Help Takes Over

This manual and the American Red Cross First Aid/ CPR/AED courses provide you with the confidence, knowledge and skills you need to give care to a person in an emergency medical situation.

In general, you should give the appropriate care to an ill or injured person until:

- You see an obvious sign of life, such as breathing.
- Another trained responder or EMS personnel take over.
- You are too exhausted to continue.
- The scene becomes unsafe.

If you are prepared for unforeseen emergencies, you can help to ensure that care begins as soon as possible for yourself, your family and your fellow citizens. If you are trained in first aid, you can give help that can save a life in the first few minutes of an emergency. First aid can be the difference between life and death. Often, it makes the difference between complete recovery and permanent disability. By knowing what to do and acting on that knowledge, you can make a difference.

Getting Permission to Give Care

People have a basic right to decide what can and cannot be done to their bodies. They have the legal right to accept or refuse emergency care. Therefore, before giving care to an injured or ill person, you must obtain the person's permission.

To get permission from a conscious person, you must first tell the person who you are, how much training you have (such as training in first aid, CPR and/or AED), what you think is wrong and what you plan to do. You also must ask if you may give care. When a conscious person who understands your questions and what you plan to do gives you permission to give care, this is called *expressed consent*. Do not touch or give care to a conscious person who refuses it. If the person refuses care or withdraws consent at any time, step back and call for more advanced medical personnel.

Sometimes, adults may not be able to give expressed consent. This includes people who are unconscious or unable to respond, confused, mentally impaired, seriously injured or seriously ill. In these cases, the law assumes that if the person could respond, he or she would agree to care. This is called *implied consent*.

If the conscious person is a child or an infant, permission to give care must be obtained from a parent or guardian when one is available. If the condition is life threatening, permission—or consent—is implied if a parent or guardian is not present. If the parent or guardian is present but does not give consent, do not give care. Instead, call 9-1-1 or the local emergency number.

DISEASE TRANSMISSION AND PREVENTION

Infectious diseases—those that can spread from one person to another—develop when germs invade the body and cause illness.

How Disease Spreads

The most common germs are bacteria and viruses. Bacteria can live outside of the body and do not depend on other organisms for life. The number of bacteria that infect humans is small, but some cause serious infections. These can be treated with medications called *antibiotics*.

Viruses depend on other organisms to live. Once in the body, it is hard to stop their progression. Few medications can fight viruses. The body's immune system is its number one protection against infection.

Bacteria and viruses spread from one person to another through direct or indirect contact. *Direct contact* occurs when germs from the person's blood or other body fluids pass directly into your body through breaks or cuts in your skin or through the lining of your mouth, nose or eyes.

Some diseases, such as the common cold, are transmitted by droplets in the air we breathe. They can be passed on through *indirect contact* with shared objects like spoons, doorknobs and pencils that have been exposed to the droplets. Fortunately, exposure to these germs usually is not adequate for diseases to be transmitted.

Animals, including humans and insects, also can spread some diseases through bites. Contracting a disease from a bite is rare in any situation and uncommon when giving first aid care.

Some diseases are spread more easily than others. Some of these, like the flu, can create discomfort but often are temporary and usually not serious for healthy adults.

Other germs can be more serious, such as the Hepatitis B virus (HBV), Hepatitis C virus (HCV) and Human Immunodeficiency Virus (HIV), which causes Acquired Immune Deficiency Syndrome (AIDS) (see HIV and AIDS box in this chapter). Although serious, they are not easily transmitted and are not spread by casual contact, such as shaking hands. The primary way to transmit HBV, HCV or HIV during first aid care is through blood-to-blood contact.

Preventing Disease Transmission

By following some basic guidelines, you can greatly decrease your risk of getting or transmitting an infectious disease while giving care or cleaning up a blood spill.

While Giving Care

To prevent disease transmission when giving care, follow what are known as *standard precautions:*

- Avoid contact with blood and other body fluids or objects that may be soiled with blood and other body fluids.
- Use protective CPR breathing barriers.
- Use barriers, such as disposable gloves, between the person's blood or body fluids and yourself.
- Before putting on personal protective equipment (PPE), such as disposable gloves, cover any of your own cuts, scrapes or sores with a bandage.
- Do not eat, drink or touch your mouth, nose or eyes when giving care or before you wash your hands after care has been given.

BE PREPARED FOR AN INJURY OR ILLNESS!

Important Information

- *Keep medical information about you and your family in a handy place, such as on the refrigerator door or in your car's glove compartment. Keep medical and insurance records up to date.*

- *Wear a medical ID tag, bracelet or necklace if you have a potentially serious medical condition, such as epilepsy, diabetes, heart disease or allergies.*

- *Make sure your house or apartment number is easy to read. Numerals are easier to read than spelled-out numbers.*

Emergency Telephone Numbers

- *Keep all emergency telephone numbers in a handy place, such as by the telephone or in the first aid kit. Include home and work numbers of family members and friends. Be sure to keep both lists current.*

- *If your wireless phone came pre-programmed with the auto-dial 9-1-1 feature turned on, turn off the feature.*

- *Do not program your phone to automatically dial 9-1-1 when one button, such as the "9" key is pressed. Unintentional 9-1-1 calls, which often occur with auto-dial keys, cause problems for emergency call centers.*

- *Lock your keypad when you're not using your wireless phone. This action prevents automatic calls to 9-1-1.*

- *Most communities are served by an emergency 9-1-1 telephone number. If your community does not operate on a 9-1-1 system, look up the numbers for the police, fire department and EMS personnel. Emergency numbers usually are listed in the front of the telephone book. Know the number for the National Poison Control Center Hotline, 1-800-222-1222, and post it on or near your telephones. Teach everyone in your home how and when to use these numbers.*

- *Many 9-1-1 calls in the United States are not emergencies. For this reason, some cities have started using 3-1-1 (or similar) as a number for people to call for non-emergency situations. Find out if your area uses this number. Remember, your local emergency number is for just that— emergencies! So, please use good judgment.*

First Aid Kit

- *Keep a first aid kit in your home, car, workplace and recreation area. A well-stocked first aid kit is a handy thing to have. Carry a first aid kit with you or know where you can find one. Find out the location of first aid kits where you work or for any place where you spend a lot of time. First aid kits come in many shapes and sizes. You can purchase one from redcross.org or the local American Red Cross chapter. Your local drug store may sell them. You also may make your own. Some kits are designed for specific activities, such as hiking, camping or boating. Whether you buy a first aid kit or put one together, make sure it has all of the items you may need. Include any personal items such as medications and emergency phone numbers or other items suggested by your health care provider. Check the kit regularly. Make sure that flashlight batteries work. Check expiration dates and replace any used or out-of-date contents.*

- *The Red Cross recommends that all first aid kits for a family of four include the following:*
  - *2 absorbent compress dressings (5 x 9 inches)*
  - *25 adhesive bandages (assorted sizes)*

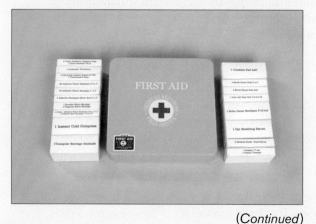

(Continued)

- 1 adhesive cloth tape (10 yards x 1 inch)
- 5 antibiotic ointment packets (approximately 1 gram each)
- 5 antiseptic wipe packets
- 2 packets of chewable aspirin (81 mg each)
- 1 blanket (space blanket)
- 1 CPR breathing barrier (with one-way valve)
- 1 instant cold compress
- 2 pairs of non-latex gloves (size: large)
- 2 hydrocortisone ointment packets (approximately 1 gram each)
- Scissors
- 1 roller bandage (3 inches wide)

- 1 roller bandage (4 inches wide)
- 5 sterile gauze pads (3 x 3 inches)
- 5 sterile gauze pads (4 x 4 inches)
- Oral thermometer (nonmercury/nonglass)
- 2 triangular bandages
- Tweezers
- First aid instruction booklet

For items to include in a workplace first aid kit, see the latest ANSI/ISEA-Z308-1 standard for minimum requirements.

Be Prepared

- Learn and practice CPR and first aid skills.
- Learn how to use an AED for victims of sudden cardiac arrest.

■ Avoid handling any of your personal items, such as pens or combs, while giving care or before you wash your hands.

■ Do not touch objects that may be soiled with blood or other body fluids.

■ Be prepared by having a first aid kit handy and stocked with PPE, such as disposable gloves, CPR breathing barriers, eye protection and other supplies.

■ Wash your hands thoroughly with soap and warm running water when you have finished giving care, even if you wore disposable gloves. Alcohol-based hand sanitizers allow you to clean your hands when soap and water are not readily available and your hands are not visibly soiled. (Keep alcohol-based hand sanitizers out of reach of children.)

■ Tell EMS personnel at the scene or your health care provider if you have come into contact with an injured or ill person's body fluids.

■ If an exposure occurs in a workplace setting, follow your company's exposure control plan for reporting incidents and follow-up (post-exposure) evaluation.

While Cleaning Up Blood Spills

To prevent disease transmission while cleaning up a blood spill:

■ Clean up the spill immediately or as soon as possible after the spill occurs (Fig. 1-3).

■ Use disposable gloves and other PPE when cleaning spills.

■ Wipe up the spill with paper towels or other absorbent material.

○ If the spill is mixed with sharp objects, such as broken glass or needles, do not pick these up with your hands. Use tongs, a broom and dustpan or two pieces of cardboard to scoop up the sharp objects.

■ After the area has been wiped up, flood the area with an appropriate disinfectant, such as a solution of approximately 1½ cups of liquid chlorine bleach

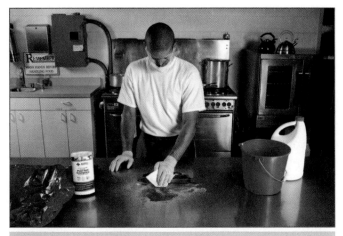

FIGURE 1-3 *Cleaning up a blood spill*

HIV AND AIDS

AIDS is a condition caused by HIV. When HIV infects the body, it damages the body's immune system and impairs its ability to fight other infections. The virus can grow quietly for months or even years. People infected with HIV might not feel or look sick. Eventually, the weakened immune system allows certain types of infections to develop. This condition is known as AIDS. People with AIDS eventually develop life-threatening infections, which can cause them to die. Because currently there is no vaccine against HIV, prevention still is the best tool.

The two most likely ways for HIV to be transmitted during care would be through:

- **Unprotected direct contact with infected blood.** This type of transmission could happen if infected blood or body fluids from one person enter another person's body at a correct entry site. For example, a responder could contract HIV if the infected person's blood splashes in the responder's eye or if the responder directly touches the infected person's body fluids.

- **Unprotected indirect contact with infected blood.** This type of transmission could happen if a person touches an object that contains the blood or other body fluids of an infected person, and that infected blood or other body fluid enters the body through a correct entry site. For example, HIV could be transmitted if a responder picks up a blood-soaked bandage with a bare hand and the infected blood enters the responder's hand through a cut in the skin.

The virus cannot enter through the skin unless there is a cut or break in the skin. Even then, the possibility of infection is very low unless there is direct contact for a lengthy period of time. Saliva is not known to transmit HIV.

The likelihood of HIV transmission during a first aid situation is very low. Always give care in ways that protect you and the person from disease transmission. For more information on preventing HIV transmission, see the Preventing Disease Transmission section in this chapter.

If you think you have put yourself at risk for an infectious disease, get tested. Tests are readily available and will tell whether your body is producing antibodies in response to the virus. If you are not sure whether you should be tested, call your health care provider, the public health department, an AIDS service organization or the AIDS hotline listed in the next paragraph.

If you have any questions about AIDS, call the Centers for Disease Control and Prevention (CDC), 24 hours a day, for information in English and Spanish at 1-800-232-4636. (TTY service is available at 1-888-232-6348.) You also can visit www.aids.gov or call your local or state health department.

---

to 1 gallon of fresh water (1 part bleach per 9 parts water), and allow it to stand for at least 10 minutes.

- Dispose of the contaminated material used to clean up the spill in a labeled biohazard container.

- Contact your worksite safety representative or your local health department regarding the proper disposal of potentially infectious material. For more information on preventing disease transmission, visit the federal Occupational Safety and Health administration: http://www.osha.gov/SLTC/bloodbornepathogens/index.html.

TAKING ACTION: EMERGENCY ACTION STEPS

In any emergency situation, follow the emergency action steps:

1. **CHECK** the scene and the person.
2. **CALL** 9-1-1 or the local emergency number.
3. **CARE** for the person.

CHECK

Before you can help an injured or ill person, make sure that the scene is safe for you and any bystanders (Fig. 1-4). Look the scene over and try to answer these questions:

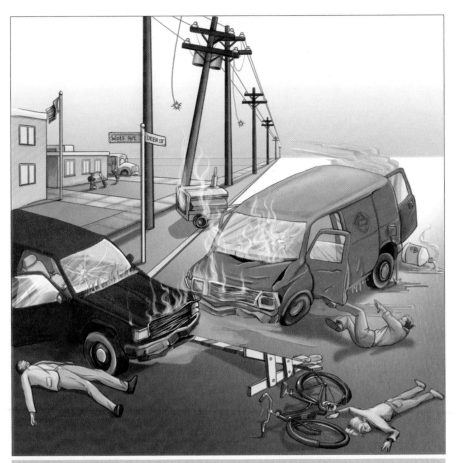

FIGURE 1-4 *Check the scene for anything that may threaten the safety of you, the injured persons and bystanders.*

- Is it safe?
- Is immediate danger involved?
- What happened?
- How many people are involved?
- Is anyone else available to help?
- What is wrong?

Is It Safe?

Check for anything unsafe, such as spilled chemicals, traffic, fire, escaping steam, downed electrical lines, smoke or extreme weather. Avoid going into confined areas with no ventilation or fresh air, places where there might be poisonous gas, collapsed structures, or places where natural gas, propane or other substances could explode. Such areas should be entered by responders who have special training and equipment, such as respirators and self-contained breathing apparatus.

If these or other dangers threaten, stay at a safe distance and call 9-1-1 or the local emergency number immediately. If the scene still is unsafe after you call, do not enter. Dead or injured heroes are no help to anyone! Leave dangerous situations to professionals like firefighters and police. Once they make the scene safe, you can offer to help.

Is Immediate Danger Involved?

Do not move a seriously injured person unless there is an immediate danger, such as fire, flood or poisonous gas; you have to reach another person who may have a more serious injury or illness; or you need to move the injured person to give proper care and you are able to do so without putting yourself in danger from the fire, flood or poisonous gas. If you must move the person, do it as quickly and carefully as possible. If there is no danger, tell the person not to move. Tell any bystanders not to move the person.

What Happened?

Look for clues to what caused the emergency and how the person might be injured. Nearby objects, such as a fallen ladder, broken glass or a spilled bottle of medicine, may give you information. Your check of the scene may be the only way to tell what happened.

If the injured or ill person is a child, keep in mind that he or she may have been moved by well-meaning adults. Be sure to ask about this when you are checking out what happened. If you find that a child has been moved, ask the adult where the child was and how he or she was found.

How Many People Are Involved?

Look carefully for more than one person. You might not spot everyone at first. If one person is bleeding or screaming, you might not notice an unconscious person. It also is easy to overlook a small child or an infant. In an emergency with more than one injured or ill person, you may need to prioritize care (in other words, decide who needs help first).

Is Anyone Else Available to Help?

You already have learned that the presence of bystanders does not mean that a person is receiving help. You may have to ask them to help. Bystanders may be able to tell you what happened or make the call for help while you provide care. If a family member, friend or co-worker is present, he or she may know if the person is ill or has a medical condition.

The injured or ill person may be too upset to answer your questions. Anyone who awakens after having been unconscious also may be frightened. Bystanders can help to comfort the person and others at the scene. A child may be especially frightened. Parents or guardians who are present may be able to calm a frightened child. They also can tell you if a child has a medical condition.

What Is Wrong?

When you reach the person, try to find out what is wrong. Look for signals that may indicate a life-threatening emergency. First, check to see if the injured or ill person is conscious (Fig. 1-5). Sometimes this is obvious. The person may be able to speak to you. He or she may be moaning, crying, making some other noise or moving around. If the person is conscious, reassure him or her and try to find out what happened.

If the person is lying on the ground, silent and not moving, he or she may be unconscious. If you are not sure whether someone is unconscious, tap him or her on the shoulder and ask if he or she is OK. Use the person's name if you know it. Speak loudly. If you are not sure whether an infant is unconscious, check by tapping the infant's shoulders and shouting or flicking the bottom of the infant's foot to see if the infant responds.

Unconsciousness is a life-threatening emergency. If the person does not respond to you in any way, assume that he or she is unconscious. Make sure that someone calls 9-1-1 or the local emergency number right away.

For purposes of first aid, an adult is defined as someone about age 12 (adolescent) or older; someone between the ages of 1 and 12 is considered to be a child; and an infant is someone younger than 1 year. When using an AED, a child is considered to be someone between the ages of 1 and 8 years or weighing less than 55 pounds.

Look for other signals of life-threatening injuries including trouble breathing, the absence of breathing or breathing that is not normal, and/or severe bleeding.

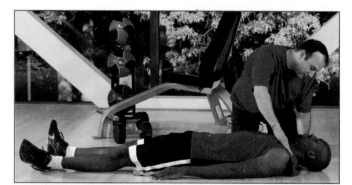

FIGURE 1-5 *When you reach the person, first check to see if he or she is conscious.*

While you are checking the person, use your senses of sight, smell and hearing. They will help you to notice anything abnormal. For example, you may notice an unusual smell that could be caused by a poison. You may see a bruise or a twisted arm or leg. You may hear the person say something that explains how he or she was injured.

Checking Children and the Elderly

Keep in mind that it is often helpful to take a slightly different approach when you check and care for children, infants and elderly people in an emergency situation. For more information on checking and caring for children, infants, the elderly and others with special needs, see Chapter 9.

Identifying Life-Threatening Conditions

At times you may be unsure if advanced medical personnel are needed. Your first aid training will help you to make this decision. The most important step you can take when giving care to a person who is unconscious or has some other life-threatening condition is to call for emergency medical help. With a life-threatening condition, the survival of a person often depends on both emergency medical help and the care you can give. You will have to use your best judgment—based on the situation, your assessment of the injured or ill person, information gained from this course and other training you may have received—to make the decision to call. When in doubt, and you think a life-threatening condition is present, make the call.

CALL

Calling 9-1-1 or the local emergency number for help often is the most important action you can take to help an injured or ill person (Fig. 1-6). It will send emergency medical help on its way as fast as possible. Make the call quickly and return to the person. If possible, ask someone else to make the call.

As a general rule, call 9-1-1 or the local emergency number if the person has any of the following conditions:

- Unconsciousness or an altered level of consciousness (LOC), such as drowsiness or confusion
- Breathing problems (trouble breathing or no breathing)
- Chest pain, discomfort or pressure lasting more than a few minutes that goes away and comes back or that radiates to the shoulder, arm, neck, jaw, stomach or back
- Persistent abdominal pain or pressure
- Severe external bleeding (bleeding that spurts or gushes steadily from a wound)
- Vomiting blood or passing blood
- Severe (critical) burns
- Suspected poisoning

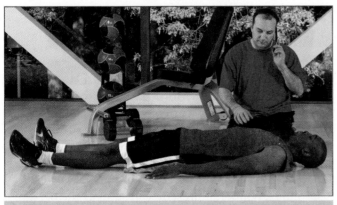

FIGURE 1-6 *Calling 9-1-1 or your local emergency number is important because getting emergency help fast greatly increases a person's chances of survival.*

- Seizures
- Stroke (sudden weakness on one side of the face/facial droop, sudden weakness on one side of the body, sudden slurred speech or trouble getting words out or a sudden, severe headache)
- Suspected or obvious injuries to the head, neck or spine
- Painful, swollen, deformed areas (suspected broken bone) or an open fracture

Also call 9-1-1 or the local emergency number immediately for any of these situations:

- Fire or explosion
- Downed electrical wires
- Swiftly moving or rapidly rising water
- Presence of poisonous gas
- Serious motor-vehicle collisions
- Injured or ill persons who cannot be moved easily

Deciding to Call First or Care First

If you are ALONE:

- *Call First* (call 9-1-1 or the local emergency number before giving care) for:
  - Any adult or child about 12 years of age or older who is unconscious.
  - A child or an infant who you witnessed suddenly collapse.
  - An unconscious child or infant known to have heart problems.
- *Care First* (give 2 minutes of care, then call 9-1-1 or the local emergency number) for:
  - An unconscious child (younger than about 12 years of age) who you did not see collapse.
  - Any drowning victim.

Call First situations are likely to be cardiac emergencies, where time is a critical factor. In Care First situations, the conditions often are related to breathing emergencies.

CARE

Once you have checked the scene and the person and have made a decision about calling 9-1-1 or the local emergency number, you may need to give care until EMS personnel take over. After making the 9-1-1 call, immediately go back to the injured or ill person. Check the person for life-threatening conditions and give the necessary care (see Checking a Conscious and Unconscious Person section in this chapter). To do so, follow these general guidelines:

- Do no further harm.
- Monitor the person's breathing and consciousness.
- Help the person rest in the most comfortable position.
- Keep the person from getting chilled or overheated.
- Reassure the person.
- Give any specific care as needed.

Transporting the Person Yourself

In some cases, you may decide to take the injured or ill person to a medical facility yourself instead of waiting for EMS personnel. *NEVER* transport a person:

- When the trip may aggravate the injury or illness or cause additional injury.
- When the person has or may develop a life-threatening condition.
- If you are unsure of the nature of the injury or illness.

If you decide it is safe to transport the person, ask someone to come with you to keep the person comfortable. Also, be sure you know the quickest route to the nearest medical facility capable of handling emergency care. Pay close attention to the injured or ill person and watch for any changes in his or her condition.

Discourage an injured or ill person from driving him- or herself to the hospital. An injury may restrict movement, or the person may become groggy or faint. A sudden onset of pain may be distracting. Any of these conditions can make driving dangerous for the person, passengers, other drivers and pedestrians.

Moving an Injured or Ill Person

One of the most dangerous threats to a seriously injured or ill person is unnecessary movement. Moving an injured person can cause additional injury and pain and may complicate his or her recovery. Generally, you should not move an injured or ill person while giving care. However, it would be appropriate in the following three situations:

1. When you are faced with immediate danger, such as fire, lack of oxygen, risk of explosion or a collapsing structure.
2. When you have to get to another person who may have a more serious problem. In this case, you may have to move a person with minor injuries to reach someone needing immediate care.

3. When it is necessary to give proper care. For example, if someone needed CPR, he or she might have to be moved from a bed because CPR needs to be performed on a firm, flat surface. If the surface or space is not adequate to give care, the person should be moved.

Techniques for Moving an Injured or Ill Person

Once you decide to move an injured or ill person, you must quickly decide how to do so. Carefully consider your safety and the safety of the person. Move an injured or ill person only when it is safe for you to do so and there is an immediate life threat. Base your decision on the dangers you are facing, the size and condition of the person, your abilities and physical condition, and whether you have any help.

To improve your chances of successfully moving an injured or ill person without injuring yourself or the person:

- Use your legs, not your back, when you bend.
- Bend at the knees and hips and avoid twisting your body.
- Walk forward when possible, taking small steps and looking where you are going.
- Avoid twisting or bending anyone with a possible head, neck or spinal injury.
- Do not move a person who is too large to move comfortably.

You can move a person to safety in many different ways, but no single way is best for every situation. The objective is to move the person without injuring yourself or causing further injury to the person. The following common types of emergency moves can all be done by one or two people and with minimal to no equipment.

Types of Non-Emergency Moves

Walking Assist

The most basic emergency move is the walking assist. Either one or two responders can use this method with a conscious person. To perform a walking assist, place the injured or ill person's arm across your shoulders and hold it in place with one hand. Support the person with your other hand around the person's waist (Fig. 1-7, A). In this way, your body acts as a crutch, supporting the person's weight while you both walk. A second responder, if present, can support the person in the same way on the other side (Fig. 1-7, B). Do not use this assist if you suspect that the person has a head, neck or spinal injury.

Two-Person Seat Carry

The two-person seat carry requires a second responder. This carry can be used for any person who is conscious and not seriously injured. Put one arm behind the person's thighs and the other across the person's back. Interlock your arms with those of a second responder behind the person's legs and across his or her back. Lift the person in the "seat" formed by the responders' arms (Fig. 1-8). Responders should coordinate their movement so they walk together. Do not use this assist if you suspect that the person has a head, neck or spinal injury.

Types of Emergency Moves

Pack-Strap Carry

The pack-strap carry can be used with conscious and unconscious persons. Using it with an unconscious person requires a second responder to help position the injured or ill person on your back. To perform the

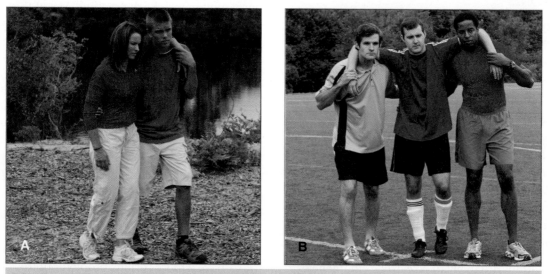

FIGURE 1-7, A–B **A,** *In a walking assist, your body acts as a crutch, supporting the person's weight while you both walk.* **B,** *Two responders may be needed for the walking assist.*

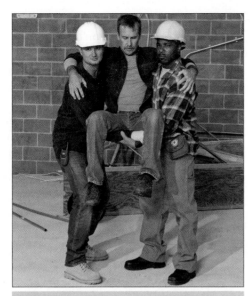

FIGURE 1-8 *The two-person seat carry*

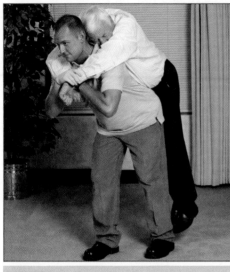

FIGURE 1-9 *The pack-strap carry*

neck and back stabilized. Grasp the person's clothing behind the neck, gathering enough to secure a firm grip. Using the clothing, pull the person (headfirst) to safety (Fig. 1-10).

During this move, the person's head is cradled by clothing and the responder's arms. Be aware that this move is exhausting and may cause back strain for the responder, even when done properly.

Blanket Drag

The blanket drag can be used to move a person in an emergency situation when equipment is limited. Keep the person between you and the blanket. Gather half of the blanket and place it against the person's side. Roll the person as a unit toward you. Reach over and place the blanket so that it is positioned under the person, then roll the person onto the blanket. Gather the blanket at the head and move the person (Fig. 1-11).

Ankle Drag

Use the ankle drag (also known as the foot drag) to move a person who is too large to carry or move in any other way. Firmly grasp the person's ankles and move backward. The person's arms should be crossed on his

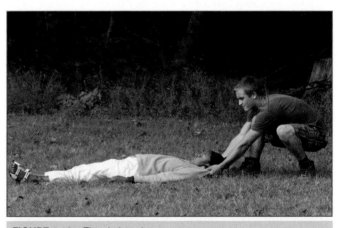

FIGURE 1-10 *The clothes drag*

pack-strap carry, have the person stand or have a second responder support the person. Position yourself with your back to the person, back straight, knees bent, so that your shoulders fit into the person's armpits.

Cross the person's arms in front of you and grasp the person's wrists. Lean forward slightly and pull the person up and onto your back. Stand up and walk to safety (Fig. 1-9). Depending on the size of the person, you may be able to hold both of his or her wrists with one hand, leaving your other hand free to help maintain balance, open doors and remove obstructions. Do not use this assist if you suspect that the person has a head, neck or spinal injury.

Clothes Drag

The clothes drag can be used to move a conscious or unconscious person with a suspected head, neck or spinal injury. This move helps keep the person's head,

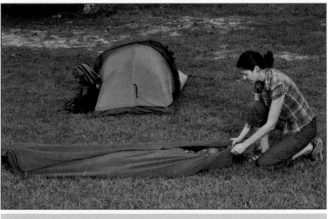

FIGURE 1-11 *The blanket drag*

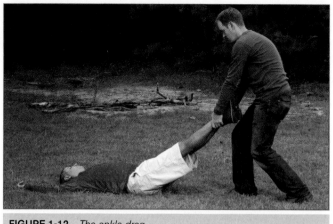

FIGURE 1-12 *The ankle drag*

or her chest. Pull the person in a straight line, being careful not to bump the person's head (Fig. 1-12).

Reaching a Person in the Water

Do not enter the water unless you are specifically trained to perform in-water rescues. Get help from a trained responder, such as a lifeguard, to get the person out of the water as quickly and safely as possible. You can help a person in trouble in the water from a safe position by using *reaching assists*, *throwing assists* or *wading assists*.

When possible, start by talking to the person. Let the person know that help is coming. If noise is a problem or if the person is too far away to hear you, use nonverbal communication. Direct the person what to do, such as grasping a line, ring buoy or other object that floats. Ask the person to move toward you, which may be done by using the back float with slight leg movements or small strokes. Some people can reach safety by themselves with the calm and encouraging assistance of someone calling to them.

- *Reaching Assists.* Firmly brace yourself on a pool deck, pier or shoreline and reach out to the person with any object that will extend your reach, such as a pole, oar or paddle, tree branch, shirt, belt or towel. If no equipment is available, you can still perform a reaching assist by lying down and extending your arm or leg for the person to grab.
- *Throwing Assists.* An effective way to rescue someone beyond your reach is to throw a floating object out to the person with a line attached. Once the person grasps the object, pull the individual to safety. Throwing equipment includes heaving lines, ring buoys, throw bags or any floating object available, such as a picnic jug, small cooler, buoyant cushion, kickboard or extra life jacket.

- *Wading Assists.* If the water is safe and shallow enough (not over your chest), you can wade in to reach the person. If there is a current or the bottom is soft or unknown, making it dangerous to wade, do *not* go in the water. If possible, wear a life jacket and take something with you to extend your reach, such as a ring buoy, buoyant cushion, kickboard, life jacket, tree branch, pole, air mattress, plastic cooler, picnic jug, paddle or water exercise belt.

CHECKING A CONSCIOUS PERSON

If you determine that an injured or ill person is conscious and has no immediate life-threatening conditions, you can begin to check for other conditions that may need care. Checking a conscious person with no immediate life-threatening conditions involves two basic steps:

- Interview the person and bystanders.
- Check the person from head to toe.

Conducting Interviews

Ask the person and bystanders simple questions to learn more about what happened. Keep these interviews brief (Fig. 1-13). Remember to first identify yourself and to get the person's consent to give care. Begin by asking the person's name. This will make him or her feel more comfortable. Gather additional information by asking the person the following questions:

- What happened?
- Do you feel pain or discomfort anywhere?
- Do you have any allergies?
- Do you have any medical conditions or are you taking any medication?

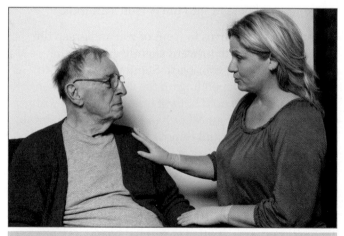

FIGURE 1-13 *Ask simple questions and keep interviews brief.*

If the person feels pain, ask him or her to describe it and to tell you where it is located. Descriptions often include terms such as burning, crushing, throbbing, aching or sharp pain. Ask when the pain started and what the person was doing when it began. Ask the person to rate his or her pain on a scale of 1 to 10 (1 being mild and 10 being severe).

Sometimes an injured or ill person will not be able to give you the information that you need. The person may not speak your language. In some cases, the person may not be able to speak because of a medical condition. Known as a *laryngectomee*, a person whose larynx (voice box) was surgically removed breathes through a permanent opening, or *stoma,* in the neck and may not be able to speak. Remember to question family members, friends or bystanders as well. They may be able to give you helpful information or help you to communicate with the person. You will learn more about communicating with people with special needs in Chapter 9.

Children or infants may be frightened. They may be fully aware of you but still unable to answer your questions. In some cases, they may be crying too hard and be unable to stop. Approach slowly and gently, and give the child or infant some time to get used to you. Use the child's name, if you know it. Get down to or below the child's eye level.

Write down the information you learn during the interviews or, preferably, have someone else write it down for you. Be sure to give the information to EMS personnel when they arrive. It may help them to determine the type of medical care that the person should receive.

Checking from Head to Toe

Next you will need to thoroughly check the injured or ill person so that you do not overlook any problems. Visually check from head to toe. When checking a conscious person:

- Do not move any areas where there is pain or discomfort, or if you suspect a head, neck or spinal injury.
- Check the person's head by examining the scalp, face, ears, mouth and nose.
- Look for cuts, bruises, bumps or depressions. Think of how the body usually looks. If you are unsure if a body part or limb looks injured, check it against the opposite limb or the other side of the body.
- Watch for changes in consciousness. Notice if the person is drowsy, confused or is not alert.
- Look for changes in the person's breathing. A healthy person breathes easily, quietly, regularly and without discomfort or pain. Young children and infants generally breathe faster than adults. Breathing that is not normal includes noisy breathing, such as gasping for air; rasping, gurgling or whistling sounds; breathing that is unusually fast or slow; and breathing that is painful.
- Notice how the skin looks and feels. Skin can provide clues that a person is injured or ill. Feel the person's forehead with the back of your hand to determine if the skin feels unusually damp, dry, cool or hot (Fig. 1-14). Note if it is red, pale or ashen.
- Look over the body. Ask again about any areas that hurt. Ask the person to move each part of the body that does not hurt. Ask the person to gently move his or her head from side to side. Check the shoulders by asking the person to shrug them. Check the chest and abdomen by asking the person to take a deep breath. Ask the person to move his or her fingers, hands and arms; and then the toes, legs and hips in the same way. Watch the person's face and listen for signals of discomfort or pain as you check for injuries.
- Look for a medical identification (ID) tag, bracelet or necklace (Fig. 1-15) on the person's wrist, neck or ankle. A tag will provide medical information about the person, explain how to care for certain conditions

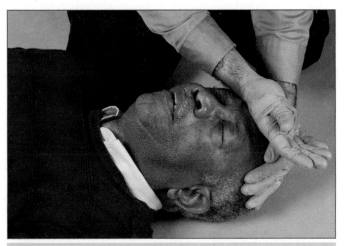

FIGURE 1-14 *Feel the forehead with the back of your hand to determine its temperature.*

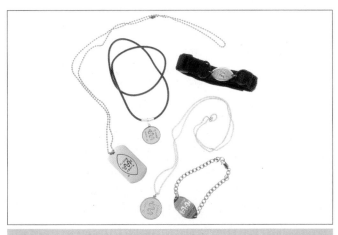

FIGURE 1-15 *Medical ID tags and bracelets can provide important information about an injured or ill person.* Courtesy of the Canadian Red Cross.

and list whom to call for help. For example, a person with diabetes may have some form of medical ID tag, bracelet or necklace identifying this condition.

If a child or an infant becomes extremely upset, conduct a toe-to-head check of the child or infant. This will be less emotionally threatening. Parents or guardians who are present may be able to calm a frightened child. In fact, it often is helpful to check a young child while he or she is seated in his or her parent's or guardian's lap. Parents also can tell you if a child has a medical condition.

When you have finished checking, determine if the person can move his or her body without any pain. If the person can move without pain and there are no other signals of injury, have him or her attempt to rest in a sitting position or other comfortable position (Fig. 1-16). When the person feels ready, help him or her to stand up. Determine what additional care is needed and whether to call 9-1-1 or the local emergency number.

SHOCK

When the body is healthy, three conditions are needed to keep the right amount of blood flowing:

- The heart must be working well.
- An adequate amount of oxygen-rich blood must be circulating in the body.
- The blood vessels must be intact and able to adjust blood flow.

Shock is a condition in which the circulatory system fails to deliver enough oxygen-rich blood to the body's tissues and vital organs. The body's organs, such as the brain, heart and lungs, do not function properly without this blood supply. This triggers a series of responses that produce specific signals known as shock. These responses are the body's attempt to maintain adequate blood flow.

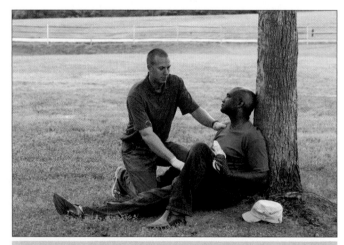

FIGURE 1-16 *If there are no signals of obvious injuries, help the person into a comfortable position.*

When someone is injured or becomes suddenly ill, these normal body functions may be interrupted. In cases of minor injury or illness, this interruption is brief because the body is able to compensate quickly. With more severe injuries or illnesses, however, the body may be unable to adjust. When the body is unable to meet its demand for oxygen because blood fails to circulate adequately, shock occurs.

What to Look For

The signals that indicate a person may be going into shock include:

- Restlessness or irritability.
- Altered level of consciousness.
- Nausea or vomiting.
- Pale, ashen or grayish, cool, moist skin.
- Rapid breathing and pulse.
- Excessive thirst.

Be aware that the early signals of shock may not be present in young children and infants. However, because children are smaller than adults, they have less blood volume and are more susceptible to shock.

When to Call 9-1-1

In cases where the person is going into shock, call 9-1-1 or the local emergency number immediately. Shock cannot be managed effectively by first aid alone. A person suffering from shock requires emergency medical care as soon as possible.

What to Do Until Help Arrives

Caring for shock involves the following simple steps:

- Have the person lie down. This often is the most comfortable position. Helping the person rest in a more comfortable position may lessen any pain. Helping the person to rest comfortably is important because pain can intensify the body's stress and speed up the progression of shock.
- Control any external bleeding.
- Since you may not be sure of the person's condition, leave him or her lying flat.
- Help the person maintain normal body temperature (Fig. 1-17). If the person is cool, try to cover him or her to avoid chilling.
- Do not give the person anything to eat or drink, even though he or she is likely to be thirsty. The person's condition may be severe enough to require surgery, in which case it is better if the stomach is empty.
- Reassure the person.

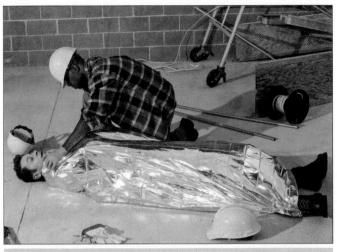

FIGURE 1-17 *Help the person going into shock to lie down and keep him or her from getting chilled or overheated.*

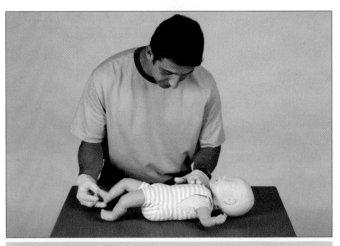

FIGURE 1-18 *If you are not sure whether an infant is unconscious, check by tapping the infant's shoulder or flicking the bottom of the infant's foot.*

■ Continue to monitor the person's breathing and for any changes in the person's condition. Do not wait for signals of shock to develop before caring for the underlying injury or illness.

CHECKING AN UNCONSCIOUS PERSON

If you think someone is unconscious, tap him or her on the shoulder and ask if he or she is OK. Use the person's name if you know it. Speak loudly. If you are not sure whether an infant is unconscious, check by tapping the infant's shoulder and shouting or by flicking the bottom of the infant's foot to see if the infant responds (Fig. 1-18).

If the person does not respond, call 9-1-1 or the local emergency number and check for other life-threatening conditions.

Always check to see if an unconscious person:

■ Has an open airway and is breathing normally.
■ Is bleeding severely.

Consciousness, effective (normal) breathing and circulation and skin characteristics sometimes are referred to as *signs of life.*

Airway

Once you or someone else has called 9-1-1 or the local emergency number, check to see if the person has an open airway and is breathing. An open airway allows air to enter the lungs for the person to breathe. If the airway is blocked, the person cannot breathe. A blocked airway is a life-threatening condition.

■ When someone is unconscious and lying on his or her back, the tongue may fall to the back of the throat and block the airway. To open an unconscious person's airway, push down on his or her forehead while pulling up on the bony part of the chin with two or three fingers of your other hand (Fig. 1-19). This procedure, known as the *head-tilt/chin-lift technique,* moves the tongue away from the back of the throat, allowing air to enter the lungs.

○ For a child: Place one hand on the forehead and tilt the head slightly past a *neutral position*

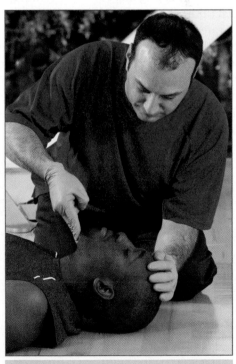

FIGURE 1-19 *Open an unconscious person's airway using the head-tilt/chin-lift technique.*

(the head and chin are neither flexed downward toward the chest nor extended backward).

- ○ For an infant: Place one hand on the forehead and tilt the head to a neutral position while pulling up on the bony part of the chin with two or three fingers of your other hand.

■ If you suspect that a person has a head, neck or spinal injury, carefully tilt the head and lift the chin just enough to open the airway.

Check the person's neck to see if he or she breathes through an opening. A person whose larynx was removed may breathe partially or entirely through a stoma instead of through the mouth (Fig. 1-20). The person may breathe partially or entirely through this opening instead of through the mouth and nose. It is important to recognize this difference in the way a person breathes. This will help you give proper care.

Breathing

After opening the airway, quickly check an unconscious person for breathing. Position yourself so that you can *look* to see if the person's chest clearly rises and falls, *listen* for escaping air and *feel* for it against the side of your face. Do this for no more than 10 seconds (Fig. 1-21). If the person needs CPR, chest compressions must not be delayed.

Normal breathing is regular, quiet and effortless. A person does not appear to be working hard or struggling when breathing normally. This means that the person is not making noise when breathing, breaths are not fast (although it should be noted that normal breathing rates in children and infants are faster than normal breathing rates in adults) and breathing does not cause discomfort or pain. In an unconscious adult you may detect an irregular, gasping or shallow breath. This is known as an *agonal breath*. Do not confuse this with normal breathing. Care for the person as if there is no breathing at all. Agonal breaths do not occur frequently in children.

If the person is breathing normally, his or her heart is beating and is circulating blood containing oxygen. In this case, maintain an open airway by using the head-tilt/chin-lift technique as you continue to look for other life-threatening conditions.

If an adult is not breathing normally, this person most likely needs immediate CPR.

If a child or an infant is not breathing, give 2 rescue breaths. Tilt the head back and lift chin up. Pinch the nose shut then make a complete seal over the child's mouth and blow in for about 1 second to make the chest clearly rise (Fig. 1-22, A). For an infant, seal your mouth over the infant's mouth and nose (Fig. 1-22, B). Give rescue breaths one after the other.

If you witness the sudden collapse of a child, assume a cardiac emergency. Do not give 2 rescue breaths. CPR needs to be started immediately, just as with an adult.

Sometimes you may need to remove food, liquid or other objects that are blocking the person's airway. This may prevent the chest from rising when you attempt rescue breaths. You will learn how to recognize an obstructed airway and give care to the person in Chapter 4.

Circulation

It is important to recognize breathing emergencies in children and infants and to act before the heart stops beating. Adults' hearts frequently stop beating because of disease. Children's and infants' hearts, however, are usually healthy. When a child's or an infant's heart stops, it usually is the result of a breathing emergency.

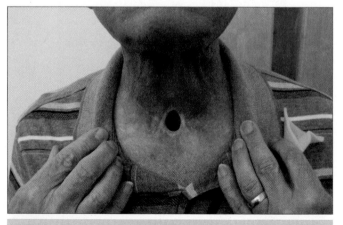

FIGURE 1-20 *A stoma is an opening in the neck that allows a person to breathe after certain surgeries on the airway.* Courtesy of the International Association of Laryngectomees.

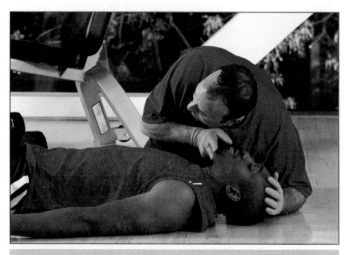

FIGURE 1-21 *Check for breathing for no more than 10 seconds.*

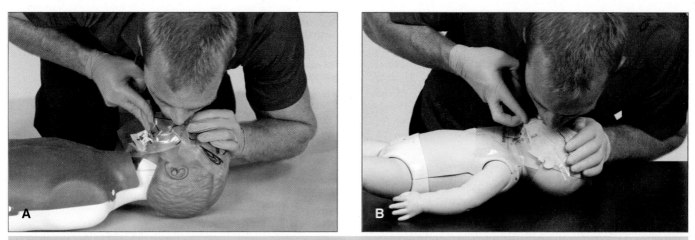

FIGURE 1-22, A–B **A,** *Give a child 2 rescue breaths with each breath lasting about 1 second.* **B,** *For an infant, cover the mouth and nose.*

If an adult is not breathing or is not breathing normally and if the emergency is not the result of non-fatal drowning or other respiratory cause such as a drug overdose, assume that the problem is a cardiac emergency.

Quickly look for severe bleeding by looking over the person's body from head to toe for signals such as blood-soaked clothing or blood spurting out of a wound (Fig. 1-23). Bleeding usually looks worse than it is. A small amount of blood on a slick surface or mixed with water usually looks like a large volume of blood. It is not always easy to recognize severe bleeding.

What to Do Next

■ If an unconscious person is breathing normally, keep the person lying face-up and maintain an open airway with the head-tilt/chin-lift technique. If the person vomits, fluids block the airway, or if you must leave the person to get help, place him or her into a modified high arm in endangered spine (H.A.IN.E.S.) recovery position. (Placing an Unconscious Person in a Recovery Position is discussed in this chapter.)

■ If an unconscious adult has irregular, gasping or shallow breaths (agonal breathing) or is not breathing at all, begin CPR. You will learn how to perform CPR in Chapter 2.

■ If an unconscious child or infant is not breathing, after giving 2 rescue breaths, perform CPR (see Chapter 2).

■ If the person is bleeding severely, control the bleeding by applying direct pressure (see Chapter 7).

Using CPR Breathing Barriers

You might not feel comfortable with giving rescue breaths, especially to someone whom you do not know. Disease transmission is an understandable worry, even though the chance of getting a disease from giving rescue breaths is extremely small.

CPR breathing barriers, such as face shields and resuscitation masks, create a barrier between your mouth and nose and those of the injured or ill person (Fig. 1-24). This barrier can help to protect you from contact with blood and other body fluids, such as saliva, as you give rescue breaths. These devices also protect you from breathing the air that the person exhales. Some devices are small enough to fit in your pocket or in the glove compartment of your car. You also can keep one in your first aid kit. If a face shield is used, switch to a resuscitation mask, if available, or when one becomes available. However, you should *not delay* rescue breaths while searching

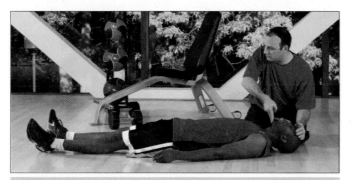

FIGURE 1-23 *Check for severe bleeding by quickly looking over the person from head to toe.*

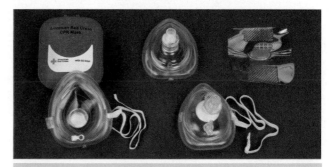

FIGURE 1-24 *CPR breathing barriers, such as face shields and resuscitation masks, create a barrier between your mouth and nose and the injured or ill person's mouth.*

for a CPR breathing barrier or by trying to learn how to use one.

Pediatric CPR breathing barriers are available and should be used to care for children and infants. Always use the appropriate equipment for the size of the injured or ill person.

Special Situations

When giving rescue breaths while performing CPR, you may encounter certain special situations. These include air in the stomach; vomiting; mouth-to-nose breathing; mouth-to-stoma breathing; persons with suspected head, neck or spinal injuries; and drowning victims.

■ Air in the Stomach: When you are giving rescue breaths, be careful to avoid forcing air into the person's stomach instead of the lungs. This may happen if you breathe too long, breathe too hard or do not open the airway far enough.

   ○ To avoid forcing air into the person's stomach, keep the person's head tilted back. Take a normal breath and blow into the person's mouth, blowing just enough to make the chest clearly rise. Each rescue breath should last about 1 second for an adult, a child or an infant. Pause between breaths long enough for the air in the person to come out and for you to take another breath.

   ○ Air in the stomach can make the person vomit and cause complications. When an unconscious person vomits, the contents of the stomach can get into the lungs and block breathing. Air in the stomach also makes it harder for the diaphragm— the large muscle that controls breathing—to move. This makes it harder for the lungs to fill with air.

■ Vomiting. Even when you are giving rescue breaths properly, the person may vomit.

   ○ If this happens, roll the person onto one side and wipe the mouth clean (Fig. 1-25). If possible, use a protective barrier, such as disposable gloves, gauze or even a handkerchief when cleaning out the mouth.

   ○ Then roll the person on his or her back again and continue giving care as necessary.

■ Mouth-to-Nose Breathing. If you are unable to make a tight enough seal over the person's mouth, you can blow into the nose (Fig. 1-26).

   ○ With the head tilted back, close the mouth by pushing on the chin.

   ○ Seal your mouth around the person's nose and breathe into the nose.

   ○ If possible, open the person's mouth between rescue breaths to let the air out.

■ Mouth-to-Stoma Breathing. Check the person's neck to see if he or she breathes through a stoma.

   ○ If you discover that the person needing rescue breaths has a stoma, expose his or her entire neck down to the breastbone. Remove anything covering the stoma that blocks the person's airway. Also, wipe away any secretions or blockages.

   ○ Keep the airway in a neutral position; do not allow the chin or head to flex forward toward the chest or extend backward as you look, listen and feel for normal breathing with your ear over the stoma. To give rescue breaths, make an airtight seal with your lips around the stoma or tracheostomy tube and blow in for about 1 second to make the chest clearly rise.

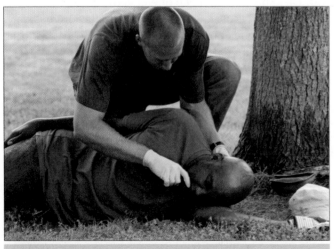

FIGURE 1-25 *If the person vomits, roll him or her onto one side and wipe the mouth clean.*

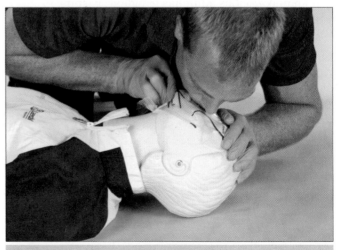

FIGURE 1-26 *If you are unable to make a tight enough seal over the person's mouth, you can blow into the nose.*

- Give rescue breaths into the stoma at the same rate you would breathe into the mouth when performing CPR. Your rescue breaths are successful if you see the chest rise and fall and you hear and feel air escape from the stoma.

- If the chest does not rise and fall, the person's tracheostomy tube may be blocked. If this happens, remove the inner tube and give rescue breaths again.

- If you hear or feel air escaping from the person's mouth or nose, the person is a partial neck breather. In order to give rescue breaths to a partial neck breather, the responder must seal the person's mouth and nose with either his or her hand or a tight-fitting face mask so that air does not escape out of the mouth or nose when you give rescue breaths into the stoma or tracheostomy tube.

- You might feel uncomfortable with the thought of giving mouth-to-stoma rescue breaths. An alternative method is to use a barrier device (see Using CPR Breathing Barriers section in this chapter). For a neck breather or partial neck breather, a round pediatric mask may provide a better seal around a stoma or tracheostomy tube neck plate (Fig. 1-27).

■ Head, Neck and Spinal Injuries. Be especially careful with a person who may have a head, neck or spinal injury. These kinds of injuries can result from a fall from a height greater than the person's height, an automobile collision or a diving mishap. If you suspect such an injury, try not to move the person's head, neck and back. If a child is strapped into a car seat, do not remove him or her from it. To give rescue breaths to a person whom you suspect has a head, neck or spinal injury:

- Minimize movement of the head and neck when opening the airway.

- Carefully tilt the head and lift the chin just enough to open the airway.

■ Drowning Victims. For an adult, give 2 rescue breaths as you would for a child or an infant once you determine there is no breathing. If alone, you should give 2 minutes of care before calling 9-1-1 (Care First) for an unconscious person who has been submerged. Do not enter the water unless you are specifically trained to perform in-water rescues. Get help from a trained responder, such as a lifeguard, to get the person out of the water as quickly and safely as possible. If the person is not breathing, you will have to give proper care.

Placing an Unconscious Person in a Recovery Position

In some cases, the person may be unconscious but breathing normally. Generally, that person should not be moved from a face-up position, especially if there is a suspected spinal injury. However, there are a few situations when you should move a person into a recovery position whether or not a spinal injury is suspected. Examples include situations where you are alone and have to leave the person (e.g., to call for help), or you cannot maintain an open and clear airway because of fluids or vomit. Fig. 1-28, A–B shows how to place a person, whether or not a spinal injury is suspected, in a modified H.A.IN.E.S. recovery position. Placing a person in this position will help to keep the airway open and clear.

To place an adult or a child in a modified H.A.IN.E.S. recovery position:

■ Kneel at the person's side.

■ Reach across the body and lift the arm farthest from you up next to the head with the person's palm facing up.

■ Take the person's arm closest to you and place it next to his or her side.

■ Grasp the leg farthest from you and bend it up.

■ Using your hand that is closest to the person's head, cup the base of the skull in the palm of your hand and carefully slide your forearm under the person's shoulder closest to you. Do not lift or push the head or neck.

■ Place your other hand under the arm and hip closest to you.

■ Using a smooth motion, roll the person away from you by lifting with your hand and forearm. Make sure the person's head remains in contact with the extended arm and be sure to support the head and neck with your hand.

■ Stop all movement when the person is on his or her side.

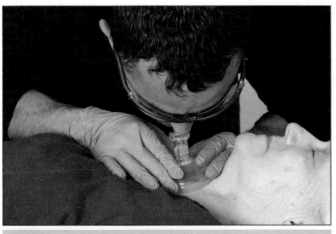

FIGURE 1-27 *To give rescue breaths into a stoma, make an airtight seal with your lips around the stoma or use a round pediatric resuscitation mask and blow in to make chest clearly rise.*

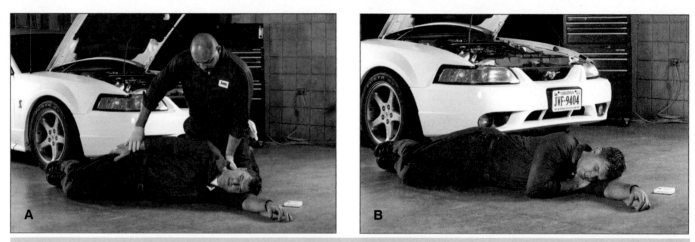

FIGURE 1-28, A–B **A,** *Placing a person in a modified H.A.IN.E.S. recovery position.* **B,** *Placing a person in a modified H.A.IN.E.S if you must leave to call 9-1-1.*

■ Bend the knee closest to you and place it on top of the other knee so that both knees are in a bent position.

■ Make sure the arm on top is in line with the upper body.

   ○ If you must leave the person to get help, place the hand of the upper arm palm side down with the fingers under the head at the armpit of the extended lower arm.

An infant can be placed in a recovery position as would be done for an older child. You can also hold an infant in a recovery position (Fig. 1-29) by:

■ Carefully positioning the infant face-down along your forearm.

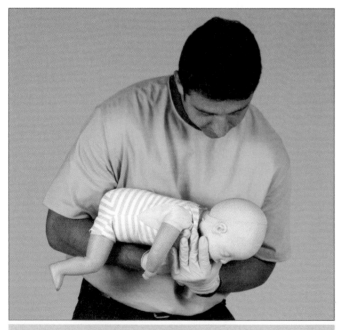

FIGURE 1-29 *An infant recovery position*

■ Supporting the infant's head and neck with your other hand while keeping the infant's mouth and nose clear.

■ Keeping the head and neck slightly lower than the chest.

INCIDENT STRESS

After responding to an emergency involving a serious injury, illness or death, it is not unusual to experience acute stress. Sometimes, people who have given first aid or performed CPR in these situations feel that they are unable to cope with the stress. This feeling is known as *incident stress*. If not appropriately managed, this acute stress may lead to a serious condition called post-traumatic stress disorder.

Signals of Incident Stress Reactions

Some effects may appear right away whereas others may take longer to develop. Signals of incident stress include:

■ Anxiousness and inability to sleep.

■ Nightmares.

■ Restlessness and other problems.

■ Confusion.

■ Lower attention span.

■ Poor concentration.

■ Denial.

■ Guilt.

■ Depression.

■ Anger.

■ Nausea.

■ Change in interactions with others.

■ Increased or decreased eating.

- Uncharacteristic, excessive humor or silence.
- Unusual behavior.
- Difficulty performing one's job.

Guidelines for Coping with Incident Stress

Incident stress may require professional help to prevent post-traumatic stress from developing. Other things that you may do to help reduce stress include using relaxation techniques, eating a balanced diet, avoiding alcohol and drugs, getting enough rest and participating in some type of physical exercise or activity.

PUTTING IT ALL TOGETHER

Given the large number of injuries and sudden illnesses that occur in the United States each year, it is likely that you might have to deal with an emergency situation someday.

Remember that you have a vital role to play in the EMS system. This includes following the emergency action steps of **CHECK—CALL—CARE**, which will help you to react quickly and calmly in any emergency situation. Emergencies happen every day. Be prepared, respond immediately and make a difference.

REMOVING GLOVES

AFTER GIVING CARE AND MAKING SURE TO NEVER TOUCH THE BARE SKIN WITH THE OUTSIDE OF EITHER GLOVE:

1 PINCH GLOVE

Pinch the palm side of one glove near the wrist. Carefully pull the glove off so that it is inside out.

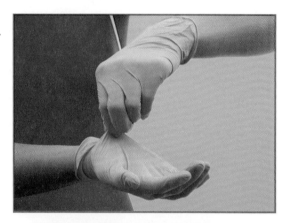

2 SLIP TWO FINGERS UNDER GLOVE

Hold the glove in the palm of the remaining gloved hand. Slip two fingers under the glove at the wrist of the remaining gloved hand.

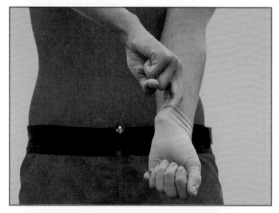

3 PULL GLOVE OFF

Pull the glove until it comes off, inside out, so that the first glove ends up inside the glove just removed.

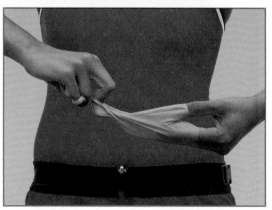

4 DISPOSE OF GLOVES AND WASH HANDS

After removing the gloves:

- Dispose of gloves in the appropriate biohazard container.
- Wash hands thoroughly with soap and warm running water, if available.
- Otherwise, use an alcohol-based hand sanitizer to clean the hands if they are not visibly soiled.

CHECKING AN INJURED OR ILL ADULT
APPEARS TO BE UNCONSCIOUS

TIP: *Use disposable gloves and other PPE.*

AFTER CHECKING THE SCENE FOR SAFETY, CHECK THE PERSON.

1 CHECK FOR RESPONSIVENESS

Tap the shoulder and shout, "Are you okay?"

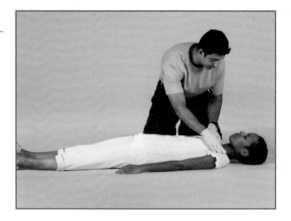

2 CALL 9-1-1

If no response, **CALL** 9-1-1 or the local emergency number.

- If an unconscious person is face-down, roll him or her face-up keeping the head, neck and back in a straight line.

If the person responds, obtain consent and **CALL** 9-1-1 or the local emergency number for any life-threatening conditions.

CHECK the person from head to toe and ask questions to find out what happened.

3 OPEN THE AIRWAY

Tilt head, lift chin.

4 CHECK FOR BREATHING

CHECK for no more than **10** seconds.

- Occasional gasps are not breathing.

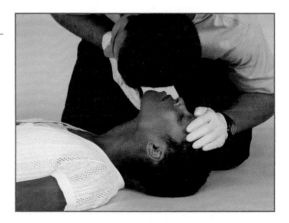

Continued on next page

5 QUICKLY SCAN FOR SEVERE BLEEDING

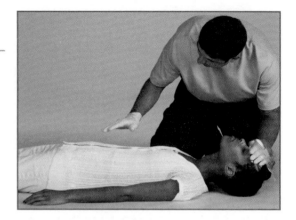

WHAT TO DO NEXT

- IF THERE IS NO BREATHING—Perform CPR or use an AED (if AED is immediately available).
- IF BREATHING—Maintain an open airway and monitor breathing and for any changes in condition.

CHECKING AN INJURED OR ILL CHILD OR INFANT

APPEARS TO BE UNCONSCIOUS

TIP: *Use disposable gloves and other PPE. Get consent from a parent or guardian, if present.*

AFTER CHECKING THE SCENE FOR SAFETY, CHECK THE CHILD OR INFANT.

1 CHECK FOR RESPONSIVENESS

Tap the shoulder and shout, "Are you okay?"
For an infant, you may flick the bottom of the foot.

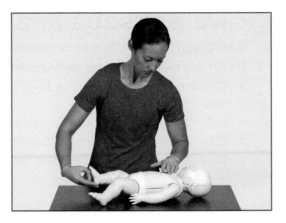

2 CALL 9-1-1

If no response, **CALL** 9-1-1 or the local emergency number.

- If an unconscious infant is face-down, roll him or her face-up supporting the head, neck and back in a straight line.

If **ALONE**, give about **2** minutes of **CARE**, then **CALL** 9-1-1.

If the child or infant responds, **CALL** 9-1-1 or the local emergency number for any life-threatening conditions and obtain consent to give **CARE**.

CHECK the child from head to toe and ask questions to find out what happened.

3 OPEN THE AIRWAY

Tilt head back slightly, lift chin.

Continued on next page

4 CHECK FOR BREATHING

CHECK for no more than **10** seconds.

- Occasional gasps are not breathing.
- Infants have periodic breathing, so changes in breathing pattern are normal for infants.

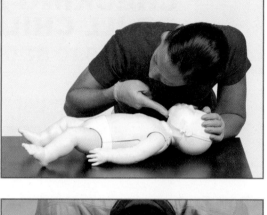

5 GIVE 2 RESCUE BREATHS

If no breathing, give **2** rescue breaths.

- Tilt the head back and lift the chin up.
- **Child:** pinch the nose shut, then make a complete seal over child's mouth.
- **Infant:** Make complete seal over infant's mouth and nose.
- Blow in for about **1** second to make the chest clearly rise.
- Give rescue breaths, one after the other.

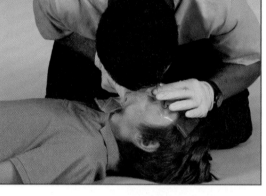

> **TIPS:**
> - *If you witnessed the child or infant suddenly collapse, skip rescue breaths and start CPR.*
> - *If the chest does not rise with rescue breaths, retilt the head and give another rescue breath.*

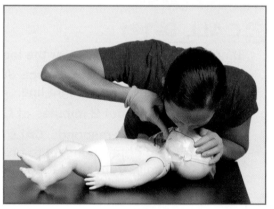

6 QUICKLY SCAN FOR SEVERE BLEEDING

WHAT TO DO NEXT

- IF THE CHEST DOES NOT RISE AFTER RETILTING THE HEAD—Give **CARE** for unconscious choking.
- IF THERE IS NO BREATHING—Perform CPR or use an AED (if AED is immediately available).
- IF BREATHING—Maintain an open airway. Monitor breathing and for any changes in condition.

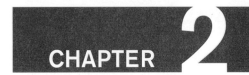
Cardiac Emergencies and CPR

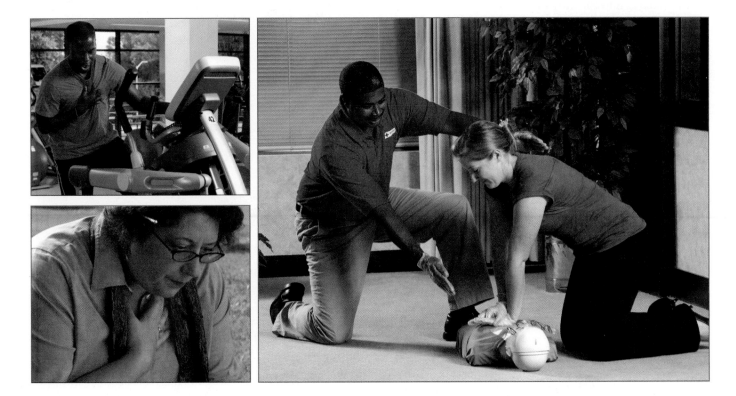

Cardiac emergencies are life threatening. Heart attack and cardiac arrest are major causes of illness and death in the United States. Every day in U.S. homes, parks and workplaces someone will have a heart attack or go into cardiac arrest. Recognizing the signals of a heart attack and cardiac arrest, calling 9-1-1 or the local emergency number and giving immediate care in a cardiac emergency saves lives. Performing CPR and using an automated external defibrillator (AED) immediately after a person goes into cardiac arrest can greatly increase his or her chance of survival.

In this chapter you will find out what signals to look for if you suspect a person is having a heart attack or has gone into cardiac arrest. This chapter also discusses how to care for a person having a heart attack and how to perform CPR for a person in cardiac arrest. In addition, this chapter covers the important links in the Cardiac Chain of Survival.

Although cardiac emergencies occur more commonly in adults, they also occur in infants and children. This chapter discusses the causes of cardiac arrest and how to provide care for all age groups.

BACKGROUND

The heart is a fascinating organ. It beats more than 3 billion times in an average lifetime. The heart is about the size of a fist and lies between the lungs in the middle of the chest. It pumps blood throughout the body. The ribs, breastbone and spine protect it from injury. The heart is separated into right and left halves (Fig. 2-1).

Blood that contains little or no oxygen enters the right side of the heart and is pumped to the lungs. The blood picks up oxygen in the lungs when you breathe. The oxygen-rich blood then goes to the left side of the heart and is pumped from the heart's blood vessels, called the *arteries*, to all other parts of the body. The heart and your body's vital organs need this constant supply of oxygen-rich blood.

Cardiovascular disease is an abnormal condition that affects the heart and blood vessels. An estimated 80 million Americans suffer from some form of the disease. It remains the number one killer in the United States and is a major cause of disability. The most common conditions caused by cardiovascular disease include *coronary heart disease*, also known as *coronary artery disease*, and stroke, also called a *brain attack*.

Coronary heart disease occurs when the arteries that supply blood to the heart muscle harden and narrow. This process is called *atherosclerosis*. The damage occurs gradually, as cholesterol and fatty deposits called *plaque* build up on the inner artery walls (Fig. 2-2). As this

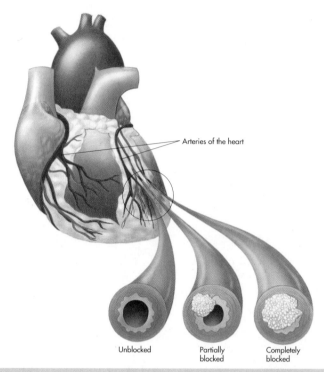

FIGURE 2-2 *Build-up of fatty materials on the inner walls of the arteries reduces blood flow to the heart muscle and may cause a heart attack.*

build-up worsens, the arteries become narrower. This reduces the amount of blood that can flow through them and prevents the heart from getting the blood and oxygen it needs. If the heart does not get blood containing oxygen, it will not work properly. Coronary heart disease accounts for about half of the greater than 800,000 adults who die each year from cardiovascular disease.

When the heart is working normally, it beats evenly and easily, with a steady rhythm. When damage to the heart causes it to stop working effectively, a person can experience a heart attack or other damage to the heart muscle. A heart attack can cause the heart to beat in an irregular way. This may prevent blood from circulating effectively.

When the heart does not work properly, normal breathing can be disrupted or stopped. A heart attack also can cause the heart to stop beating entirely. This condition is called *cardiac arrest*. The number one cause of heart attack and cardiac arrest in adults is coronary heart disease. Other significant causes of cardiac arrest are non-heart related (e.g., poisoning or drowning).

HEART ATTACK

When blood flow to the heart muscle is reduced, people experience chest pain. This reduced blood flow usually is caused by coronary heart disease. When the blood and oxygen supply to the heart is reduced, a heart attack may result.

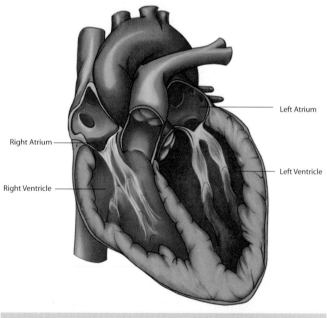

FIGURE 2-1 *The heart is separated into right and left halves. Blood that contains little or no oxygen enters the right side of the heart and is pumped to the lungs. The blood picks up oxygen in the lungs when you breathe. The oxygen-rich blood then goes to the left side of the heart and is pumped to all parts of the body.*

What to Look For

A heart attack can be indicated by common signals. Even people who have had a heart attack may not recognize the signals, because each heart attack may not show the same signals. You should be able to recognize the following signals of a heart attack so that you can give prompt and proper care:

■ *Chest pain, discomfort or pressure*. The most common signal is persistent pain, discomfort or pressure in the chest that lasts longer than 3 to 5 minutes or goes away and comes back. Unfortunately, it is not always easy to distinguish heart attack pain from the pain of indigestion, muscle spasms or other conditions. This often causes people to delay getting medical care. Brief, stabbing pain or pain that gets worse when you bend or breathe deeply usually is not caused by a heart problem.

  ○ The pain associated with a heart attack can range from discomfort to an unbearable crushing sensation in the chest.

  ○ The person may describe it as pressure, squeezing, tightness, aching or heaviness in the chest.

  ○ Many heart attacks start slowly as mild pain or discomfort.

  ○ Often the person feels pain or discomfort in the center of the chest (Fig. 2-3).

  ○ The pain or discomfort becomes constant. It usually is not relieved by resting, changing position or taking medicine.

  ○ Some individuals may show no signals at all.

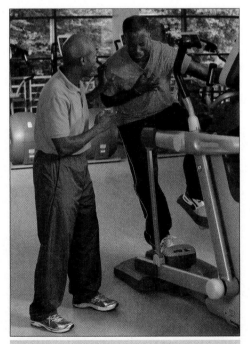

FIGURE 2-3 *Heart attack pain or pressure is often felt in the center of the chest. It may spread to the shoulder, arm, neck or jaw.*

■ *Discomfort in other areas of the upper body in addition to the chest*. Discomfort, pain or pressure may also be felt in or spread to the shoulder, arm, neck, jaw, stomach or back.

■ *Trouble breathing*. Another signal of a heart attack is trouble breathing. The person may be breathing faster than normal because the body tries to get the much-needed oxygen to the heart. The person may have noisy breathing or shortness of breath.

■ *Other signals*. The person's skin may be pale or ashen (gray), especially around the face. Some people suffering from a heart attack may be damp with sweat or may sweat heavily, feel dizzy, become nauseous or vomit. They may become fatigued, lightheaded or lose consciousness. These signals are caused by the stress put on the body when the heart does not work as it should. Some individuals may show no signals at all.

■ *Differences in signals between men and women*. Both men and women experience the most common signal for a heart attack: chest pain or discomfort. However, it is important to note that women are somewhat more likely to experience some of the other warning signals, particularly shortness of breath, nausea or vomiting, back or jaw pain and unexplained fatigue or malaise. When they do experience chest pain, women may have a greater tendency to have atypical chest pain: sudden, sharp but short-lived pain outside of the breastbone.

When to Call 9-1-1

Remember, the key signal of a heart attack is persistent chest pain or discomfort that lasts more than 3 to 5 minutes or goes away and comes back. If you suspect the person is having a heart attack based on his or her signals, call 9-1-1 or the local emergency number immediately. A person having a heart attack probably will deny that any signal is serious. Do not let this influence you. If you think the person might be having a heart attack, act quickly.

What to Do Until Help Arrives

It is important to recognize the signals of a heart attack and to act on those signals. Any heart attack might lead to cardiac arrest, but prompt action may prevent further damage to the heart. A person suffering from a heart attack, and whose heart is still beating, has a far better chance of living than does a person whose heart has stopped. Most people who die of a heart attack die within 2 hours of the first signal. Many could have been saved if people on the scene or the person having the heart attack had been aware of the signals and acted promptly.

Many people who have heart attacks delay seeking care. Nearly half of all heart attack victims wait for 2 hours or more before going to the hospital. Often they do not realize they are having a heart attack. They may say the signals are just muscle soreness, indigestion or heartburn.

CORONARY HEART DISEASE

Recognizing a heart attack and getting the necessary care at once may prevent a person from going into cardiac arrest. However, preventing a heart attack in the first place is even more effective. There is no substitute for prevention.

Heart attacks usually result from disease of the heart and blood vessels. Although a heart attack may seem to strike suddenly, many people's lifestyles are gradually putting their hearts in danger. Because coronary heart disease develops slowly, some individuals may not be aware of it for many years. Fortunately, it is possible to slow the progression of the disease by making lifestyle changes.

Many things increase a person's chances of developing coronary heart disease. These are called risk factors. Some of them cannot be changed. For instance, although more women than men die each year from coronary heart disease in the United States, heart disease generally affects men at younger ages than it does women.

Besides gender, ethnicity also plays an important role in determining the risk for heart disease. African Americans and Native Americans have higher rates of heart disease than do other U.S. populations. A family history of heart disease also increases your risk.

Reducing Risk Factors

There are some risk factors that can be reduced. Cigarette smoking, a poor diet, uncontrolled high blood cholesterol or high blood pressure, being overweight and lack of regular exercise all increase your risk of heart disease. When you combine one risk factor, like smoking, with others, such as high blood pressure and lack of exercise, your risk of heart attack is much greater.

By taking steps to control your risk factors, you can improve your chances for living a long and healthy life. Remember, it is never too late.

The best way to deal with a heart attack or cardiac arrest is to prevent it. Begin to reduce your risk of heart disease today.

Early treatment with certain medications—including aspirin—can help minimize damage to the heart after a heart attack. To be most effective, these medications need to be given within 1 hour of the start of heart attack signals.

If you suspect that someone might be having a heart attack, you should:

- Call 9-1-1 or the local emergency number immediately.
- Have the person stop what he or she is doing and rest comfortably (Fig. 2-4). This will ease the heart's need for oxygen. Many people experiencing a heart attack find it easier to breathe while sitting.
- Loosen any tight or uncomfortable clothing.
- Closely watch the person until advanced medical personnel take over. Notice any changes in the person's appearance or behavior. Monitor the person's condition.
- Be prepared to perform CPR and use an AED, if available, if the person loses consciousness and stops breathing.
- Ask the person if he or she has a history of heart disease. Some people with heart disease take

prescribed medication for chest pain. You can help by getting the medication for the person and assisting him or her with taking the prescribed medication.

- Offer aspirin, if medically appropriate and local protocols allow, and if the patient can swallow and has no known contraindications (see the following section). Be sure that the person has not been

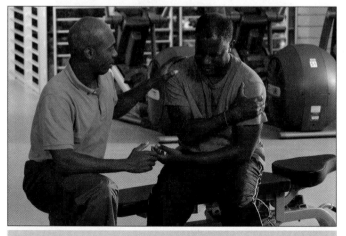

FIGURE 2-4 *Comforting the person helps to reduce anxiety and eases some of the discomfort.*

told by his or her health care provider to avoid taking aspirin.

■ Be calm and reassuring. Comforting the person helps to reduce anxiety and eases some of the discomfort.

■ Talk to bystanders and if possible the person to get more information.

■ Do not try to drive the person to the hospital yourself. He or she could quickly get worse on the way.

Giving Aspirin to Lessen Heart Attack Damage

You may be able to help a conscious person who is showing early signals of a heart attack by offering him or her an appropriate dose of aspirin when the signals first begin. However, you should never delay calling 9-1-1 or the local emergency number to do this. Always call for help as soon as you recognize the signals of a heart attack. Then help the person to be comfortable before you give the aspirin.

If the person is able to take medicine by mouth, ask:

■ Are you allergic to aspirin?

■ Do you have a stomach ulcer or stomach disease?

■ Are you taking any blood thinners, such as warfarin (Coumadin™)?

■ Have you ever been told by a doctor to avoid taking aspirin?

If the person answers **no** to *all* of these questions, you may offer him or her two chewable (81 mg each) baby aspirins, or one 5-grain (325 mg) adult aspirin tablet with a small amount of water. Do not use coated aspirin products or products meant for multiple uses such as for cold, fever and headache. You also may offer these doses of aspirin if the person regains consciousness while you are giving care and is able to take the aspirin by mouth.

Be sure that you offer only aspirin and not Tylenol®, acetaminophen or *nonsteroidal anti-inflammatory drugs* (NSAIDs), such as ibuprofen, Motrin®, Advil®, naproxen and Aleve®.

CARDIAC ARREST

Cardiac arrest occurs when the heart stops beating or beats too ineffectively to circulate blood to the brain and other vital organs. The beats, or contractions, of the heart become ineffective if they are weak, irregular or uncoordinated, because at that point the blood no longer flows through the arteries to the rest of the body.

When the heart stops beating properly, the body cannot survive. Breathing will soon stop, and the body's organs will no longer receive the oxygen they need to function. Without oxygen, brain damage can begin in about

4 to 6 minutes, and the damage can become irreversible after about 10 minutes.

A person in cardiac arrest is unconscious, not breathing and has no heartbeat. The heart has either stopped beating or is beating weakly and irregularly so that a pulse cannot be detected.

Cardiovascular disease is the primary cause of cardiac arrest in adults. Cardiac arrest also results from drowning, choking, drug abuse, severe injury, brain damage and electrocution.

Causes of cardiac arrest in children and infants include airway and breathing problems, traumatic injury, a hard blow to the chest, congenital heart disease and sudden infant death syndrome (SIDS).

Cardiac arrest can happen suddenly, without any of the warning signs usually seen in a heart attack. This is known as *sudden cardiac arrest* or *sudden cardiac death* and accounts for more than 300,000 deaths annually in the United States. Sudden cardiac arrest is caused by abnormal, chaotic electrical activity of the heart (known as *arrhythmias*). The most common life-threatening abnormal arrhythmia is *ventricular fibrillation* (V-fib).

Cardiac Chain of Survival

CPR alone may not be enough to help someone survive cardiac arrest. Advanced medical care is needed as soon as possible. A person in cardiac arrest will have the greatest chance of survival if you follow the four links in the Cardiac Chain of Survival:

1. **Early recognition and early access to the emergency medical services (EMS) system.** The sooner someone calls 9-1-1 or the local emergency number, the sooner EMS personnel will take over.

2. **Early CPR.** CPR helps supply blood containing oxygen to the brain and other vital organs. This helps to keep the person alive until an AED is used or advanced medical care is provided.

3. **Early defibrillation.** An electrical shock, called *defibrillation,* may help to restore an effective heart rhythm.

4. **Early advanced medical care.** EMS personnel provide more advanced medical care and transport the person to a hospital.

For each minute that CPR and defibrillation are delayed, the chance for survival is reduced by about 10 percent.

In the Cardiac Chain of Survival, each link of the chain depends on, and is connected to, the other links. Taking quick action by calling 9-1-1 or the local emergency number, starting CPR immediately and using an AED, if one is available, makes it more likely that a person in cardiac arrest will survive. Remember, you are the first link in the Cardiac Chain of Survival. By acting quickly, you can make a positive difference for someone experiencing a cardiac emergency.

What to Look For

The main signals of cardiac arrest in an adult, a child and an infant are unconsciousness and no breathing.

The presence of these signals means that no blood and oxygen are reaching the person's brain and other vital organs.

When to Call 9-1-1

Call 9-1-1 or the local emergency number *immediately* if you suspect that a person is in cardiac arrest or you witness someone suddenly collapse.

What to Do Until Help Arrives

Perform CPR until an AED is available and ready to use or advanced medical personnel take over.

Early CPR and Defibrillation

A person in cardiac arrest needs immediate CPR and defibrillation. The cells of the brain and other important organs continue to live for a short time—until all of the oxygen in the blood is used.

CPR is a combination of chest compressions and rescue breaths. When the heart is not beating, chest compressions are needed to circulate blood containing oxygen. Given together, rescue breaths and chest compressions help to take over for the heart and lungs. CPR increases the chances of survival for a person in cardiac arrest.

In many cases, however, CPR alone cannot correct the underlying heart problem: defibrillation delivered

by an AED is needed. This shock disrupts the heart's electrical activity long enough to allow the heart to spontaneously develop an effective rhythm on its own. Without *early* CPR and *early* defibrillation, the chances of survival are greatly reduced. (Using an AED is discussed in detail in Chapter 3.)

CPR for Adults

To determine if an unconscious adult needs CPR, follow the emergency action steps (**CHECK—CALL—CARE**) that you learned in Chapter 1.

- **CHECK** the scene and the injured or ill person.
- **CALL** 9-1-1 or the local emergency number.
- **CHECK** for breathing for no more than 10 seconds.
- Quickly **CHECK** for severe bleeding.
- If the person is not breathing, give **CARE** by beginning CPR.

For chest compressions to be the most effective, the person should be on his or her back on a firm, flat surface. If the person is on a soft surface like a sofa or bed, quickly move him or her to a firm, flat surface before you begin.

To perform CPR on an adult:

- Position your body correctly by kneeling beside the person's upper chest, placing your hands in the correct position, and keeping your arms and elbows as straight as possible so that your shoulders are directly over your hands (Fig. 2-5). Your body position is important when giving chest compressions. Compressing the person's chest straight down will help you reach the necessary depth. Using the correct body position also will be less tiring for you.
- Locate the correct hand position by placing the heel of one hand on the person's sternum (breastbone) at the center of his or her chest (Fig. 2-6). Place

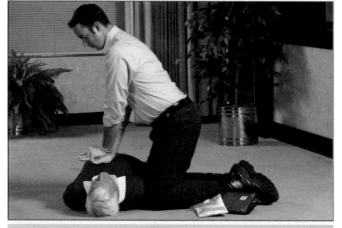

FIGURE 2-5 *Position yourself so that your shoulders are directly over your hands.*

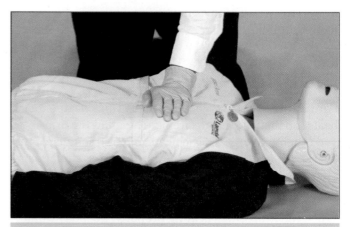

FIGURE 2-6 *Locate the correct hand position by placing the heel of one hand on the person's sternum (breastbone) in the center of the person's chest.*

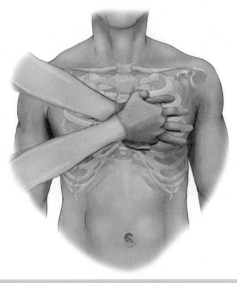

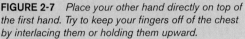

FIGURE 2-7 *Place your other hand directly on top of the first hand. Try to keep your fingers off of the chest by interlacing them or holding them upward.*

your other hand directly on top of the first hand and try to keep your fingers off of the chest by interlacing them or holding them upward (Fig. 2-7). If you feel the notch at the end of the sternum, move your hands slightly toward the person's head. If you have arthritis in your hands, you can give compressions by grasping the wrist of the hand positioned on the chest with your other hand (Fig. 2-8). The person's clothing should not interfere with finding the proper hand position or your ability to give effective compressions. If it does, loosen or remove enough clothing to allow deep compressions in the center of the person's chest.

■ Give 30 chest compressions. Push hard, push fast at a rate of at least 100 compressions per minute. Note that the term "100 compressions per minute" refers to the *speed of compressions,* not the *number of compressions* given in a minute. As you give compressions, count out loud, "One and two and three and four and five and six and..." up to 30. Push down as you say the number and come up as you say "and." This will help you to keep a steady, even rhythm.

■ Give compressions by pushing the sternum down at least 2 inches (Fig. 2-9, A). The downward and upward movement should be smooth, not jerky. Push straight down with the weight of your upper body, not with your arm muscles. This way, the weight of your upper body will create the force needed to compress the chest. Do not rock back and forth. Rocking results in less-effective compressions and wastes much-needed energy. If your arms and shoulders tire quickly, you are not using the correct body position.

■ After each compression, release the pressure on the chest without removing your hands or changing hand position (Fig. 2-9, B). Allow the chest to return to its normal position before starting the next compression. Maintain a steady down-and-up rhythm and do not pause between compressions. Spend half of the time pushing down and half of the time coming up. When you press down, the walls of the heart squeeze together, forcing the blood to empty out of the heart. When you come up, you should release all pressure on the chest, but do not take hands off the chest. This allows the heart's chambers to fill with blood between compressions.

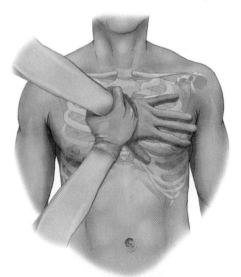

FIGURE 2-8 *If you have arthritis in your hands, you can give compressions by grasping the wrist of the hand positioned on the chest with your other hand.*

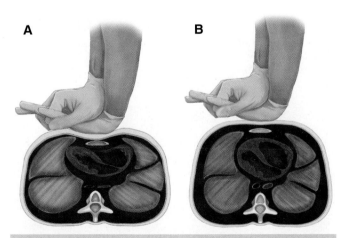

FIGURE 2-9, A–B *To give chest compressions:* **A,** *Push straight down with the weight of your body.* **B,** *Release, allowing the chest to return to its normal position.*

- Once you have given 30 compressions, open the airway using the head-tilt/chin-lift technique and give 2 rescue breaths. Each rescue breath should last about 1 second and make the chest clearly rise.
  - Open the airway and give rescue breaths, one after the other.
  - Tilt the head back and lift the chin up.
  - Pinch the nose shut then make a complete seal over the person's mouth.
  - Blow in for about 1 second to make the chest clearly rise.
- Continue cycles of chest compressions and rescue breaths. Each cycle of chest compressions and rescue breaths should take about 24 seconds. Minimize the interruption of chest compressions.

If Two Responders Are Available

If two responders trained in CPR are at the scene, both should identify themselves as being trained. One should call 9-1-1 or the local emergency number for help while the other performs CPR. If the first responder is tired and needs help:

- The first responder should tell the second responder to take over.
- The second responder should immediately take over CPR, beginning with chest compressions.

When to Stop CPR

Once you begin CPR, do not stop except in one of these situations:

- You notice an obvious sign of life, such as breathing.
- An AED is available and ready to use.
- Another trained responder or EMS personnel take over (Fig. 2-10).

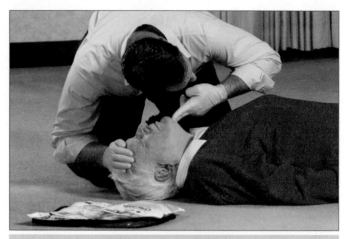

FIGURE 2-11 *Monitor breathing until help arrives.*

- You are too exhausted to continue.
- The scene becomes unsafe.

If at any time you notice that the person is breathing, stop CPR. Keep his or her airway open and continue to monitor the person's breathing and for any changes in the person's condition until EMS personnel take over (Fig. 2-11).

Cardiac Emergencies in Children and Infants

It is rare for a child or an infant to initially suffer a cardiac emergency. Usually, a child or an infant has a respiratory emergency first and then a cardiac emergency develops.

Causes of cardiac arrest in children and infants include:

- Airway and breathing problems.
- Traumatic injury or an accident (e.g., motor-vehicle collision, drowning, electrocution or poisoning).
- A hard blow to the chest.
- Congenital heart disease.
- Sudden infant death syndrome (SIDS).

If you recognize that a child or an infant is not breathing, begin CPR.

CPR for Children and Infants

Follow the emergency action steps (**CHECK—CALL—CARE**) to determine if you will need to perform CPR for a child or an infant. The principles of CPR (compressing the chest and giving rescue breaths) are the same for children and infants as for adults. However, the CPR techniques are slightly different since children's and infants' bodies are smaller.

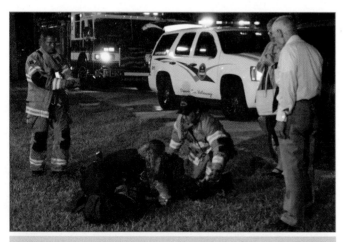

FIGURE 2-10 *Perform CPR until an AED becomes available and is ready to use or EMS personnel take over.* Courtesy of Terry Georgia.

ADVANCE DIRECTIVES

Your 85-year-old grandfather is living with your family. He has a terminal illness and is frequently in the hospital.

One afternoon, you go to his room to give him lunch. As you start to talk to him, you realize that he is unconscious. You check for breathing. He is not breathing. What should you do?

No one but you can answer that question. No one can advise you. No one can predict the outcome of your decision. You alone must decide whether or not to give your grandfather CPR.

Endless questions race through your mind. Can I face the fact I am losing someone I love? Should I always try to perform CPR? What would his life be like after resuscitation? What would my grandfather want? Your mind tells you to perform CPR, yet your heart says no.

It is important to realize that it is okay to withhold CPR when a terminally ill person is dying. Nature takes its course, and in some cases people feel they have lived full lives and are prepared for death.

Advance Directives

Fortunately, this type of heart-wrenching, last-second decision sometimes can be avoided if loved ones talk to each other in advance about their preferences regarding lifesaving treatments.

Instructions that describe a person's wishes about medical treatment are called advance directives. *These instructions make known a person's intentions while he or she is still capable of doing so and are used when the person can no longer make his or her own health-care decisions.*

As provided by the Federal Patient Self-Determination Act, adults who are admitted to a hospital or a health-care facility or who receive assistance from certain organizations that receive funds from Medicare and Medicaid have the right to make fundamental choices about their own care. They must be told about their right to make decisions about the level of life support that would be provided in an emergency situation. They are supposed to be offered the opportunity to make these choices at the time of admission.

Conversations with relatives, friends or health care providers while the person is still capable of making decisions are the most common form of advance directives. However, because conversations may not be recalled accurately or may not have taken into account the illness or emergency now facing the person, the courts consider written directives to be more reliable.

Two examples of written advance directives are living wills and durable powers of attorney for health care. The types of health-care decisions covered by these documents vary by state. Talking with a legal professional can help to determine which advance directive options are available in your state and what they cover.

If a person establishes a living will, directions for health care would be in place before he or she became unable to communicate his or her wishes. Instructions that can be included in this document vary from state to state. A living will generally allows a person to refuse only medical care that "merely prolongs the process of dying," such as resuscitating a person with a terminal illness.

If a person has established a durable power of attorney for health care, the document would authorize someone else to make medical decisions for that person in any situation in which the person could no longer make them for him- or herself. This authorized person is called a health care surrogate *or* proxy. *This surrogate, with the information given by the person's health care provider, may consent to or refuse medical treatment on the person's behalf.*

Do Not Resuscitate or Do Not Attempt Resuscitation

A doctor could formalize the person's preferences by writing Do Not Resuscitate (DNR) or Do Not Attempt Resuscitation (DNAR) orders in his or her medical records. Such orders would state that if the person's heart or breathing stops, he or she should not be resuscitated. DNR/DNAR orders may be covered in a living will or in the durable power of attorney for health care.

(Continued)

Appointing someone to act as a health care surrogate, along with writing down your instructions, is the best way to formalize your wishes about medical care. Some of these documents can be obtained through a personal physician, attorney or various state and health care organizations. A lawyer is not always needed to execute advance directives. However, if you have any questions concerning advance directives, it is wise to obtain legal advice.

Talk in Advance

Copies of advance directives should be provided to all personal physicians, family members and the person chosen as the health care surrogate. Tell them which documents have been prepared and where the original and other copies are located.

Discuss the document with all parties so that they understand the intent of all requests. Keep these documents updated.

Keep in mind that advance directives are not limited to elderly people or people with terminal illnesses. Advance directives should be considered by anyone who has decided on the care he or she would like to have provided. An unexpected injury or illness could create a need for decisions at any time.

Knowing about living wills, durable powers of attorney for health care and DNR/DNAR orders can help you prepare for difficult decisions. For more information about your rights and the options available to you in your state, contact a legal professional.

CPR for a Child

If during the unconscious check you find that the child is not breathing, place the child face-up on a firm, flat surface. Begin CPR by following these steps:

- Locate the proper hand position on the middle of the breastbone as you would for an adult (Fig. 2-12, A). If you feel the notch at the end of the sternum, move your hands slightly toward the child's head.

- Position your body as you would for an adult, kneeling next to the child's upper chest, positioning your shoulders over your hands and keeping your arms and elbows as straight as possible.

- Give 30 chest compressions. Push hard, push fast to a depth of about 2 inches and at a rate of at least 100 compressions per minute. Lift up, allowing the chest to fully return to its normal position, but keep contact with the chest.

- After giving 30 chest compressions, open the airway and give 2 rescue breaths (Fig. 2-12, B). Each rescue breath should last about 1 second and make the chest clearly rise. Use the head-tilt/chin-lift technique to ensure that the child's airway is open.

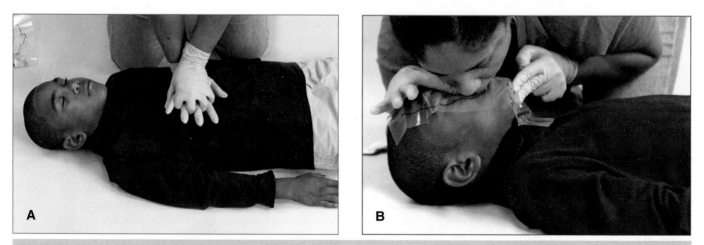

A **B**

FIGURE 2-12, A–B *To perform CPR on a child:* **A,** *Locate the proper hand position in the center of the child's chest by placing 2 hands on the center of the child's chest.* **B,** *After giving 30 chest compressions, open the airway and give 2 rescue breaths.*

Continue cycles of 30 chest compressions and 2 rescue breaths. Do not stop CPR except in one of these situations:

- You find an obvious sign of life, such as breathing.
- An AED is ready to use.
- Another trained responder or EMS personnel take over.
- You are too exhausted to continue.
- The scene becomes unsafe.

If at any time you notice the child begin to breathe, stop CPR, keep the airway open and monitor breathing and for any changes in the child's condition until EMS personnel take over.

CPR for an Infant

If during your check you find that the infant is not breathing, begin CPR by following these steps:

- Find the correct location for compressions. Keep one hand on the infant's forehead to maintain an open airway. Use the pads of two or three fingers of your other hand to give chest compressions on the center of the chest, just below the nipple line (toward the infant's feet). If you feel the notch at the end of the infant's sternum, move your fingers slightly toward the infant's head.
- Give 30 chest compressions using the pads of these fingers to compress the chest. Compress the chest about 1½ inches. Push hard, push fast (Fig. 2-13, A). Your compressions should be smooth, not jerky. Keep a steady rhythm. Do not pause between each compression.

When your fingers are coming up, release pressure on the infant's chest completely but do not let your fingers lose contact with the chest. Compress at a rate of at least 100 compressions per minute.

- After giving 30 chest compressions, give 2 rescue breaths, covering the infant's mouth and nose with your mouth (Fig. 2-13, B). Each rescue breath should last about 1 second and make the chest clearly rise.

Continue cycles of 30 chest compressions and 2 rescue breaths. Do not stop CPR except in one of these situations:

- You find an obvious sign of life, such as breathing.
- An AED is ready to use.
- Another trained responder or EMS personnel take over.
- You are too exhausted to continue.
- The scene becomes unsafe.

If at any time you notice the infant begin to breathe, stop CPR, keep the airway open and monitor breathing and for any changes in the infant's condition until EMS personnel take over.

Continuous Chest Compressions (Hands-Only CPR)

If you are unable or unwilling for any reason to perform full CPR (with rescue breaths), give continuous chest compressions after calling 9-1-1 or the local emergency number. Continue giving chest compressions until EMS personnel take over or you notice an obvious sign of life, such as breathing.

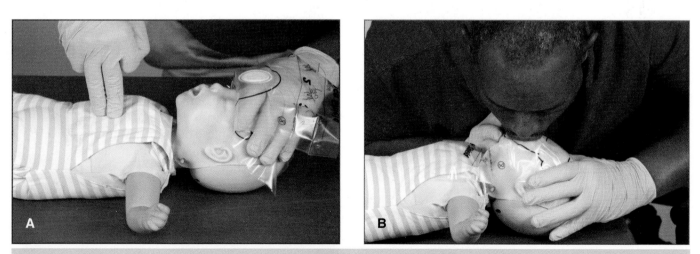

FIGURE 2-13, A–B *To perform CPR on an infant:* **A,** *Place the pads of two or three fingers in the center of the infant's chest and compress the chest about 1½ inches.* **B,** *Give 2 rescue breaths, covering the infant's mouth and nose with your mouth.*

TABLE 2-1   CPR SKILL COMPARISON

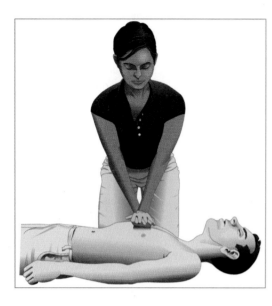
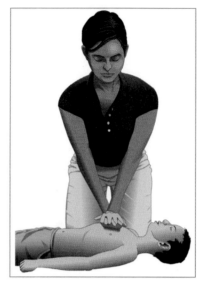
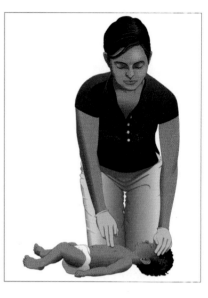

Skill Components	Adult	Child	Infant
HAND POSITION	Two hands in center of chest (on lower half of sternum)	Two hands in center of chest (on lower half of sternum)	Two or three fingers in center of chest (on lower half of sternum, just below nipple line)
CHEST COMPRESSIONS **RESCUE BREATHS**	At least 2 inches Until the chest clearly rises (about 1 second per breath)	About 2 inches Until the chest clearly rises (about 1 second per breath)	About 1½ inches Until the chest clearly rises (about 1 second per breath)
CYCLE	30 chest compressions and 2 rescue breaths	30 chest compressions and 2 rescue breaths	30 chest compressions and 2 rescue breaths
RATE	30 chest compressions in about 18 seconds (at least 100 compressions per minute)	30 chest compressions in about 18 seconds (at least 100 compressions per minute)	30 chest compressions in about 18 seconds (at least 100 compressions per minute)

PUTTING IT ALL TOGETHER

Cardiac emergencies are life threatening. Every day someone will have a heart attack or go into cardiac arrest. These cardiac emergencies usually happen in the home. If you know the signals of a heart attack and cardiac arrest, you will be able to respond immediately. Call 9-1-1 or the local emergency number and give care until help takes over. If the person is in cardiac arrest, perform CPR. Use an AED if one is available. These steps will increase the chances of survival for the person having a cardiac emergency.

CPR—ADULT
NO BREATHING

AFTER CHECKING THE SCENE AND THE INJURED OR ILL PERSON:

1 GIVE 30 CHEST COMPRESSIONS

Push hard, push fast in the center of the chest at least **2** inches deep and at least **100** compressions per minute.

> **TIP:** *The person must be on a firm, flat surface.*

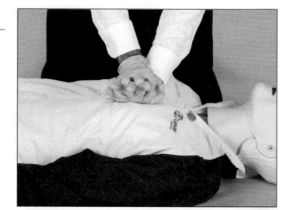

2 GIVE 2 RESCUE BREATHS

- Tilt the head back and lift the chin up.
- Pinch the nose shut then make a complete seal over the person's mouth.
- Blow in for about **1** second to make the chest clearly rise.
- Give rescue breaths, one after the other.
- If chest does not rise with rescue breaths, retilt the head and give another rescue breath.

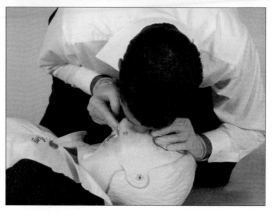

3 DO NOT STOP

Continue cycles of CPR. Do not stop except in one of these situations:
- You find an obvious sign of life, such as breathing.
- An AED is ready to use.
- Another trained responder or EMS personnel take over.
- You are too exhausted to continue.
- The scene becomes unsafe.

> **TIP:** *If at any time you notice an obvious sign of life, stop CPR and monitor breathing and for any changes in condition.*

WHAT TO DO NEXT

- USE AN AED AS SOON AS ONE IS AVAILABLE.
- IF BREATHS DO NOT MAKE CHEST RISE AFTER RETILTING THE HEAD—Give CARE for unconscious choking.

CPR–CHILD
NO BREATHING

AFTER CHECKING THE SCENE AND THE INJURED OR ILL CHILD:

1 GIVE 30 CHEST COMPRESSIONS

Push hard, push fast in the center of the chest about **2** inches deep and at least **100** compressions per minute.

> **TIP:** *The child must be on a firm, flat surface.*

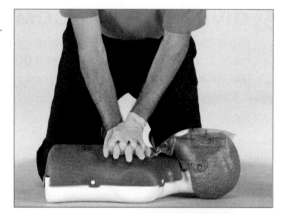

2 GIVE 2 RESCUE BREATHS

- Tilt the head back and lift the chin up.
- Pinch the nose shut then make a complete seal over the child's mouth.
- Blow in for about **1** second to make the chest clearly rise.
- Give rescue breaths, one after the other.
- If chest does not rise with rescue breaths, retilt the head and give another rescue breath.

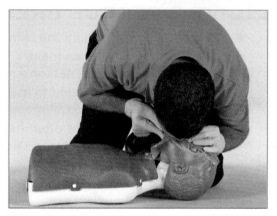

3 DO NOT STOP

Continue cycles of CPR. Do not stop except in one of these situations:

- You find an obvious sign of life, such as breathing.
- An AED is ready to use.
- Another trained responder or EMS personnel take over.
- You are too exhausted to continue.
- The scene becomes unsafe.

> **TIP:** *If at any time you notice an obvious sign of life, stop CPR and monitor breathing and for any changes in condition.*

WHAT TO DO NEXT

- USE AN AED AS SOON AS ONE IS AVAILABLE.
- IF BREATHS DO NOT MAKE CHEST RISE AFTER RETILTING THE HEAD—Give **CARE** for unconscious choking.

CPR–INFANT
NO BREATHING

AFTER CHECKING THE SCENE AND THE INJURED OR ILL INFANT:

1 GIVE 30 CHEST COMPRESSIONS

Push hard, push fast in the center of the chest about **1½** inches deep and at least **100** compressions per minute.

> **TIP:** *The infant must be on a firm, flat surface.*

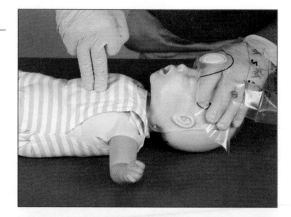

2 GIVE 2 RESCUE BREATHS

- Tilt the head back and lift the chin up.
- Make a complete seal over the infant's mouth and nose.
- Blow in for about **1** second to make the chest clearly rise.
- Give rescue breaths, one after the other.
- If chest does not rise with rescue breaths, retilt the head and give another rescue breath.

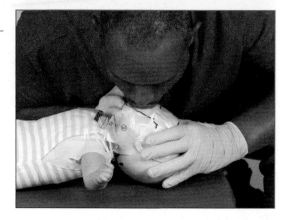

3 DO NOT STOP

Continue cycles of CPR. Do not stop except in one of these situations:

- You find an obvious sign of life, such as breathing.
- An AED is ready to use.
- Another trained responder or EMS personnel take over.
- You are too exhausted to continue.
- The scene becomes unsafe.

> **TIP:** *If at any time you notice an obvious sign of life, stop CPR and monitor breathing and for any changes in condition.*

WHAT TO DO NEXT

- USE AN AED AS SOON AS ONE IS AVAILABLE.
- IF BREATHS DO NOT MAKE CHEST RISE AFTER RETILTING THE HEAD—Give **CARE** for unconscious choking.

CHAPTER 3

AED

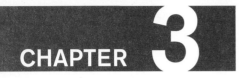

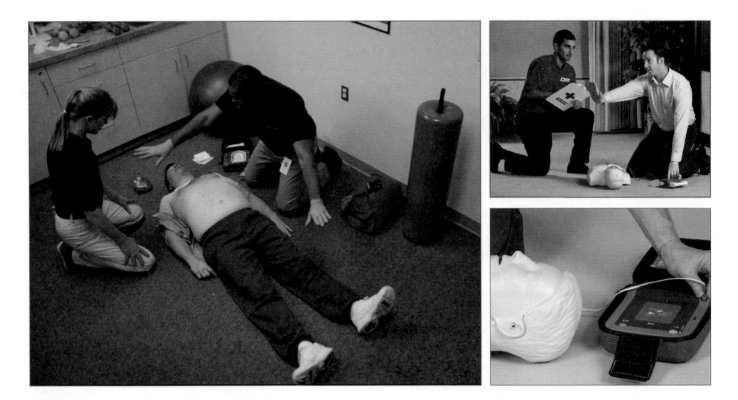

Sudden cardiac arrest occurs when the heart suddenly stops beating normally because of abnormal electrical activity of the heart. Every year in the United States more than 300,000 people die of sudden cardiac arrest. Sudden cardiac arrest can happen to anyone, anytime without warning but usually occurs in adults. Most cardiac arrests happen in the home. Therefore, knowing how to activate the emergency medical services (EMS) system, perform CPR and use an automated external defibrillator (AED) could help you save a life—most likely someone you love.

This chapter further discusses the third link in the Cardiac Chain of Survival: early defibrillation, including what it is and how it works in the case of life-threatening abnormal electrical activity of the heart. You also will read about the steps to follow when using an AED. This knowledge will give you the confidence to give care to anyone who experiences sudden cardiac arrest.

WHEN THE HEART SUDDENLY FAILS

The heart's electrical system sends out signals that tell the heart to pump blood. These signals travel through the upper chambers of the heart, called the *atria*, to the lower chambers, called the *ventricles*.

When the heart is normal and healthy, these electrical signals cause the ventricles to squeeze together, or contract. These contractions force blood out of the heart. The blood then circulates throughout the body. When the ventricles relax between contractions, blood flows back into the heart. The pause that you notice between heart beats when taking a person's pulse are the pauses between contractions.

If the heart is damaged by disease or injury, its electrical system can be disrupted. This can cause an abnormal heart rhythm that can stop the blood from circulating. The most common abnormal heart rhythm that causes sudden cardiac arrest occurs when the ventricles simply quiver, or *fibrillate*, without any organized rhythm. This condition is called *ventricular fibrillation* (V-fib). In V-fib, the electrical impulses fire at random, creating chaos and preventing the heart from pumping and circulating blood. The person may suddenly collapse unconscious, and stop breathing.

Another abnormal rhythm found during sudden cardiac arrest is *ventricular tachycardia*, or V-tach. With V-tach, the electrical system tells the ventricles to contract too quickly. As a result, the heart cannot pump blood properly. As with V-fib, during V-tach the person may collapse, become unconscious and stop breathing.

In many cases, V-fib and V-tach can be corrected by an electrical shock delivered by an AED. AEDs are portable electronic devices that analyze the heart's rhythm and deliver an electrical shock, known as *defibrillation*, which helps the heart to re-establish an effective rhythm (Fig. 3-1). For each minute that CPR and defibrillation are delayed, the person's chance for survival is reduced by about 10 percent. However, by learning how to perform CPR and use an AED, you can make a difference before EMS personnel take over.

USING AN AED

When a cardiac arrest in an adult occurs, call 9-1-1 or local emergency number and begin CPR immediately. Also, use an AED as soon as it is available and ready to use (Fig. 3-2). If CPR is in progress, do not interrupt until the AED is turned on and the defibrillation pads are applied. Always follow *local protocols*, which are

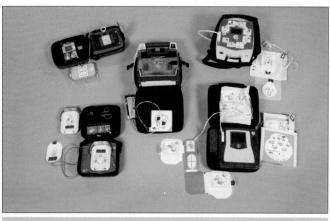

FIGURE 3-1 *There are several types of AEDs.*

guidelines provided by the facility's medical director or EMS system, when using an AED. Be thoroughly familiar with the manufacturer's operating instructions. Also, be familiar with maintenance guidelines for the device that you will be using.

AED PRECAUTIONS

When operating an AED, follow these general precautions:

- Do *not* use alcohol to wipe the person's chest dry. Alcohol is flammable.
- Do *not* use an AED and/or pads designed for adults on a child younger than 8 years or weighing less than 55 pounds unless pediatric AED pads specific to the device are not available.
- Do *not* use pediatric AED pads on an adult or on a child older than 8 years, or on a person weighing more than 55 pounds. AEDs equipped with pediatric AED pads deliver lower levels of energy that are considered appropriate only for children

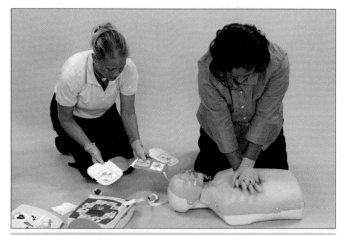

FIGURE 3-2 *Defibrillation may help the heart to re-establish an effective heart rhythm.*

and infants up to 8 years old or weighing less than 55 pounds.

- Do *not* touch the person while the AED is analyzing. Touching or moving the person may affect analysis.
- Before shocking a person with an AED, make sure that *no one* is touching or is in contact with the person or any resuscitation equipment.
- Do *not* touch the person while the device is defibrillating. You or someone else could be shocked.
- Do *not* defibrillate someone when around flammable or combustible materials, such as gasoline or free-flowing oxygen.
- Do *not* use an AED in a moving vehicle. Movement may affect the analysis.
- Do *not* use an AED on a person who is in contact with water. Move the person and AED away from puddles of water or swimming pools or out of the rain before defibrillating.
- Do *not* use an AED on a person wearing a nitroglycerin patch or other medical patch on the chest. With a gloved hand, remove any patches from the chest before attaching the device.
- Do *not* use a mobile phone or radio within 6 feet of the AED. Radiofrequency interference (RFI) and electromagnetic interference (EMI), as well as infrared interference, generated by radio signals can disrupt analysis.

HOW TO USE AN AED—ADULTS

Different types of AEDs are available, but all are similar to operate and have some common features, such as electrode (AED or defibrillation) pads, voice prompts, visual displays and/or lighted buttons to guide the responder through the steps of the AED operation. Most AEDs can be operated by following these simple steps:

- Turn on the AED.
- Expose the person's chest and wipe the bare chest dry with a small towel or gauze pads. This ensures that the AED pads will stick to the chest properly.
- Apply the AED pads to the person's *bare, dry* chest. (Make sure to peel the backing off each pad, one at a time, to expose the adhesive surface of the pad before applying it to the person's bare chest.) Place one pad on the upper right chest and the other pad on the left side of the chest (Fig. 3-3, A).
- Plug the connector into the AED, if necessary.
- Let the AED analyze the heart rhythm (or push the button marked "analyze," if indicated and prompted by the AED). Advise all responders and bystanders to "stand clear" (Fig. 3-3, B). No one should touch the person while the AED is analyzing because this could result in faulty readings.
- If the AED advises that a shock is needed:
  - Make sure that no one, including you, is touching the person.
  - Say, "EVERYONE, STAND CLEAR."
  - Deliver the shock by pushing the "shock" button, if necessary. (Some models can deliver the shock automatically while others have a "shock" button that must be manually pushed to deliver the shock.)
- After delivering the shock, or if no shock is advised:
  - Perform about 2 minutes (or 5 cycles) of CPR.
  - Continue to follow the prompts of the AED.

If at any time you notice an obvious sign of life, such as breathing, stop performing CPR and monitor the person's breathing and any changes in the person's condition.

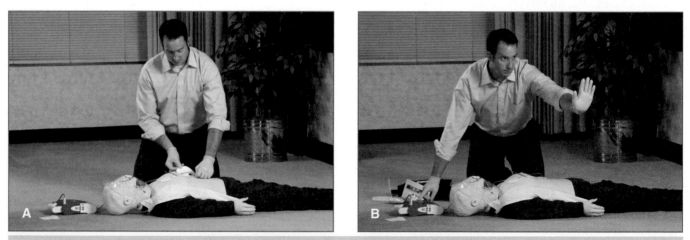

FIGURE 3-3, A–B *To use an AED on an adult: Turn on the AED.* **A,** *Apply the pads to the person's bare, dry chest. Place one pad on the upper right chest and the other pad on the left side of the chest.* **B,** *Advise everyone to "stand clear" while the AED analyzes the heart rhythm. Deliver a shock by pushing the shock button if indicated and prompted by the AED.*

HOW TO USE AN AED—CHILDREN AND INFANTS

While the incidence of cardiac arrest is relatively low compared with adults, sudden cardiac arrest resulting from V-fib does happen to young children and infants. However, most cases of cardiac arrest in children and infants are not sudden and may be caused by:

- Airway and breathing problems.
- Traumatic injuries or accidents (e.g., motor-vehicle collision, drowning, electrocution or poisoning).
- A hard blow to the chest.
- Congenital heart disease.
- Sudden infant death syndrome (SIDS).

Use an AED as soon as it is available, ready to use and is safe to do so. However, as you learned in the Cardiac Chain of Survival, in a cardiac emergency, you should always call 9-1-1 or the local emergency number *first*.

AEDs equipped with pediatric AED pads can deliver lower levels of energy considered appropriate for children and infants up to 8 years of age or weighing less than 55 pounds. Use pediatric AED pads and/or equipment if available. If pediatric-specific equipment is not available, use an AED designed for adults on children and infants. Always follow local protocols (i.e., guidelines provided by the facility's medical director or EMS) and the manufacturer's instructions. Follow the same general steps and precautions that you would when using an AED on an adult in cardiac arrest.

- Turn on the AED.
- Expose the child's or infant's chest and wipe it dry.
- Apply the pediatric pads to the child's or infant's bare, dry chest. Place one pad on the child's upper right chest and the other pad on the left side of the chest. Make sure that the pads are not touching. If the pads risk touching each other, such as with a small child or an infant, place one pad in the middle of the child's or infant's chest and the other pad on the child's or infant's back, between the shoulder blades (Fig. 3-4, A–B).
- Plug the connector into the AED, if necessary.
- Let the AED analyze the heart rhythm (or push the button marked "analyze," if indicated and prompted by the AED). Advise all responders and bystanders to "Stand clear." No one should touch the child or infant while the AED is analyzing because this could result in faulty reading.
- If the AED advises that a shock is needed:
  ○ Make sure that no one, including you, is touching the child or infant.
  ○ Say, "EVERYONE, STAND CLEAR."
  ○ Deliver the shock by pushing the "shock" button, if necessary.
- After delivering the shock, or if no shock is advised:
  ○ Perform about 2 minutes (or 5 cycles) of CPR.
  ○ Continue to follow the prompts of the AED.

If at any time you notice an obvious sign of life, such as breathing, stop performing CPR and monitor breathing and for any changes in the child's or infant's condition.

SPECIAL AED SITUATIONS

Some situations require you to pay special attention when using an AED. These include using AEDs around water and on people with implantable devices, transdermal patches, hypothermia, trauma and jewelry or body piercings. Or, you may need to determine what

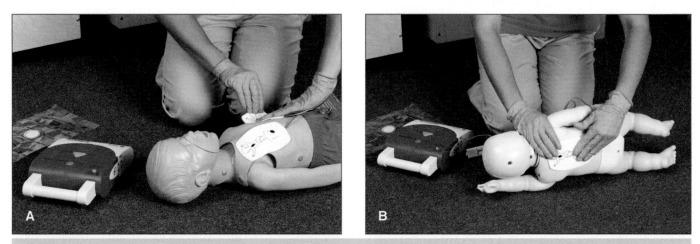

FIGURE 3-4, A–B **A,** *Place one pediatric pad on the upper right chest and the other pad on the left side of the chest.* **B,** *If the pads risk touching each other, place one on the chest and the other on the back of the child or infant.*

to do if local protocols or the AED's instructions differ from those you have learned. Familiarize yourself with these situations as much as possible so that you know how to respond appropriately, should the situation arise. Always use common sense when using an AED and follow the manufacturer's recommendations.

AEDs Around Water

If the person is in water, remove him or her from the water before defibrillation. A shock delivered in water could harm responders or bystanders. Once you have removed the person from the water, be sure there are no puddles of water around you, the person or the AED. Remove wet clothing to place the pads properly, if necessary. Dry the person's chest and attach the AED pads.

If it is raining, take steps to make sure that the person is as dry as possible and sheltered from the rain. Ensure that the person's chest is wiped dry. Do not delay defibrillation when taking steps to create a dry environment. AEDs are safe when all precautions and manufacturer's operating instructions are followed, even in rain and snow. Avoid getting the AED or defibrillation pads wet.

Pacemakers and Implantable Cardioverter-Defibrillators

Some people whose hearts are weak, beat too slowly, skip beats or beat in a rhythm that is too fast may have had a *pacemaker* implanted. These small, implantable devices are usually located in the area below the person's left collar bone, although they can be placed elsewhere. Typically they feel like a small lump under the skin. Other people may have an *implantable cardioverter-defibrillator* (ICD), a miniature version of an AED. ICDs automatically recognize and restore abnormal heart rhythms. Sometimes a person's heart beats irregularly, even if the person has a pacemaker or ICD.

If the implanted device is visible or you know that the person has one, do *not* place the defibrillation pads directly over the device (Fig. 3-5). This may interfere with the delivery of the shock. Adjust pad placement if necessary and continue to follow the AED instructions. If you are not sure whether the person has an implanted device, use the AED if needed. It will not harm the person or responder.

The responder should be aware that it is possible to receive a mild shock if an implantable ICD delivers a shock to the person during CPR. However, this risk of injury to responders is minimal, and the amount of electrical energy involved is low. Follow any special precautions associated with ICDs but do not delay in performing CPR and using an AED.

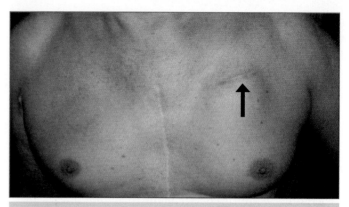

FIGURE 3-5 *Look for an ICD before defibrillation.* Courtesy of Ted Crites.

Transdermal Medication Patches

Some people have a patch on their skin that automatically delivers medication through the skin, called a *transdermal medication patch*. A common medication patch is the nitroglycerin patch, which is used by people with a history of cardiac problems. Because a responder can absorb medication through the skin, remove patches with a gloved hand before defibrillation. Nicotine patches used to stop smoking look similar to nitroglycerin patches. Do not waste time trying to identify patches. Instead remove any patch that you see on the person's chest with a gloved hand. *Never* place AED electrode pads directly on top of medication patches.

Hypothermia

Hypothermia is a life-threatening condition in which the entire body cools because its ability to keep warm fails. Some people who have experienced hypothermia have been resuscitated successfully, even after prolonged exposure to the cold. If the person is not breathing, begin CPR until an AED becomes readily available. Follow local protocols as to whether you should use an AED in this situation.

If the person is wet, remove wet clothing and dry his or her chest. Attach the AED pads. If a shock is indicated, deliver it, following the instructions of the AED. If the person still is not breathing, continue CPR and protect the person from further heat loss. Follow local protocols as to whether additional shocks should be delivered. Do not withhold CPR or defibrillation to re-warm the person. Be careful not to unnecessarily shake a person who has experienced hypothermia as this could result in V-fib.

Trauma

If a person is in cardiac arrest as a result of traumatic injuries, you still can use an AED. Administer defibrillation according to local protocols.

Chest Hair

Some men have excessive chest hair that may interfere with AED pad-to-skin contact, although it's a rare occurrence. Since time is critical in a cardiac arrest situation and chest hair rarely interferes with pad adhesion, attach the pads and analyze the heart's rhythm as soon as possible. Press firmly on the pads to attach them to the person's chest.

If you get a "check pads" or similar message from the AED, remove the pads and replace them with new ones. The pad adhesive may pull out some of the chest hair, which may solve the problem. If you continue to get the "check pads" message, remove the pads, shave the person's chest where the pads should be placed, and attach new pads to the person's chest. (There should be spare defibrillation pads and a safety razor included in the AED kit.) Be careful not to cut the person while shaving the chest, as cuts and scrapes can interfere with rhythm analysis.

Metal Surfaces

It is safe to deliver a shock to a person in cardiac arrest when he or she is lying on a metal surface, such as bleachers, as long as appropriate safety precautions are taken. Specifically, care should be taken that defibrillation electrode pads do not contact the conductive (metal) surface and that no one is touching the person when the shock button is pressed.

Jewelry and Body Piercings

You *do not* need to remove jewelry and body piercings when using an AED. Leaving them on the person will do no harm. Taking time to remove them will delay giving the first shock. Therefore, do *not* delay the use of an AED to remove jewelry or body piercings. However, do *not* place the AED pads directly over metallic jewelry or body piercings. Adjust AED pad placement if necessary.

OTHER AED PROTOCOLS

Other AED protocols, such as delivering three shocks and then performing CPR, are neither wrong nor harmful to the person. However, improved methods, based on scientific evidence, make it easier to coordinate performing CPR and using the AED. Follow the instructions of the AED device you are using.

AED MAINTENANCE

For defibrillators to perform properly, they must be maintained like any other machine. AEDs require minimal maintenance. They have a variety of self-testing features. However, it is important to be familiar with any visual or audible warning prompts on the AED that warn of malfunction or a low battery. Read the operator's manual thoroughly and check with the manufacturer to obtain all necessary information regarding maintenance.

In most cases, if the machine detects any malfunction, contact the manufacturer. You may need to return the device to the manufacturer for service. Although AEDs require minimal maintenance, it is important to remember the following:

- Follow the manufacturer's specific recommendations and your facility's schedule for periodic equipment checks, including checking the batteries and defibrillation pads.
- Make sure that the batteries have enough energy for one complete rescue. (A fully charged backup battery should be readily available.)
- Make sure that the correct defibrillation pads are in the package and are properly sealed.
- Check any expiration dates on defibrillation pads and batteries and replace as needed.
- After use, make sure that all accessories are replaced and that the machine is in proper working order.
- If at any time the machine fails to work properly or warning indicators are recognized, stop using it and contact the manufacturer immediately. If the AED stops working during an emergency continue performing CPR until EMS personnel take over.

PUTTING IT ALL TOGETHER

Sudden cardiac arrest is a life-threatening emergency that happens when the heart suddenly stops beating or circulating blood because of abnormal electrical activity of the heart. You must act quickly to help. For a person to survive cardiac arrest, responders must recognize the cardiac emergency, call 9-1-1 immediately, perform CPR and use an AED as soon as one becomes available. These actions will keep blood containing oxygen flowing throughout the body, stop the abnormal heart rhythm and ensure that advanced medical care arrives as quickly as possible. The sooner the EMS system is activated, CPR is started and a defibrillation shock from an AED is delivered, the greater are the chances for survival. By following the four links of the Cardiac Chain of Survival you can help save a life.

AED–ADULT OR CHILD
OLDER THAN 8 YEARS OR WEIGHING MORE THAN 55 POUNDS
NO BREATHING

> **TIP:** *Do not use pediatric AED pads or equipment on an adult or on a child older than 8 years or weighing more than 55 pounds.*

AFTER CHECKING THE SCENE AND THE INJURED OR ILL PERSON:

1 TURN ON AED

Follow the voice and/or visual prompts.

2 WIPE BARE CHEST DRY

> **TIP:** *Remove any medication patches with a gloved hand.*

3 ATTACH PADS

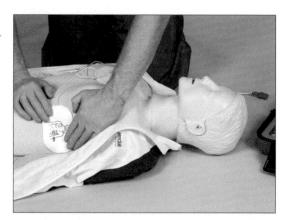

4 PLUG IN CONNECTOR, IF NECESSARY

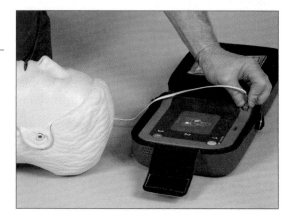

5 STAND CLEAR

Make sure no one, including you, is touching the person.

- Say, "EVERYONE STAND CLEAR."

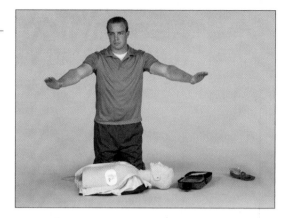

6 ANALYZE HEART RHYTHM

Push the "analyze" button, if necessary. Let the AED analyze the heart rhythm.

7 DELIVER SHOCK

IF A SHOCK IS ADVISED:

- Make sure no one, including you, is touching the person.
- Say, "EVERYONE STAND CLEAR."
- Push the "shock" button, if necessary.

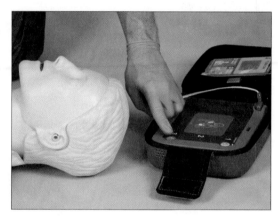

8 PERFORM CPR

After delivering the shock, or if no shock is advised:

- Perform about **2** minutes (or **5** cycles) of CPR.
- Continue to follow the prompts of the AED.

TIPS:

- *If at any time you notice an obvious sign of life, stop CPR and monitor breathing and for any changes in condition.*

- *If two trained responders are present, one should perform CPR while the second responder operates the AED.*

AED–CHILD AND INFANT
YOUNGER THAN 8 YEARS OR WEIGHING LESS THAN 55 POUNDS
NO BREATHING

> **TIP:** *When available, use pediatric settings or pads when caring for children and infants. If pediatric equipment is not available, rescuers may use AEDs configured for adults.*

AFTER CHECKING THE SCENE AND THE INJURED OR ILL CHILD OR INFANT:

1 TURN ON AED

Follow the voice and/or visual prompts.

2 WIPE BARE CHEST DRY

3 ATTACH PADS

If the pads risk touching each other, use the front-to-back pad placement.

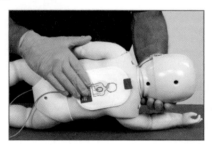
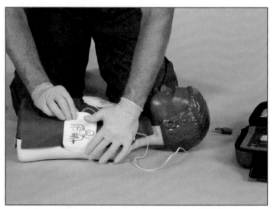

4 PLUG IN CONNECTOR, IF NECESSARY

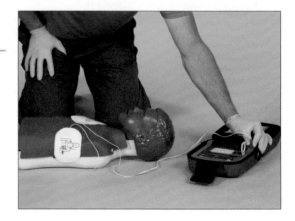

5 STAND CLEAR

Make sure no one, including you, is touching the child or infant.

- Say, "EVERYONE STAND CLEAR."

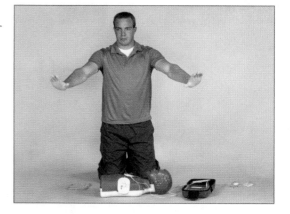

6 ANALYZE HEART RHYTHM

Push the "analyze" button, if necessary. Let the AED analyze the heart rhythm.

7 DELIVER SHOCK

IF A SHOCK IS ADVISED:

- Make sure no one, including you, is touching the child or infant.
- Say, "EVERYONE STAND CLEAR."
- Push the "shock" button.

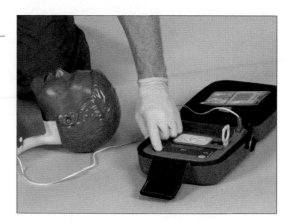

8 PERFORM CPR

After delivering the shock, or if no shock is advised:

- Perform about **2** minutes (or **5** cycles) of CPR.
- Continue to follow the prompts of the AED.

TIPS:

- *If at any time you notice an obvious sign of life, stop CPR and monitor breathing and for any changes in condition.*

- *If two trained responders are present, one should perform CPR while the second responder operates the AED.*

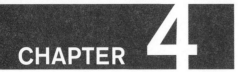

CHAPTER 4

Breathing Emergencies

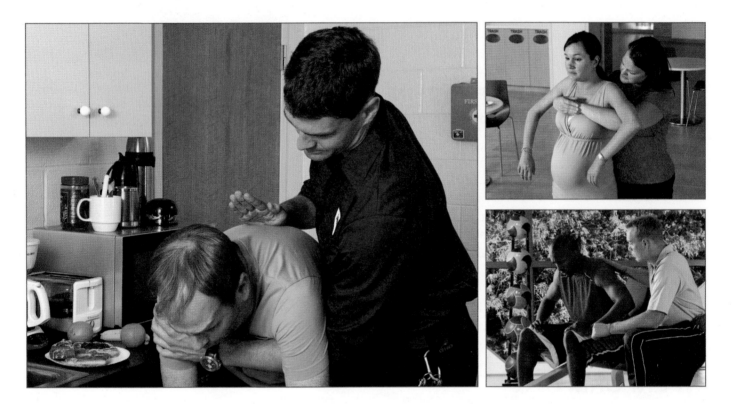

A *breathing emergency* is any respiratory problem that can threaten a person's life. Breathing emergencies happen when air cannot travel freely and easily into the lungs. Respiratory distress, respiratory arrest and choking are examples of breathing emergencies. In a breathing emergency, seconds count so you must react at once. This chapter discusses how to recognize and care for breathing emergencies.

BACKGROUND

The human body needs a constant supply of oxygen to survive. When you breathe through your mouth and nose, air travels down your throat, through your windpipe and into your lungs. This pathway from the mouth and nose to the lungs is called the *airway*.

As you might imagine, the airway, mouth and nose are smaller in children and infants than they are in adults (Fig. 4-1, A–B). As a result, they can be blocked more easily by small objects, blood, fluids or swelling.

In a breathing emergency, air must reach the lungs. For any person, regardless of age, it is important to keep the airway open when giving care.

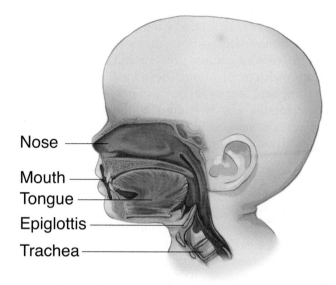

Nose
Mouth
Tongue
Epiglottis
Trachea

FIGURE 4-1, A *A child's airway*

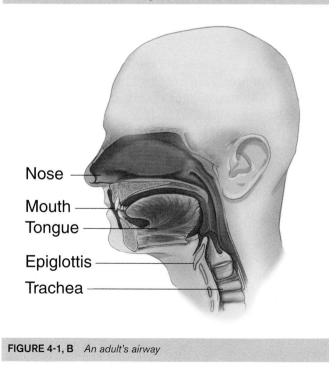

Nose
Mouth
Tongue
Epiglottis
Trachea

FIGURE 4-1, B *An adult's airway*

Once air reaches the lungs, oxygen in the air is transferred to the blood. The heart pumps the blood throughout the body. The blood flows through the blood vessels, delivering oxygen to the brain, heart and all other parts of the body.

In some breathing emergencies the oxygen supply to the body is greatly reduced, whereas in others the oxygen supply is cut off entirely. As a result, the heart soon stops beating and blood no longer moves through the body. Without oxygen, brain cells can begin to die within 4 to 6 minutes (Fig. 4-2). Unless the brain receives oxygen within minutes, permanent brain damage or death will result.

It is important to recognize breathing emergencies in children and infants and act before the heart stops beating. Frequently, an adult's heart stops working (known as *cardiac arrest*) because of heart disease. However, children and infants usually have healthy hearts. When the heart stops in a child or infant, it usually is the result of a breathing emergency.

No matter what the age of the person, trouble breathing can be the first signal of a more serious emergency, such as a heart problem. Recognizing the signals of breathing problems and giving care often are the keys to preventing these problems from becoming more serious emergencies.

If the injured or ill person is conscious, he or she may be able to indicate what is wrong by speaking or gesturing to you and may be able to answer questions. However, if you are unable to communicate with a

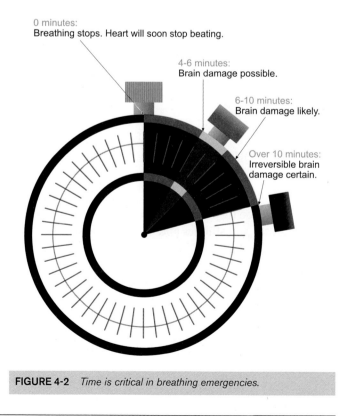

0 minutes:
Breathing stops. Heart will soon stop beating.

4-6 minutes:
Brain damage possible.

6-10 minutes:
Brain damage likely.

Over 10 minutes:
Irreversible brain damage certain.

FIGURE 4-2 *Time is critical in breathing emergencies.*

person, it can be difficult to determine what is wrong. Therefore, it is important to recognize the signals of breathing emergencies, know when to call 9-1-1 or the local emergency number and know what to do until help arrives and takes over.

RESPIRATORY DISTRESS AND RESPIRATORY ARREST

Respiratory distress and respiratory arrest are types of breathing emergencies. *Respiratory distress* is a condition in which breathing becomes difficult. It is the most common breathing emergency. Respiratory distress can lead to *respiratory arrest*, which occurs when breathing has stopped.

Normal breathing is regular, quiet and effortless. A person does not appear to be working hard or struggling when breathing normally. This means that the person is not making noise when breathing, breaths are not fast and breathing does not cause discomfort or pain. However, it should be noted that normal breathing rates in children and infants are faster than normal breathing rates in adults. Infants have periodic breathing, so changes in breathing patterns are normal for infants.

You usually can identify a breathing problem by watching and listening to the person's breathing and by asking the person how he or she feels.

Causes of Respiratory Distress and Respiratory Arrest

Respiratory distress and respiratory arrest can be caused by:

- Choking (a partially or completely obstructed airway).
- Illness.
- Chronic conditions (long-lasting or frequently recurring), such as asthma.
- Electrocution.
- Irregular heartbeat.
- Heart attack.
- Injury to the head or brain stem, chest, lungs or abdomen.
- Allergic reactions.
- Drug overdose (especially alcohol, narcotic painkillers, barbiturates, anesthetics and other depressants).
- Poisoning.
- Emotional distress.
- Drowning.

Asthma

Asthma is the inflammation of the air passages that results in a temporary narrowing of the airways that carry oxygen to the lungs. An asthma attack happens when a trigger, such as exercise, cold air, allergens or other irritants, causes the airway to swell and narrow. This makes breathing difficult.

The Centers for Disease Control and Prevention (CDC) estimate that in 2005, nearly 22.2 million Americans were affected by asthma. Asthma is more common in children and young adults than in older adults, but its frequency and severity is increasing in all age groups in the United States. Asthma is the third-ranking cause of hospitalization among those younger than 15 years.

You often can tell when a person is having an asthma attack by the hoarse whistling sound that he or she makes while exhaling. This sound, known as *wheezing*, occurs because air becomes trapped in the lungs. Trouble breathing, shortness of breath, tightness in the chest and coughing after exercise are other signals of an asthma attack. Usually, people diagnosed with asthma prevent and control their attacks with medication. These medications reduce swelling and mucus production in the airways. They also relax the muscle bands that tighten around the airways, making breathing easier. For more information on asthma, see Chapter 10.

Chronic Obstructive Pulmonary Disease

Chronic obstructive pulmonary disease (COPD) is a long-term lung disease encompassing both chronic bronchitis and emphysema. COPD causes a person to have trouble breathing because of damage to the lungs. In a person with COPD, the airways become partly blocked and the air sacs in the lungs lose their ability to fill with air. This makes it hard to breathe in and out. There is no cure for COPD, and it worsens over time.

The most common cause of COPD is cigarette smoking, but breathing in other types of lung irritants, pollution, dust or chemicals over a long period also can cause COPD. It usually is diagnosed when a person is middle aged or older. It is the fourth-ranking cause of death in the United States and a major cause of illness.

Common signals of COPD include:

- Coughing up a large volume of mucus.
- Tendency to tire easily.
- Loss of appetite.
- Bent posture with shoulders raised and lips pursed to make breathing easier.
- A fast pulse.
- Round, barrel-shaped chest.
- Confusion (caused by lack of oxygen to the brain).

Emphysema

Emphysema is a type of COPD. *Emphysema* is a disease that involves damage to the air sacs in the lungs. It is a chronic (long-lasting or frequently recurring) disease that worsens over time. The most common signal of emphysema is shortness of breath. Exhaling is extremely difficult. In advanced cases, the affected person may feel restless, confused and weak, and even may go into respiratory or cardiac arrest.

Bronchitis

Bronchitis is an inflammation of the main air passages to the lungs. It can be acute (short-lasting) or chronic. Chronic bronchitis is a type of COPD. To be diagnosed with chronic bronchitis, a person must have a cough with mucus on most days of the month for at least 3 months.

Acute bronchitis is *not* a type of COPD; it develops after a person has had a viral respiratory infection. It first affects the nose, sinuses and throat and then spreads to the lungs. Those most at risk for acute bronchitis include children, infants, the elderly, people with heart or lung disease and smokers.

Signals of both types of bronchitis include:

- Chest discomfort.
- Cough that produces mucus.
- Fatigue.
- Fever (usually low).
- Shortness of breath that worsens with activity.
- Wheezing.

Additional signals of chronic bronchitis include:

- Ankle, feet and leg swelling.
- Blue lips.
- Frequent respiratory infections, such as colds or the flu.

Hyperventilation

Hyperventilation occurs when a person's breathing is faster and more shallow than normal. When this happens, the body does not take in enough oxygen to meet its demands. People who are hyperventilating feel as if they cannot get enough air. Often they are afraid and anxious or seem confused. They may say that they feel dizzy or that their fingers and toes feel numb and tingly.

Hyperventilation often results from fear or anxiety and usually occurs in people who are tense and nervous. However, it also can be caused by head injuries, severe bleeding or illnesses, such as high fever, heart failure, lung disease and diabetic emergencies. Asthma and exercise also can trigger hyperventilation.

Hyperventilation is the body's way of compensating when there is a lack of enough oxygen. The result is a decrease in carbon dioxide, which alters the acidity of the blood.

Allergic Reactions

An *allergic reaction* is the response of the immune system to a foreign substance that enters the body. Common allergens include bee or insect venom, antibiotics, pollen, animal dander, sulfa and some foods such as nuts, peanuts, shellfish, strawberries and coconut oils.

Allergic reactions can cause breathing problems. At first the reaction may appear to be just a rash and a feeling of tightness in the chest and throat, but this condition can become life threatening. The person's face, neck and tongue may swell, closing the airway.

A severe allergic reaction can cause a condition called *anaphylaxis,* also known as *anaphylactic shock.* During anaphylaxis, air passages swell and restrict a person's breathing. Anaphylaxis can be brought on when a person with an allergy comes into contact with allergens via insect stings, food, certain medications or other substances. Signals of anaphylaxis include a rash, tightness in the chest and throat, and swelling of the face, neck and tongue. The person also may feel dizzy or confused. Anaphylaxis is a life-threatening emergency.

Some people know that they are allergic to certain substances or to insect stings. They may have learned to avoid these things and may carry medication to reverse the allergic reaction. People who have severe allergic reactions may wear a medical identification (ID) tag, bracelet or necklace.

Croup

Croup is a harsh, repetitive cough that most commonly affects children younger than 5 years. The airway constricts, limiting the passage of air, which causes the child to produce an unusual-sounding cough that can range from a high-pitched wheeze to a barking cough. Croup mostly occurs during the evening and nighttime.

Most children with croup can be cared for at home using mist treatment or cool air. However, in some cases, a child with croup can progress quickly from respiratory distress to respiratory arrest.

Epiglottitis

Epiglottitis is a far less common infection than croup that causes severe swelling of the epiglottis. The epiglottis is a piece of cartilage at the back of the tongue.

When it swells, it can block the windpipe and lead to severe breathing problems. Epiglottitis usually is caused by infection with *Haemophilus influenzae* bacteria.

The signals of epiglottitis may be similar to croup, but it is a more serious illness and can result in death if the airway is blocked completely.

In the past, epiglottitis was a common illness in children between 2 and 6 years of age. However, epiglottitis in children has dropped dramatically in the United States since the 1980s when children began routinely receiving the H. influenzae type B (Hib) vaccine.

For children and adults, epiglottitis begins with a high fever and sore throat. A person with epiglottitis may need to sit up and lean forward, perhaps with the chin thrust out in order to breathe. Other signals include drooling, difficulty swallowing, voice changes, chills, shaking and fever.

Seek medical care immediately for a person who may have epiglottitis. This condition is a medical emergency.

What to Look For

Although breathing problems have many causes, you do not need to know the exact cause of a breathing emergency to care for it. You do need to be able to recognize when a person is having trouble breathing or is not breathing at all. Signals of breathing emergencies include:

- Trouble breathing or no breathing.
- Slow or rapid breathing.
- Unusually deep or shallow breathing.
- Gasping for breath.
- Wheezing, gurgling or making high-pitched noises.
- Unusually moist or cool skin.
- Flushed, pale, ashen or bluish skin.
- Shortness of breath.
- Dizziness or light-headedness.
- Pain in the chest or tingling in the hands, feet or lips.
- Apprehensive or fearful feelings.

When to Call 9-1-1

If a person is not breathing or if breathing is too fast, too slow, noisy or painful, call 9-1-1 or the local emergency number immediately.

What to Do Until Help Arrives

If an adult, child or infant is having *trouble breathing*:

- Help the person rest in a comfortable position. Usually, sitting is more comfortable than lying down because breathing is easier in that position (Fig. 4-3).

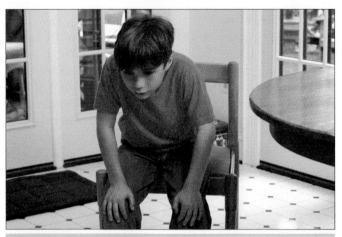

FIGURE 4-3 *A person who is having trouble breathing may breathe more easily in a sitting position.*

- If the person is conscious, check for other conditions.
- Remember that a person having breathing problems may find it hard to talk. If the person cannot talk, ask him or her to nod or to shake his or her head to answer yes-or-no questions. Try to reassure the person to reduce anxiety. This may make breathing easier.
- If bystanders are present and the person with trouble breathing is having difficulty answering your questions, ask them what they know about the person's condition.
- If the person is hyperventilating and you are sure whether it is caused by emotion, such as excitement or fear, tell the person to relax and breathe slowly. A person who is hyperventilating from emotion may resume normal breathing if he or she is reassured and calmed down. If the person's breathing still does not slow down, the person could have a serious problem.

If an adult is unconscious and *not* breathing, the cause is most likely a cardiac emergency. Immediately begin CPR starting with chest compressions. If an adult is not breathing because of a respiratory cause, such as drowning, or drug overdose, give 2 rescue breaths after checking for breathing and before quickly scanning for severe bleeding and beginning CPR.

Remember, a nonbreathing person's greatest need is for oxygen. If breathing stops or is restricted long enough, a person will become unconscious, the heart will stop beating and body systems will quickly fail.

If a child or an infant is unconscious and *not breathing*, give 2 rescue breaths after checking for breathing and before quickly scanning for severe bleeding and beginning CPR.

CHOKING

Choking is a common breathing emergency. It occurs when the person's airway is partially or completely blocked. If a conscious person is choking, his or her airway has been blocked by a foreign object, such as a piece of food or a small toy; by swelling in the mouth or throat; or by fluids, such as vomit or blood. With a partially blocked airway, the person usually can breathe with some trouble. A person with a partially blocked airway may be able to get enough air in and out of the lungs to cough or to make wheezing sounds. The person also may get enough air to speak. A person whose airway is completely blocked cannot cough, speak, cry or breathe at all.

Causes of Choking in Adults

Causes of choking in an adult include:

- Trying to swallow large pieces of poorly chewed food.
- Drinking alcohol before or during meals. (Alcohol dulls the nerves that aid swallowing.)
- Wearing dentures. (Dentures make it difficult to sense whether food is fully chewed before it is swallowed.)
- Eating while talking excitedly or laughing, or eating too fast.
- Walking, playing or running with food or objects in the mouth.

Causes of Choking in Children and Infants

Choking is a common cause of injury and death in children younger than 5 years. Because young children put nearly everything in their mouths, small, nonfood items, such as safety pins, small parts from toys and coins, often cause choking. However, food is responsible for most of the choking incidents in children.

The American Academy of Pediatrics (AAP) recommends that young children not be given hard, smooth foods such as raw vegetables. These foods must be chewed with a grinding motion, which is a skill that children do not master until 4 years of age; therefore, children may attempt to swallow these foods whole. For this same reason, the AAP recommends not giving children peanuts until they are 7 years of age or older.

The AAP also recommends that young children not be given round, firm foods such as hot dogs and carrot sticks unless they are chopped into small pieces no larger than ½ inch. Since choking remains a significant danger to children younger than 5 years, the AAP further recommends keeping the following foods, and other items meant to be chewed or swallowed, away from young children:

- Hard, gooey or sticky candy
- Grapes
- Popcorn

FOCUS ON PREVENTION

CHOKING IN CHILDREN AND INFANTS

- *Supervise mealtimes for young children and infants.*
- *Do not let children eat while playing or running.*
- *Teach children to chew and swallow food before talking or laughing.*
- *Do not give chewing gum to young children.*
- *Do not give young children smooth, hard food such as peanuts and raw vegetables.*
- *Do not give young children round, firm foods such as hot dogs and carrot sticks unless chopped into pieces ½ inch or smaller.*
- *Do not allow small children to play with un-inflated balloons. (The U.S. Consumer Product Safety Commission recommends keeping these away from children younger than 8 years of age.)*
- *Keep small objects such as safety pins, small parts from toys and coins away from small children.*
- *Make sure that toys are too large to be swallowed.*
- *Make sure that toys have no small parts that could be pulled off.*

If you are unsure whether an object is safe for young children, test it by trying to pass it through a toilet paper roll. If it fits through the 1¾-inch diameter roll, it is not safe for young children.

- Chewing gum
- Vitamins

Although food items cause most of the choking injuries in children, toys and household items also can be hazardous. Balloons, when broken or un-inflated, can choke or suffocate young children who try to swallow them. According to the Consumer Product Safety Commission (CPSC), more children have suffocated on non-inflated balloons and pieces of broken balloons than any other type of toy. Other nonfood items that can cause choking include:

- Baby powder.
- Objects from the trash, such as eggshells and pop-tops from beverage cans.
- Safety pins.
- Coins.
- Marbles.
- Pen and marker caps.
- Small button-type batteries.

What to Look For

Signals of choking include:

- Coughing, either forcefully or weakly.
- Clutching the throat with one or both hands (Fig. 4-4).
- Inability to cough, speak, cry or breathe.
- Making high-pitched noises while inhaling or noisy breathing.
- Panic.
- Bluish skin color.
- Losing consciousness if blockage is not removed.

When to Call 9-1-1

If the person continues to cough without coughing up the object, have someone call 9-1-1 or the local emergency number. A partially blocked airway can quickly become completely blocked.

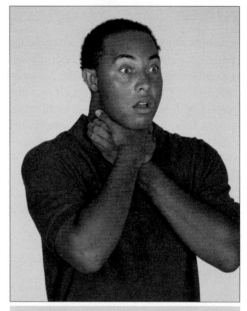

FIGURE 4-4 *Clutching the throat with one or both hands is universally recognized as a signal for choking.*

A person whose airway is completely blocked cannot cough, speak, cry or breathe. Sometimes the person may cough weakly or make high-pitched noises. This tells you that the person is not getting enough air to stay alive. Act at once! If a bystander is available, have him or her call 9-1-1 or the local emergency number while you begin to give care.

What to Do Until Help Arrives
Caring for a Conscious Choking Adult or Child

If the choking person is coughing forcefully, let him or her try to cough up the object. A person who is getting enough air to cough or speak is getting enough air to breathe. Stay with the person and encourage him or her to continue coughing.

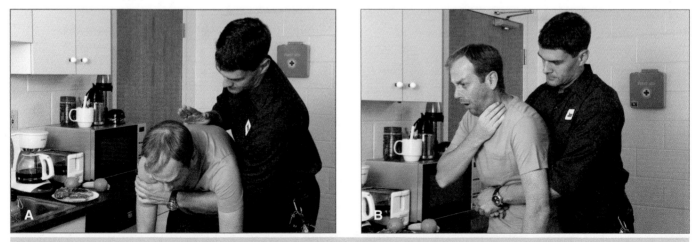

FIGURE 4-5, A–B *If a conscious adult has a completely blocked airway:* **A,** *Give back blows.* **B,** *Then give abdominal thrusts.*

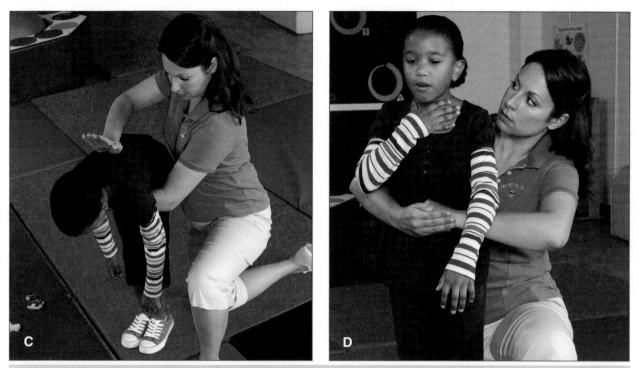

FIGURE 4-5, C–D   *If a conscious child has a completely blocked airway:* **C,** *Give back blows.* **D,** *Then give abdominal thrusts, as you would for an adult.*

A conscious adult or child who has a completely blocked airway needs immediate care. Using more than one technique often is necessary to dislodge an object and clear a person's airway. A combination of 5 back blows followed by 5 abdominal thrusts provides an effective way to clear the airway obstruction (Fig. 4-5, A–D).

To give back blows, position yourself slightly behind the person. Provide support by placing one arm diagonally across the chest and bend the person forward at the waist until the upper airway is at least parallel to the ground. Firmly strike the person between the shoulder blades with the heel of your other hand.

To give abdominal thrusts to a conscious choking adult or child:

■ Stand or kneel behind the person and wrap your arms around his or her waist.

■ Locate the navel with one or two fingers of one hand. Make a fist with the other hand and place the thumb side against the middle of the person's abdomen, just above the navel and well below the lower tip of the breastbone.

■ Grab your fist with your other hand and give quick, upward thrusts into the abdomen.

Each back blow and abdominal thrust should be a separate and distinct attempt to dislodge the obstruction. Continue sets of 5 back blows and 5 abdominal thrusts until the object is dislodged; the person can cough forcefully, speak or breathe; or the person becomes unconscious. For a conscious child, use less force when

giving back blows and abdominal thrusts. Using too much force may cause internal injuries.

A person who has choked and has been given back blows, abdominal thrusts and/or chest thrusts to clear the airway requires a medical evaluation. Internal injuries and damage to the airway may not be evident immediately.

Special Situations in Caring for the Conscious Choking Adult or Child

Special situations include:

■ **A large or pregnant person.** If a conscious choking person is too large for you to reach around, is obviously pregnant or is known to be pregnant, give chest thrusts instead (Fig. 4-6). Chest thrusts

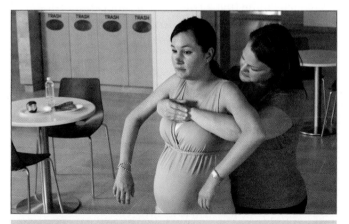

FIGURE 4-6   *Give chest thrusts to a choking person who is obviously pregnant or known to be pregnant or is too large for you to reach around.*

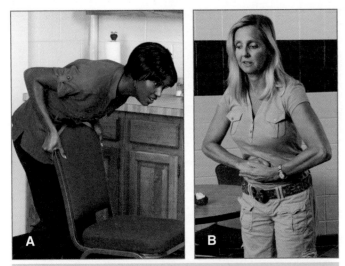

FIGURE 4-7, A–B *If you are alone and choking; A, Bend over and press your abdomen against any firm object, such as the back of a chair. B, Or, give yourself abdominal thrusts by using your hands, just as you would do to another person.*

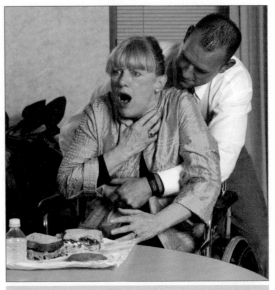

FIGURE 4-8 *For a choking person in a wheelchair, give abdominal thrusts.*

for a conscious adult are like abdominal thrusts, except for the placement of your hands. For chest thrusts, place your fist against the center of the person's breastbone. Then grab your fist with your other hand and give quick thrusts into the chest.

■ **Being alone and choking.** If you are alone and choking, bend over and press your abdomen against any firm object, such as the back of a chair, a railing or the kitchen sink (Fig. 4-7, A). Do not bend over anything with a sharp edge or corner that might hurt you, and be careful when leaning on a rail that is elevated. Alternatively, give yourself abdominal thrusts, using your hands, just as if you were administering the abdominal thrusts to another person (Fig. 4-7, B).

■ **A person in a wheelchair.** For a choking person in a wheelchair, give abdominal thrusts (Fig. 4-8).

Caring for a Conscious Choking Infant

If you determine that a conscious infant cannot cough, cry or breathe, you will need to give a combination of 5 back blows followed by 5 chest thrusts.

To give back blows:

■ Position the infant face-up on your forearm.
  ○ Place one hand and forearm on the child's back, cradling the back of the head, and one hand and forearm on the front of the infant. Use your thumb and fingers to hold the infant's jaw while sandwiching the infant between your forearms.
  ○ Turn the infant over so that he or she is face-down along your forearm (Fig. 4-9, A).
■ Lower your arm onto your thigh so that the infant's head is lower than his or her chest. Then give 5 firm

back blows with the heel of your hand between the shoulder blades (Fig. 4-9, B). Each back blow should be a separate and distinct attempt to dislodge the object.

■ Maintain support of the infant's head and neck by firmly holding the jaw between your thumb and forefinger.

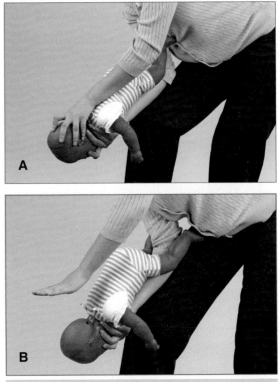

FIGURE 4-9, A–B *A, To give back blows, position the infant so that he or she is face-down along your forearm. B, Give 5 firm back blows with the heel of your hand while supporting the arm that is holding the infant on your thigh.*

To give chest thrusts:

- Place the infant in a face-up position.
  - Place one hand and forearm on the child's back, cradling the back of the head, while keeping your other hand and forearm on the front of the infant. Use your thumb and fingers to hold the infant's jaw while sandwiching the infant between your forearms (Fig. 4-10, A).
  - Turn the infant onto his or her back.
- Lower your arm that is supporting the infant's back onto your opposite thigh. The infant's head should be lower than his or her chest, which will assist in dislodging the object.
- Place the pads of two or three fingers in the center of the infant's chest just below the nipple line (toward the infant's feet).
- Use the pads of these fingers to compress the breastbone. Compress the breastbone 5 times about 1½ inches and then let the breastbone return to its normal position. Keep your fingers in contact with the infant's breastbone (Fig. 4-10, B).

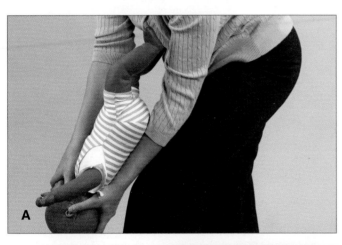

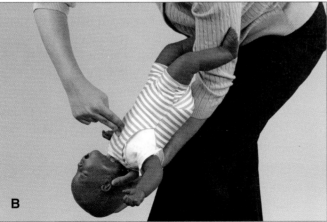

FIGURE 4-10, A–B **A,** *To give chest thrusts, sandwich the infant between your forearms. Continue to support the infant's head.* **B,** *Turn the infant onto his or her back keeping the infant's head lower than the chest. Give 5 chest thrusts.*

Continue giving sets of 5 back blows and 5 chest thrusts until the object is forced out; the infant begins to cough forcefully, cry or breathe on his or her own; or the infant becomes unconscious.

You can give back blows and chest thrusts effectively whether you stand, kneel or sit, as long as the infant is supported on your thigh and the infant's head is lower than the chest. If the infant is large or your hands are too small to adequately support it, you may prefer to sit.

Use less force when giving back blows and chest thrusts to an infant than for a child or an adult. Using too much force may cause internal injuries.

Caring for a Conscious Choking Adult or Child Who Becomes Unconscious

If a conscious choking adult or child becomes unconscious, carefully lower the person to the ground, open the mouth and look for an object. If an object is seen, remove it with your finger. If no object is seen, open the person's airway by tilting the head and try to give 2 rescue breaths. If the chest does not clearly rise, begin the modified CPR technique used for an unconscious choking person, which is described next.

Caring for an Unconscious Choking Adult or Child

If you determine that an adult or a child is unconscious, not breathing and the chest does not rise with rescue breaths, retilt the head and try another rescue breath. If the chest still does not rise, assume that the airway is blocked.

To care for an unconscious choking adult or child, perform a modified CPR technique:

- Locate the correct hand position for chest compressions. Use the same technique that is used for CPR.
- Give chest compressions. Compress an adult's chest 30 times to a depth of at least 2 inches (Fig. 4-11, A). Compress a child's chest 30 times to a depth of about 2 inches. Compress at a rate of at least 100 chest compressions per minute; the 30 chest compressions should take about 18 seconds to complete.
- Look for a foreign object (Fig. 4-11, B). Open the person's mouth. (Remove the CPR breathing barrier if you are using one.) If you see an object, remove it with a finger (Fig. 4-11, C).

- Give 2 rescue breaths (Fig. 4-11, D). If the chest does not clearly rise, repeat cycles of chest compressions, foreign object check/removal and 2 rescue breaths. Do not stop except in one of these situations:
  - The object is removed and the chest clearly rises with rescue breaths.
  - The person starts to breathe on his or her own.
  - Another trained responder or EMS personnel take over.
  - You are too exhausted to continue.
  - The scene becomes unsafe.

If the breaths make the chest clearly rise, quickly check for breathing. Care for the conditions you find.

Caring for a Conscious Choking Infant Who Becomes Unconscious

If a conscious choking infant becomes unconscious, carefully lower the infant to the ground, open the mouth and look for an object. If an object is seen, remove it with your little finger. If no object is seen, open the infant's airway by retilting the head and try to give 2 rescue breaths. If the chest does not clearly rise, begin a modified CPR technique used for an unconscious choking infant, which is described next.

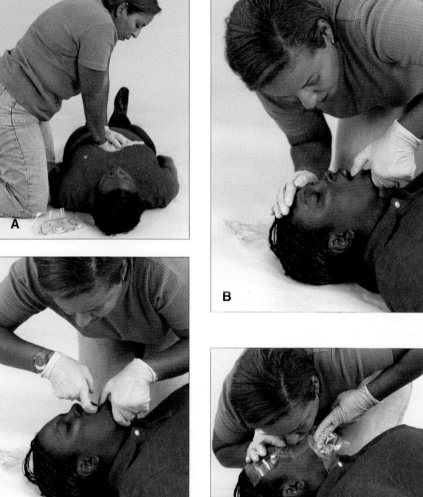

FIGURE 4-11, A–D *For an unconscious choking adult or child:* **A,** *Give 30 chest compressions.* **B,** *Look for an object.* **C,** *If you see one, remove it with a finger.* **D,** *Give 2 rescue breaths.*

Caring for an Unconscious Choking Infant

If you determine that an infant is unconscious, not breathing and the chest does not rise with rescue breaths, retilt the head and try another rescue breath. If the chest still does not rise, assume that the airway is blocked.

To care for an unconscious choking infant:

- Locate the correct hand and finger position for chest compressions. Use the same technique that is used for CPR.
- Give 30 chest compressions at a rate of at least 100 chest compressions per minute (Fig. 4-12, A). Each compression should be about 1½ inches deep.

- Look for a foreign object (Fig. 4-12, B). If the object is seen, remove it with your little finger (Fig. 4-12, C).
- Give 2 rescue breaths (Fig. 4-12, D). If the breaths do not make the chest clearly rise, repeat cycles of chest compressions, foreign object check/removal and rescue breaths. Do not stop except in one of these situations:
  - The object is removed and the chest clearly rises with rescue breaths.
  - The infant starts to breathe on his or her own.
  - Another trained responder or EMS personnel take over.
  - You are too exhausted to continue.
  - The scene becomes unsafe.

If the breaths make the chest clearly rise, quickly check for breathing. Care for the conditions you find.

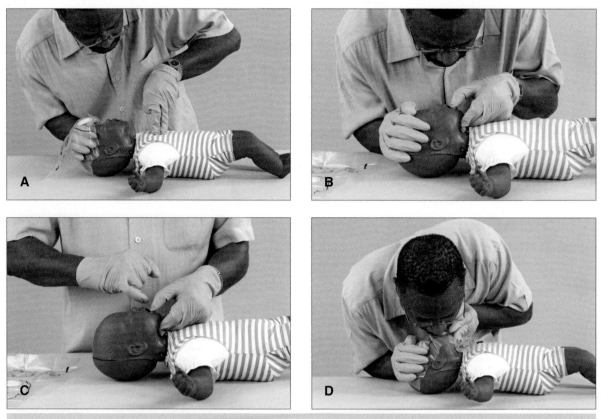

FIGURE 4-12, A–D *For an unconscious choking infant:* **A,** *Give 30 chest compressions.* **B,** *Look for an object.* **C,** *If you see one, remove it with a smaller finger.* **D,** *Give 2 rescue breaths.*

PUTTING IT ALL TOGETHER

In a breathing emergency, seconds count so it is important to act at once. Breathing emergencies include respiratory distress, respiratory arrest and choking. Look for signals that indicate a person is having trouble breathing, is not breathing or is choking. When you recognize that an adult, a child or an infant is having trouble breathing, is not breathing or is choking, call 9-1-1 or the local emergency number immediately. Then give care for the condition until help arrives and takes over. You could save a life.

CONSCIOUS CHOKING–ADULT
CANNOT COUGH, SPEAK OR BREATHE

AFTER CHECKING THE SCENE AND THE INJURED OR ILL PERSON, HAVE SOMEONE CALL 9-1-1 AND GET CONSENT.

1 GIVE 5 BACK BLOWS

Bend the person forward at the waist and give **5** back blows between the shoulder blades with the heel of one hand.

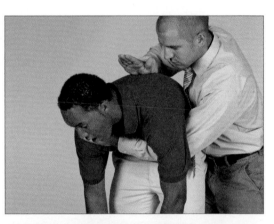

2 GIVE 5 ABDOMINAL THRUSTS

- Place a fist with the thumb side against the middle of the person's abdomen, just above the navel.
- Cover your fist with your other hand.
- Give **5** quick, upward abdominal thrusts.

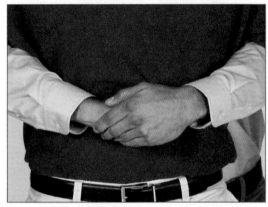

3 CONTINUE CARE

Continue sets of **5** back blows and **5** abdominal thrusts until the:

- Object is forced out.
- Person can cough forcefully or breathe.
- Person becomes unconscious.

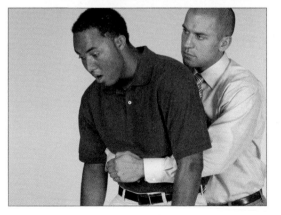

WHAT TO DO NEXT

- IF PERSON BECOMES UNCONSCIOUS—**CALL** 9-1-1, if not already done.
- Carefully lower the person to the ground and give **CARE** for an unconscious choking adult, beginning with looking for an object.

CONSCIOUS CHOKING—CHILD
CANNOT COUGH, SPEAK OR BREATHE

TIP: *Stand or kneel behind the child, depending on his or her size.*

AFTER CHECKING THE SCENE AND THE INJURED OR ILL CHILD, HAVE SOMEONE CALL 9-1-1 AND GET CONSENT FROM THE PARENT OR GUARDIAN, IF PRESENT.

1 GIVE 5 BACK BLOWS

Bend the child forward at the waist and give **5** back blows between the shoulder blades with the heel of one hand.

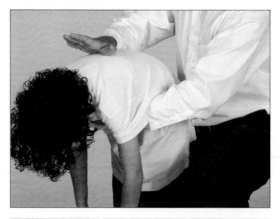

2 GIVE 5 ABDOMINAL THRUSTS

- Place a fist with the thumb side against the middle of the child's abdomen, just above the navel.
- Cover your fist with your other hand.
- Give **5** quick, upward abdominal thrusts.

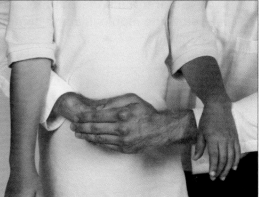

3 CONTINUE CARE

Continue sets of **5** back blows and **5** abdominal thrusts until the:

- Object is forced out.
- Child can cough forcefully or breathe.
- Child becomes unconscious.

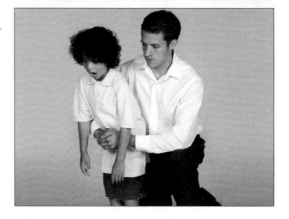

WHAT TO DO NEXT

- IF CHILD BECOMES UNCONSCIOUS—**CALL** 9-1-1, if not already done.
- Carefully lower the child to the ground and give **CARE** for an unconscious choking child, beginning with looking for an object.

CONSCIOUS CHOKING–INFANT
CANNOT COUGH, CRY OR BREATHE

AFTER CHECKING THE SCENE AND THE INJURED OR ILL INFANT, HAVE SOMEONE CALL 9-1-1 AND GET CONSENT FROM PARENT OR GUARDIAN, IF PRESENT.

1 GIVE 5 BACK BLOWS

Give firm back blows with the heel of one hand between the infant's shoulder blades.

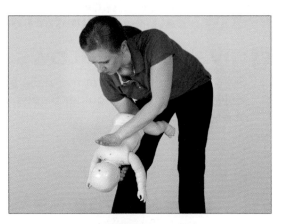

2 GIVE 5 CHEST THRUSTS

Place two or three fingers in the center of the infant's chest just below the nipple line and compress the breastbone about **1½ inches**.

> **TIP:** *Support the head and neck securely when giving back blows and chest thrusts. Keep the head lower than the chest.*

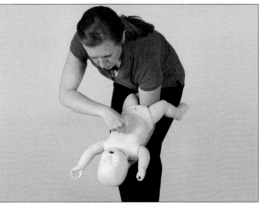

3 CONTINUE CARE

Continue sets of **5** back blows and **5** chest thrusts until the:

- Object is forced out.
- Infant can cough forcefully, cry or breathe.
- Infant becomes unconscious.

■ WHAT TO DO NEXT

- IF INFANT BECOMES UNCONSCIOUS–**CALL** 9-1-1, if not already done.
- Carefully lower the infant onto a firm, flat surface, and give **CARE** for an unconscious choking infant, beginning with looking for an object.

UNCONSCIOUS CHOKING–ADULT
CHEST DOES NOT RISE WITH RESCUE BREATHS

IF AT ANY TIME THE CHEST DOES NOT RISE:

1 GIVE ANOTHER RESCUE BREATH

Retilt the head and give another rescue breath.

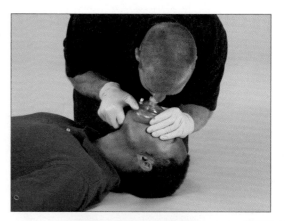

2 GIVE 30 CHEST COMPRESSIONS

If the chest still does not rise, give **30** chest compressions.

> **TIP:** *The person must be on firm, flat surface. Remove the CPR breathing barrier when giving chest compressions.*

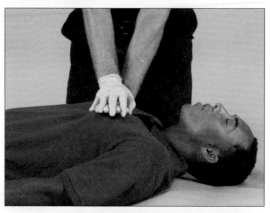

3 LOOK FOR AND REMOVE OBJECT IF SEEN

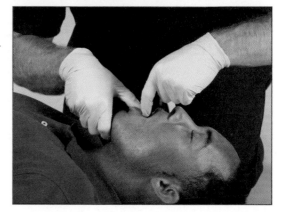

4 GIVE 2 RESCUE BREATHS

WHAT TO DO NEXT

- IF BREATHS DO NOT MAKE THE CHEST RISE–Repeat steps **2** through **4**.
- IF CHEST CLEARLY RISES–**CHECK** for breathing. Give **CARE** based on the conditions found.

UNCONSCIOUS CHOKING–CHILD AND INFANT

CHEST DOES NOT RISE WITH RESCUE BREATHS

IF AT ANY TIME THE CHEST DOES NOT RISE:

1 GIVE ANOTHER RESCUE BREATH

Retilt the head and give another rescue breath.

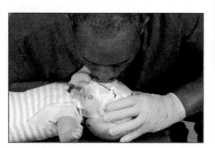

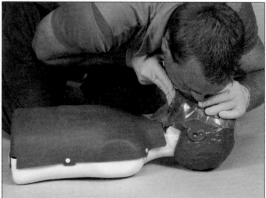

2 GIVE CHEST COMPRESSIONS

If the chest still does not rise, give **30** chest compressions.

TIP: *The child or infant must be on firm, flat surface. Remove the CPR breathing barrier when giving chest compressions.*

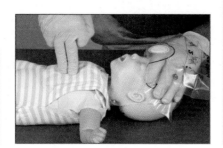

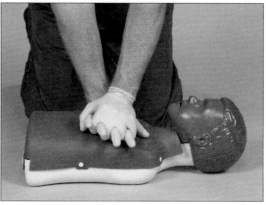

3 LOOK FOR AND REMOVE OBJECT IF SEEN

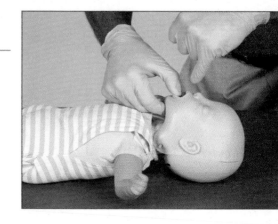

4 GIVE 2 RESCUE BREATHS

WHAT TO DO NEXT

- IF BREATHS DO NOT MAKE THE CHEST RISE—Repeat steps **2** through **4**.
- IF CHEST CLEARLY RISES—**CHECK** for breathing. Give **CARE** based on the conditions found.

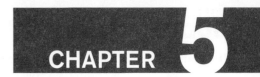

Sudden Illness

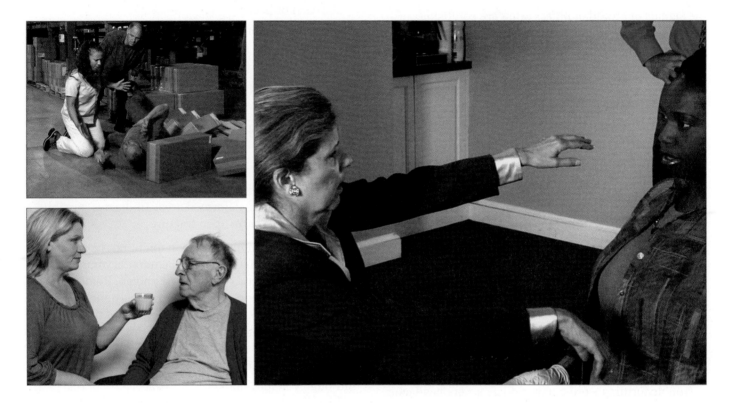

I f a person suddenly becomes ill, it is important to respond quickly and effectively. When illness happens suddenly it can be hard to determine what is wrong and what you should do to help.

In this chapter you will read about the signals of sudden illnesses including fainting, seizures, stroke, diabetic emergencies, allergic reactions, poisoning and substance abuse. This chapter also discusses how to care for specific sudden illnesses, even if you do not know the exact cause.

SUDDEN ILLNESS

It usually is obvious when someone is injured and needs care. The person may be able to tell you what happened and what hurts. Checking the person also gives you clues about what might be wrong. However, when someone becomes suddenly ill, it is not as easy to tell what is physically wrong. At times, there are no signals to give clues about what is happening. At other times, the signals only confirm that something is wrong, without being clear as to what is wrong. In either case, the signals of a sudden illness often are confusing. You may find it difficult to determine if the person's condition is an emergency and whether to call 9-1-1 or the local emergency number.

What to Look For

When a person becomes suddenly ill, he or she usually looks and feels sick. Common signals include:

- Changes in level of consciousness, such as feeling lightheaded, dizzy, drowsy or confused, or becoming unconscious.
- Breathing problems (i.e., trouble breathing or no breathing).
- Signals of a possible heart attack, including persistent chest pain, discomfort or pressure lasting more than a few minutes that goes away and comes back or that spreads to the shoulder, arm, neck, jaw, stomach or back.
- Signals of a stroke, including sudden weakness on one side of the face (facial droop); sudden weakness, often on one side of the body; sudden slurred speech or trouble forming words; or a sudden, severe headache.
- Loss of vision or blurred vision.
- Signals of shock, including rapid breathing, changes in skin appearance and cool, pale or ashen (grayish) skin.
- Sweating.
- Persistent abdominal pain or pressure.
- Nausea or vomiting.
- Diarrhea.
- Seizures.

Look around the area for clues that might tell you what is wrong with the person. This may help you to find out what the person was doing when the illness started. For example, if someone working in a hot environment suddenly becomes ill, it would make sense to conclude that the illness resulted from the heat. If someone suddenly feels ill or acts strangely and is attempting to take medication, the medication may be a clue as to what is wrong. For example, the person may need the medication for a heart condition and is trying to take it to avoid a medical emergency.

When to Call 9-1-1

Call 9-1-1 or the local emergency for any of the following conditions:

- Unconsciousness or altered level of consciousness
- Breathing problems
- No breathing
- Chest pain, discomfort or pressure lasting more than 3 to 5 minutes that goes away and comes back or that radiates to the shoulder, arm, jaw, neck, stomach or back
- Persistent abdominal pain or pressure
- Severe external bleeding (bleeding that spurts or gushes steadily from a wound)
- Vomiting blood or passing blood
- Severe (critical) burns
- Suspected poisoning
- Seizures
- Stroke
- Suspected or obvious injuries to the head, neck or spine
- Painful, swollen, deformed areas (indicates possible broken bone) or an open fracture

With some sudden illnesses, you might not be sure whether to call 9-1-1 or the local emergency number for help. Sometimes the signals come and go. Remember, if you cannot sort out the problem quickly and easily or if you have any doubts about the severity of the illness, make the call for help.

What to Do Until Help Arrives

Although you may not know the exact cause of the sudden illness, you should still give care. Initially you will care for the signals and not for any specific condition. In the few cases in which you know that the person has a medical condition, such as diabetes, epilepsy or heart disease, the care you give may be slightly different. This care may involve helping the person take medication for his or her specific illness.

Care for sudden illnesses by following the same general guidelines as you would for any emergency.

- Do no further harm.
- Check the scene for safety, and then check the person.
- First care for life-threatening conditions such as unconsciousness; trouble breathing; no breathing; severe bleeding; severe chest pain; or signals of a stroke, such as weakness, numbness or trouble with speech.
- Help the person to rest comfortably.
- Keep the person from getting chilled or overheated.
- Reassure the person because he or she may be anxious or frightened.
- Watch for changes in consciousness and breathing.

- If the person is conscious, ask if he or she has any medical conditions or is taking any medication.
- Do not give the person anything to eat or drink unless he or she is fully conscious, is able to swallow and does not show any signals of a stroke.
- If the person vomits and is unconscious and lying down, position the person on his or her side so that you can clear the mouth.
- If you know the person is having a severe allergic reaction or a diabetic emergency, assist the person with his or her prescribed medication, if asked.

SPECIFIC SUDDEN ILLNESSES

Some sudden illnesses may be linked with chronic conditions. These conditions include degenerative diseases, such as heart and lung diseases. There may be a hormone imbalance, such as in diabetes. The person could have epilepsy, a condition that causes seizures. An allergy can cause a sudden and sometimes dangerous reaction to certain substances. When checking a person, look for a medical identification (ID) tag, bracelet, necklace or anklet indicating that the person has a chronic condition or allergy.

Having to deal with a sudden illness can be frightening, especially when you do not know what is wrong. Do not hesitate to give care. Remember, you do not have to know the cause to help. Signals for sudden illnesses are similar to other conditions and the care probably involves skills that you already know.

Fainting

One common signal of sudden illness is a loss of consciousness, such as when a person faints. Fainting is a temporary loss of consciousness. When someone suddenly loses consciousness and then reawakens, he or she may simply have fainted.

Fainting occurs when there is an insufficient supply of blood to the brain for a short period of time. This condition results from a widening of the blood vessels in the body. This causes blood to drain away from the brain to the rest of the body.

Fainting usually is not harmful. The person usually recovers quickly with no lasting effects. However, what appears to be a simple case of fainting actually may be a signal of a more serious condition.

What to Look For

A person who is about to faint often becomes pale, begins to sweat and then loses consciousness and collapses. A person who feels weak or dizzy may prevent a fainting spell by lying down or sitting with his or her head level with the knees.

When to Call 9-1-1

Call 9-1-1 or the local emergency number when in doubt about the condition of a person who has fainted. It is always appropriate to seek medical care for fainting.

What to Do Until Help Arrives

Lower the person to the ground or other flat surface and position him or her on his or her back, lying flat. Loosen any tight clothing, such as a tie or collar (Fig. 5-1). Check that the person is breathing. Do not give the person anything to eat or drink. If the person vomits, roll him or her onto one side.

Seizures

When the normal functions of the brain are disrupted by injury, disease, fever, infection, metabolic disturbances or conditions causing a decreased oxygen level, a *seizure* may occur. The seizure is a result of abnormal electrical activity in the brain and causes temporary, involuntary changes in body movement, function, sensation, awareness or behavior.

Epilepsy

Epilepsy is a chronic seizure condition. Almost 3 million Americans have some form of epilepsy. The seizures that occur with epilepsy usually can be controlled with medication. Still, some people with epilepsy who take seizure medication occasionally have seizures. Others who go a long time without a seizure may think that the condition has gone away and stop taking their medication, thus putting themselves at risk for another seizure.

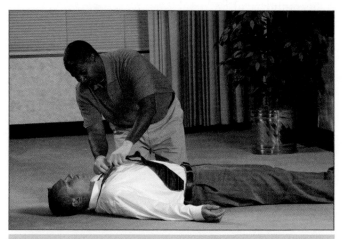

FIGURE 5-1 *To care for a person who has fainted, place the person on his or her back lying flat and loosen any restrictive clothing, such as a tie or collar.*

Febrile Seizures

Young children and infants may be at risk for *febrile seizures*, which are seizures brought on by a rapid increase in body temperature. They are most common in children younger than 5 years.

Febrile seizures often are caused by infections of the ear, throat or digestive system and are most likely to occur when a child or an infant experiences a rapid rise in temperature. A child or an infant experiencing a febrile seizure may experience some or all of the signals listed below.

What to Look For

Signals of seizures include:

- A blank stare.
- A period of distorted sensation during which the person is unable to respond.
- Uncontrolled muscular contractions, called *convulsions*, which last several minutes.

A person with epilepsy may experience something called an *aura* before the seizure occurs. An aura is an unusual sensation or feeling, such as a visual hallucination; strange sound, taste or smell; or an urgent need to get to safety. If the person recognizes the aura, he or she may have time to tell bystanders and sit down before the seizure occurs.

Febrile seizures may have some or all of the following signals:

- Sudden rise in body temperature
- Change in consciousness
- Rhythmic jerking of the head and limbs
- Loss of bladder or bowel control
- Confusion
- Drowsiness
- Crying out
- Becoming rigid
- Holding breath
- Upward rolling of the eyes

Although it may be frightening to see someone unexpectedly having a seizure, you should remember that most seizures last only for a few minutes and the person usually recovers without problems.

When to Call 9-1-1

Call 9-1-1 or the local emergency number if:

- The seizure lasts more than 5 minutes.
- The person has multiple seizures with no signs of slowing down.
- The person appears to be injured or fails to regain consciousness after the seizure.

- The cause of the seizure is unknown.
- The person is pregnant.
- The person has diabetes.
- The person is a young child or an infant and experienced a febrile seizure brought on by a high fever.
- The seizure takes place in water.
- The person is elderly and could have suffered a stroke.
- This is the person's first seizure.

If the person is known to have occasional seizures, you *may not* have to call 9-1-1 or the local emergency number. He or she usually will recover from a seizure in a few minutes.

What to Do Until Help Arrives

Although it may be frightening to watch, you can easily help to care for a person having a seizure. Remember that he or she cannot control the seizure. Do not try to stop the seizure. General principles of managing a seizure are to prevent injury, protect the person's airway and make sure that the airway is open after the seizure has ended.

Do not hold or restrain the person. Do not put anything in the person's mouth or between the teeth. People having seizures rarely bite their tongues or cheeks with enough force to cause significant bleeding; however, some blood may be present.

Make sure that the environment is as safe as possible to prevent injury to the person who is having a seizure. Remove any nearby furniture or other objects that may injure the person.

Give care to a person who has had a seizure the same way you would for an unconscious person. When the seizure is over, make sure that the person's airway is open. Usually, the person will begin to breathe normally. If there is fluid in the person's mouth, such as saliva, blood or vomit, roll him or her on one side so that the fluid drains from the mouth. If the child or infant has a febrile seizure, it is important to immediately cool the body by giving a sponge bath with lukewarm water.

The person may be drowsy and disoriented or unresponsive for a period of time. Check to see if he or she was injured during the seizure. Be comforting and reassuring. If the seizure occurred in public, the person may be embarrassed and self-conscious. Ask bystanders not to crowd around the person. He or she may be tired and want to rest. Stay on the scene with the person until he or she is fully conscious and aware of the surroundings.

For more information on epilepsy, visit the Epilepsy Foundation at epilepsyfoundation.org.

Stroke

Stroke is the third-leading killer and a leading cause of long-term disability in the United States. Nearly 800,000 Americans will have a stroke this year.

A *stroke,* also called a *brain attack*, is caused when blood flow to a part of the brain is cut off or when there is bleeding into the brain. Strokes can cause permanent brain damage, but sometimes the damage can be stopped or reversed.

A stroke usually is caused by a blockage in the arteries that supply blood to the brain. Once the blood flow is cut off, that part of the brain starts to "suffocate" and die unless the blood flow can be restored. Blockages can be caused by blood clots that travel from other parts of the body, like the heart, or they can be caused by slow damage to the arteries over time from diseases such as high blood pressure and diabetes.

In a small percentage of strokes there is bleeding into the brain. This bleeding can be from a broken blood vessel or from a bulging aneurysm that has broken open. There is no way to tell the type of stroke until the person gets to an emergency room and undergoes a thorough medical evaluation.

A *mini-stroke* is when a person has the signals of a stroke, which then completely go away. Most mini-strokes get better within a few minutes, although they can last several hours. Although the signals of a mini-stroke disappear quickly, the person is not out of danger at that point. In fact, someone who has a mini-stroke is at very high risk of having a full stroke within the next 2 days.

Risk Factors

The *risk factors* for stroke, meaning things that make a stroke more likely, are similar to those for heart disease. Some risk factors are beyond one's control, such as age, gender and family history of stroke or cardiovascular disease. Other risk factors can be controlled through diet, changes in lifestyle or medication. With a history of high blood pressure, previous stroke or mini-stroke, diabetes or heart disease one's chances of a stroke increases.

High Blood Pressure

Uncontrolled high blood pressure is the number one risk factor for stroke. If you have high blood pressure, you are approximately seven times more likely to have a stroke compared with someone who does not have high blood pressure.

High blood pressure puts added pressure on arteries and makes them stiffer. The excess pressure also damages organs, including the brain, heart and kidneys. Even mildly elevated blood pressure can increase one's risk of a stroke.

High blood pressure is the most important of the controllable risk factors. Have your blood pressure checked regularly and if it is high, follow the advice of your health care provider about how to lower it. Often, high blood pressure can be controlled by losing weight, changing diet, exercising routinely and managing stress. If those measures are not sufficient, your health care provider may prescribe medication.

Diabetes

Diabetes is a major risk factor for stroke. If you have been diagnosed with diabetes, follow the advice of your health care provider about how to control it. If uncontrolled, the resulting elevated blood sugar levels can damage blood vessels throughout the body.

Cigarette Smoking

Cigarette smoking is another major risk factor of stroke. Smoking is linked to heart disease and cancer, as well as to stroke. Smoking increases blood pressure, damages blood vessels and makes blood more likely to clot. If you smoke and would like to quit, many techniques and support systems are available to help, including seeking help from your health care provider and local health department.

The benefits of quitting smoking begin as soon as you stop, and some of the damage from smoking actually may be reversible. Approximately 10 years after a person has stopped smoking, his or her risk of stroke is about the same as the risk for a person who has never smoked. Even if you do not smoke, be aware that inhaling smoke from smokers can harm your health. Avoid long-term exposure to cigarette smoke and protect children from this danger as well.

Diet

Diets that are high in saturated fats and cholesterol can increase your risk of stroke by causing fatty materials to build up on the walls of your blood vessels. Foods high in cholesterol include egg yolks and organ meats, such as liver and kidneys. Saturated fats are found in beef, lamb, veal, pork, ham, whole milk and whole-milk products. Limiting your intake of these foods can help to prevent stroke.

Preventing Stroke

You can help prevent stroke if you:

- Control your blood pressure.
- Quit smoking.
- Eat a healthy diet.
- Exercise regularly. Regular exercise reduces your chances of stroke by strengthening the heart and improving blood circulation. Exercise also helps in weight control.

- Maintain a healthy weight. Being overweight increases the chance of developing high blood pressure, heart disease and fat deposits lining the arteries.
- Control diabetes.

What to Look For

As with other sudden illnesses, looking or feeling ill, or behaving in a strange way, are common, general signals of a stroke or mini-stroke. Other specific signals of stroke have a *sudden onset*, including:

- Weakness or numbness of the face, arm or leg. This usually happens on only one side of the body.
- Facial droop or drooling.
- Trouble with speech. The person may have trouble talking, getting words out or being understood when speaking and may have trouble understanding.
- Loss of vision or disturbed (blurred or dimmed) vision in one or both eyes. The pupils may be of unequal size.
- Sudden severe headache. The person will not know what caused the headache and may describe it as "the worst headache ever."
- Dizziness, confusion, agitation, loss of consciousness or other severe altered mental status.
- Loss of balance or coordination, trouble walking or ringing in the ears.
- Incontinence.

Think FAST for a Stroke

For a stroke, think **FAST,** which stands for the following:

- **Face**: Weakness, numbness or drooping on one side of the face. Ask the person to smile. Does one side of the face droop (Fig. 5-2, A)?

- **Arm:** Weakness or numbness in one arm. Ask the person to raise both arms. Does one arm drift downward (Fig. 5-2, B)?
- **Speech**: Slurred speech or difficulty speaking. Ask the person to repeat a simple sentence (e.g., Ask the person to say something like, "The sky is blue.") Are the words slurred? Can the person repeat the sentence correctly?
- **Time:** Try to determine when the signals began. If the person shows any signals of stroke, time is critical. Call 9-1-1 or the local emergency number right away.

The FAST mnemonic is based on the Cincinnati Pre-Hospital Stroke Scale. This scale originally was developed for EMS personnel in 1997. The scale was designed to help EMS personnel to identify strokes in the field. The FAST method for public awareness has been in use in the community in Cincinnati, Ohio, since 1999. Researchers at the University of North Carolina validated it in 2003 as an appropriate tool for helping lay persons to recognize and respond quickly to the signals of stroke.

By paying attention to the signals of stroke and reporting them to your health care provider, you can prevent damage before it occurs. Experiencing a mini-stroke is the clearest warning that a stroke may occur. Do not ignore its stroke-like signals, even if they disappear completely within minutes or hours.

When to Call 9-1-1

Call 9-1-1 or the local emergency number immediately if you encounter someone who is having or has had a stroke, if you see signals of a stroke or if the person had a mini-stroke (even if the signals have gone away). Note the time of onset of signals and report it to the call taker or EMS personnel when they arrive.

In the past, a stroke usually caused permanent brain damage. Today, new medications and medical

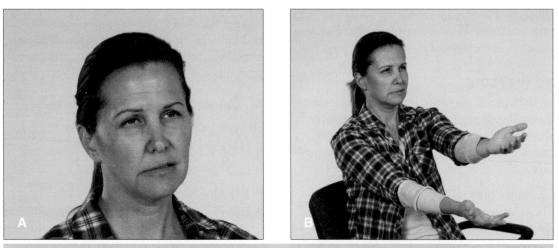

FIGURE 5-2, A–B *Signals of stroke include* **A,** *facial drooping, and* **B,** *weakness on one side of the body.*

procedures can limit or reduce the damage caused by stroke. Many of these new treatments must be given quickly to be the most helpful. It is important for the person to get the best care as quickly as possible.

What to Do Until Help Arrives

Note the time that the signals started. If the person is unconscious, make sure that he or she has an open airway and care for life-threatening conditions. If fluid or vomit is in the person's mouth, position him or her on one side to allow fluids to drain out of the mouth. Remove any material from the mouth with a finger if the person is unconscious. Stay with the person and monitor breathing and for any changes in the person's condition.

If the person is conscious, check for non-life-threatening conditions. A stroke can make the person fearful and anxious. Often, he or she does not understand what has happened. Offer comfort and reassurance. Have the person rest in a comfortable position. Do not give him or her anything to eat or drink.

Diabetic Emergencies

A total of 23.6 million people in the United States (7.8% of the population) have diabetes. Among this group, more than 5 million people are unaware that they have the disease. Diabetes was the seventh-leading cause of death listed on U.S. death certificates in 2006. Altogether, diabetes contributed to 233,619 deaths in 2005. Diabetes is likely to be underreported as a cause of death. Overall, the risk for death among people with diabetes is about twice that of people without diabetes.

The American Diabetes Association defines *diabetes* as the inability of the body to change sugar (glucose) from food into energy. This process is regulated by *insulin*, a hormone produced in the pancreas. Diabetes can lead to other medical conditions such as blindness, nerve disease, kidney disease, heart disease and stroke.

The cells in your body need *glucose* (sugar) as a source of energy. The cells receive this energy during digestion or from stored forms of sugar. The sugar is absorbed into the bloodstream with the help of insulin. Insulin is produced in the pancreas. For the body to properly function, there has to be a balance of insulin and sugar. People who have diabetes may become suddenly ill because there is too much or too little sugar in their blood.

There are two major types of diabetes: Type I and Type II diabetes.

Type I diabetes, formerly called juvenile diabetes, affects about 1 million Americans. This type of diabetes, which usually begins in childhood, occurs when the body produces little or no insulin. People with Type I diabetes must inject insulin into their bodies daily and are therefore considered to be insulin-dependent. Type I diabetes is a chronic disease that currently has no cure.

The exact cause of Type I diabetes is not known. Warning signals include:

- Frequent urination.
- Increased hunger and thirst.
- Unexpected weight loss.
- Irritability.
- Weakness and fatigue.

Type II diabetes is the most common type, affecting about 90 to 95 percent of people with diabetes. This condition usually occurs in adults but also can occur in children. With Type II diabetes, the body makes insulin but not enough to meet the body's needs or the body becomes resistant to the insulin produced. Since Type II diabetes is a progressive disease, people with this type of diabetes eventually may need to use insulin.

People from certain racial and ethnic backgrounds are known to be at greater risk for diabetes. Type II diabetes is more common among African-Americans, Latinos, Asians, certain Native Americans and Pacific Islanders. Although genetics and other factors increase risk for diabetes, being overweight or obese also is a risk factor for developing the disease in adults and children.

People with Type II diabetes often do not experience any warning signals. Possible warning signals of Type II diabetes include:

- Any signals of Type I diabetes.
- Frequent infections, especially involving the skin, gums and bladder.
- Blurred vision.
- Numbness in the legs, feet and fingers.
- Cuts or bruises that are slow to heal.
- Itching.

People with diabetes should monitor their exercise and diet. Self-monitoring for blood sugar levels is a valuable tool. Insulin-dependent diabetics also must monitor their use of insulin. If the person with diabetes does not control these factors, he or she can have a diabetic emergency.

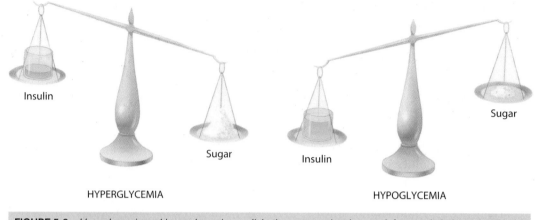

INSULIN — HYPERGLYCEMIA   INSULIN — HYPOGLYCEMIA

Insulin   Sugar   Sugar   Insulin

HYPERGLYCEMIA   HYPOGLYCEMIA

FIGURE 5-3 *Hypoglycemia and hyperglycemia are diabetic emergencies that result from an imbalance between sugar and insulin within the body.*

A diabetic emergency is caused by an imbalance between sugar and insulin in the body (Fig. 5-3). A diabetic emergency can happen when there is:

- Too much sugar in the blood (*hyperglycemia*): Among other causes, the person may not have taken enough insulin or the person is reacting adversely to a large meal or a meal that is high in carbohydrates.
- Too little sugar in the blood (*hypoglycemia*): The person may have taken too much insulin, eaten too little food, or overexerted him- or herself. Extremely low blood sugar levels can quickly become life threatening.

What to Look For

Signals of a diabetic emergency include:

- Changes in the level of consciousness.
- Changes in mood.
- Rapid breathing and pulse.
- Feeling and looking ill.
- Dizziness and headache.
- Confusion.

When to Call 9-1-1

Always call 9-1-1 or the local emergency number if:

- The person is unconscious or about to lose consciousness. In this situation, do not give the person anything by mouth. After calling 9-1-1 or the local emergency number, care for the person in the same way you would care for an unconscious person. This includes making sure the person's airway is clear of vomit, checking for breathing and giving care until advanced medical personnel take over.
- The person is conscious but unable to swallow. (In this case, *do not* put anything, liquid or solid, into the person's mouth.)
- The person does not feel better within about 5 minutes after taking some form of sugar.

- You cannot find any form of sugar immediately. Do not spend time looking for it.

What to Do Until Help Arrives

You may know the person is a diabetic or the person may tell you he or she is a diabetic. Often diabetics know what is wrong and will ask for something with sugar in it. They may carry some form of sugar with them in case they need it.

If the diabetic person is conscious and able to swallow, and advises you that he or she needs sugar, give sugar in the form of several glucose tablets or glucose paste, a 12-ounce serving of fruit juice, milk, nondiet soft drink or table sugar dissolved in a glass of water (Fig. 5-4). Most fruit juices and nondiet soft drinks have enough sugar to be effective. If the problem is too much sugar, this amount of sugar will not cause further harm. Diabetics also may carry glucagon, which they can self-administer to counter hypoglycemia. People who take insulin to control diabetes may have injectable medication with them to care for hyperglycemia.

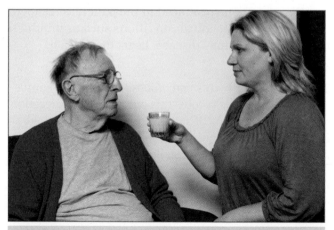

FIGURE 5-4 *If the person having a diabetic emergency is conscious and able to swallow, give him or her sugar, preferably glucose tablets or in liquid form.*

For more information about diabetes, contact the American Diabetes Association at 1-800-DIABETES, go to diabetes.org or visit the National Diabetes Education Program website at ndep.nih.gov. For specific information about Type I diabetes, contact the Juvenile Diabetes Foundation at 1-800-533-CURE or at jdrf.org.

Allergic Reactions

Allergic reactions are caused by over activity of the immune system against specific *antigens* (foreign substances). People with allergies are especially sensitive to these antigens. When their immune systems overreact to the antigens it is called an *allergic reaction*.

Antigens that often cause allergic reactions in at-risk people include the following:

- Bee or insect venom
- Antibiotics
- Pollen
- Animal dander
- Latex
- Sulfa drugs
- Certain foods (e.g., tree nuts, peanuts, shellfish and dairy products)

People who know that they are severely allergic to certain substances or bee stings may wear a medical ID tag, necklace or bracelet.

What to Look For

Allergic reactions can range from mild to severe. An example of a mild reaction is an itchy skin rash from touching poison ivy. Severe allergic reactions can cause a life-threatening condition called *anaphylaxis* (also called *anaphylactic shock*). Anaphylaxis usually occurs suddenly. It happens within seconds or minutes after contact with the substance. The skin or area of the body that comes in contact with the substance usually swells and turns red. Other signals include the following:

- Hives
- Itching
- Rash
- Weakness
- Nausea
- Stomach cramps
- Vomiting
- Dizziness
- Trouble breathing (including coughing and wheezing)

Trouble breathing can progress to a blocked airway as the lips, tongue, throat and *larynx* (voice box) swell.

Low blood pressure and shock may accompany these reactions. Death from anaphylaxis may happen quickly because the person's breathing is restricted severely.

When to Call 9-1-1

Call 9-1-1 or the local emergency number if the person:

- Has trouble breathing.
- Complains of the throat tightening.
- Explains that he or she is subject to severe allergic reactions.
- Is unconscious.

What to Do Until Help Arrives

If you suspect anaphylaxis and have called 9-1-1 or the local emergency number, follow these guidelines for giving care:

1. Monitor the person's breathing and for any changes in the person's condition.
2. Give care for life-threatening emergencies.
3. Check a conscious person to determine:
   - The substance (antigen) involved.
   - The route of exposure to the antigen.
   - The effects of the exposure.
4. Assist the person with using an epinephrine auto-injector, if available and state or local regulations allow.
5. Assist the person with taking an antihistamine, if available.
6. Document any changes in the person's condition over time.

For more information on anaphylaxis, see Chapter 11.

POISONING

A poison is any substance that causes injury, illness or death if it enters the body. In 2008, Poison Control Centers (PCCs) received more than 2.4 million calls having to do with people who had come into contact with a poison. Over 93 percent of these poisonings took place in the home. Fifty percent (1.2 million) involved children younger than 6 years. Poisoning deaths in children younger than 6 years represented about 2 percent of the total deaths from poisoning. The 20- to 59-year-old age group represented about 76 percent of all deaths from poisoning.

In recent years there has been a decrease in child poisonings. This is due partly to child-resistant packaging for medications. This packaging makes it harder for children to get into these substances. The decrease also is a result of preventive actions by parents and others who care for children. At the same time, there has been an increase in adult poisoning deaths. This increase is linked to an increase in both suicides and drug-related poisonings.

Types of Poisoning

A person can be poisoned by swallowing poison, breathing it, absorbing it through the skin and by having it injected into the body.

Swallowed Poisons

Poisons that can be swallowed include foods, such as certain mushrooms and shellfish; an overdose of drugs, such as sleeping pills, tranquilizers and alcohol; medications, such as a high quantity of aspirin; household items, such as cleaning products and pesticides; and certain plants. Many substances that are not poisonous in small amounts are poisonous in larger amounts. Combining certain substances can result in poisoning, although if taken by themselves they might not cause harm.

Inhaled Poisons

A person can be poisoned by breathing in (inhaling) toxic fumes. Examples of poisons that can be inhaled include:

- Gases, such as:
  - Carbon monoxide from an engine or car exhaust.
  - Carbon dioxide from wells and sewers.
  - Chlorine, found in many swimming pools.
- Fumes from:
  - Household products, such as glues and paints.
- Drugs, such as crack cocaine.

Absorbed Poisons

Poisons that can be absorbed through the skin come from many sources including plants, such as poison ivy, poison oak and poison sumac, and fertilizers and pesticides.

Injected Poisons

Injected poisons enter the body through the bites or stings of insects, spiders, ticks, some marine life, snakes and other animals or through drugs or medications injected with a hypodermic needle.

What to Look For

How will you know if someone who is ill has been poisoned? Look for clues about what has happened. Try to get information from the person or from bystanders. As you check the scene, be aware of unusual odors, flames, smoke, open or spilled containers, an open medicine cabinet or an overturned or a damaged plant. Also, notice if the person is showing any of the following signals of poisoning:

- Nausea and vomiting
- Diarrhea
- Chest or abdominal pain
- Trouble breathing
- Sweating
- Changes in consciousness
- Seizures
- Headache
- Dizziness
- Weakness
- Irregular pupil size
- Burning or tearing eyes
- Abnormal skin color
- Burns around the lips, tongue or on the skin

You also may suspect a poisoning based on information from or about the person. If you suspect someone has swallowed a poison, try to find out:

- The type of poison.
- The quantity taken.
- When it was taken.
- How much the person weighs.

This information can help you and others to give the most appropriate care.

When to Call 9-1-1

For life-threatening conditions (such as if a person is unconscious or is not breathing or if a change in the level of consciousness occurs), CALL 9-1-1 or local emergency number. If the person is conscious and alert, CALL the National Poison Control Center (PCC) hotline at 1-800-222-1222 and follow the advice given.

What to Do Until Help Arrives

After you have checked the scene and determined that there has been a poisoning, follow these general care guidelines:

- Remove the person from the source of poison if the scene is dangerous. Do this only if you are able to without endangering yourself.
- Check the person's level of consciousness and breathing.
- Care for any life-threatening conditions.
- If the person is conscious, ask questions to get more information.
- Look for any containers and take them with you to the telephone.
- Call the National Poison Control Center Hotline at 1-800 222-1222.
- Follow the directions of the Poison Control Center.

If the person becomes violent or threatening, move to safety and wait for help to arrive. Do not give the person anything to eat or drink unless medical professionals tell you to do so. If you do not know what the poison was and the person vomits, save some of the vomit. The hospital may analyze it to identify the poison.

POISONING

Use common sense when handling substances that could be harmful, such as chemicals and cleaners. Use them in a well-ventilated area. Wear protective clothing, such as gloves and a facemask.

Use common sense with your own medications. Read the product information and use only as directed. Ask your health care provider or pharmacist about the intended effects, side effects and possible interactions with other medications that you are taking. Never use another person's prescribed medications. What is right for one person often is wrong for another.

Always keep medications in their original containers. Make sure that this container is well marked with the original pharmacy labeling. If taking several medications, always check the label to ensure that you are taking the correct medication, and be especially aware of possible adverse drug interactions.

Over time, expired medications can become less effective and even toxic to humans if consumed. Dispose of out-of-date or unused medications properly by following the guidelines below.

Most medications should be thrown away in the household trash and not flushed down the toilet. Follow these steps to maintain safety and protect the environment from unnecessary exposure to medications:

1. Pour the medication out of its original container into a sealable plastic bag.
2. Mix the medication with something that will hide the medication or make it unpleasant (e.g., coffee grounds or kitty litter).
3. Seal the plastic bag.
4. Throw the plastic bag into your household trash.
5. Remove and destroy all *personal information and medication information (prescription label)* from the medication container. Recycle or throw away the medication container.

Another option is to check if your state or local community has a community-based household hazardous waste collection program. You may be able to take your expired and unused medications to your pharmacy or another location for disposal.

The U.S. Food and Drug Administration (FDA) website maintains a list of some of the medications that should be flushed down the toilet. These medications are especially dangerous to humans and pets. One dose could cause death if taken by someone other than the person for whom it was prescribed. Flushing these medications avoids any chance that children or pets would ingest them accidentally.

According to the FDA, any possible risk to people and the environment from flushing these few medications is small. The FDA maintains that the risk is outweighed by the possibility of someone accidentally ingesting these medications, which could be life threatening.

Preventing Poisoning in Children
Many substances found in or around the house are poisonous. Children younger than 3 years and infants that are able to crawl are especially likely to be poisoned because of their curious nature, and because they explore their world through touching and tasting things around them (Fig. 5-5). If you care for or are near young children, be warned: it only takes a moment for a small child to get into trouble.

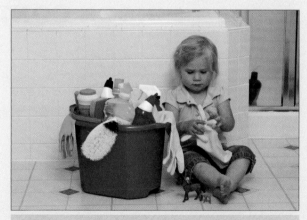

FIGURE 5-5 *Always supervise young children closely, especially in areas where common, but poisonous, household items are stored.*

(Continued)

Most child poisonings take place when a parent or guardian is watching a child.

Follow these guidelines to guard against poisoning emergencies in children:

- Always supervise children closely, especially in areas where poisons are commonly stored, such as kitchens, bathrooms and garages.
- Keep children out of your work area when you are using potentially harmful substances.
- Consider all household or drugstore products to be potentially harmful.
- Read all labels of products you use in your home. Look for these words on bottles and packages: "Caution," "Warning," "Poison," "Danger" or "Keep Out of Reach of Children."
- Be careful when using and storing household products with fruit shown on the labels. Children may think that they are okay to drink.

- Remove all medications and medical supplies from bags, purses, pockets, shelves, unlocked cabinets and drawers.
- Keep all medications, medical supplies and household products locked away, well out of the reach of children and away from food and drinks.
- Install special child safety locks to keep children from opening cabinets.
- Use childproof safety caps on all medications, chemicals and cleaning products.
- Never call medicine "candy" to get a child to take it, even if it has a pleasant candy flavor.
- Keep products in their original containers with the original labels in place.
- Use poison symbols to identify dangerous substances and teach children the meaning of the symbols.
- Dispose of outdated or unused medications and household products as recommended (see above for appropriate disposal of medications).

FOCUS ON PREPAREDNESS

POISON CONTROL CENTERS

There are 60 regional PCCs across the United States. These centers are dedicated to helping people deal with poisons. Medical professionals staff PCCs. These professionals give free, 24-hour advice to callers. PCC staff have access to information about most poisonous substances. They also can tell you what to do if a poisoning happened or is suspected.

If you think a person has been poisoned and the person is conscious, call the National Poison Control Center hotline at 1-800-222-1222 first. When you call this number, your call is automatically routed to your regional PCC based on the area code from which you called. The regional PCC staff

then will tell you what care to give. They also will tell you whether you should call 9-1-1 or the local emergency number.

In 2008, PCCs answered over 2.4 million calls about poisonings. In over 70 percent of the cases, the caller was able to get the help needed without having to call 9-1-1 or the local emergency number, or go to the hospital or health care provider. PCCs help reduce the workload of the EMS personnel and safely reduce the number of emergency room visits.

Be prepared: Keep the telephone number of the National Poison Control Center hotline posted by every telephone in your home or office!

Special Care Considerations

Toxic Fumes

It is often difficult to tell if a poisoning victim has inhaled toxic fumes. Toxic fumes come from a variety of sources. They may have an odor or be odor-free. When someone breathes in toxic fumes, the person's skin may turn pale or ashen, which indicates a lack of oxygen. If it is safe for you to do so, get the person to fresh air. Anyone who has inhaled toxic fumes needs fresh air as soon as possible.

Chemicals

In the case of poisoning with dry chemicals, such as lime, brush off the dry chemicals with gloved hands or a cloth. Carefully remove any contaminated clothing but avoid contaminating yourself or others. Then flush the area thoroughly with large amounts of water. Be careful not to get any of the chemicals in your eyes or the eyes of the person or of bystanders.

If the poisoning resulted from wet chemicals coming into contact with the skin, flush the affected area with large amounts of cool water (Fig. 5-6). Have someone else call 9-1-1 or the local emergency number. Keep flushing the area until EMS personnel arrive.

Substance Abuse

People in our society abuse numerous drugs and other substances. This substance abuse causes a wide range of psychological and physical effects.

What to Look For

Signals of possible substance abuse include:

- Behavioral changes not otherwise explained.
- Sudden mood changes.
- Restlessness, talkativeness or irritability.

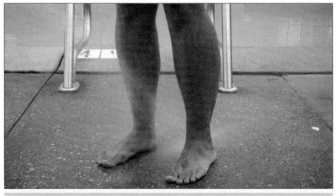

FIGURE 5-6 *If poisons such as wet chemicals get on the skin, flush the affected area with large amounts of cool water.*

- Changes in consciousness, including loss of consciousness.
- Slurred speech or poor coordination.
- Moist or flushed skin.
- Chills, nausea or vomiting.
- Dizziness or confusion.
- Irregular pulse.
- Abnormal breathing.

When to Call 9-1-1

Call 9-1-1 or the local emergency number if the person:

- Is unconscious, confused or seems to be losing consciousness.
- Has trouble breathing or is breathing irregularly.
- Has persistent chest pain or pressure.
- Has pain or pressure in the abdomen that does not go away.
- Is vomiting blood or passing blood.
- Has a seizure, severe headache or slurred speech.
- Acts violently.

Also call 9-1-1 or the local emergency number if you are unsure what to do or you are unsure about the seriousness of the problem.

What to Do Until Help Arrives

If you think that a person took an overdose or has another substance abuse problem requiring medical attention or other professional help, you should check the scene for safety and check the person. If you have good reason to suspect that a substance was taken, call the National Poison Control Center Hotline at 1-800-222-1222 and follow the call taker's directions.

In general, to care for the person, you should:

- Try to learn from others what substances may have been taken.
- Calm and reassure the person.
- Keep the person from getting chilled or overheated to minimize shock.

PUTTING IT ALL TOGETHER

When a person becomes ill suddenly, it can be frightening to that person, to you and to other bystanders. It may be difficult to determine what is causing the sudden illness, and you might not know what care to give. However, if you have learned the general signals as well as the signals of specific sudden illnesses, you can give care confidently and quickly.

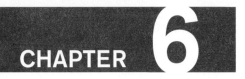

CHAPTER 6

Environmental Emergencies

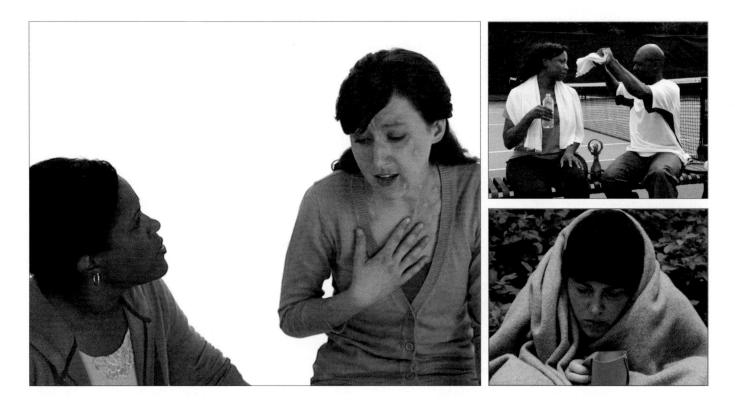

Disease, illness and injury are not the only causes of medical emergencies. Much of our environment appears to be relatively harmless. A weekend outing can bring you closer to the joys of nature: animals, mountains, rivers, blue skies. But it also can expose you to disease-carrying insects, other biting or stinging creatures and rapid changes in the weather. Whereas many environmental emergencies can be avoided, even with the best prevention efforts, emergencies do occur.

In this chapter you will discover how to prevent heat-related illnesses and cold-related emergencies, as well as bites and stings from insects, spiders and other animals. You also will find information on how to avoid contact with poisonous plants and how to avoid being struck by lightning. In addition, you will read about when to call for help and how to give care until help arrives.

HEAT-RELATED ILLNESSES AND COLD-RELATED EMERGENCIES

Exposure to extreme heat or cold can make a person seriously ill. The likelihood of illness also depends on factors such as physical activity, clothing, wind, humidity, working and living conditions, and a person's age and state of mind (Fig. 6-1).

Once the signals of a heat-related illness or cold-related emergency begin to appear, a person's condition can quickly worsen. A heat-related illness or cold-related emergency can result in death. If you see any of the signals, act quickly.

People at risk for heat-related illness or a cold-related emergency include those who work or exercise outdoors, elderly people, young children and people with health problems. Also at risk are those who have had a heat-related illness or cold-related emergency in the past, those with medical conditions that cause poor blood circulation and those who take medications to eliminate water from the body (*diuretics*).

People usually try to get out of extreme heat or cold before they begin to feel ill. However, some people do not or cannot. Athletes and those who work outdoors often keep working even after they begin to feel ill. People living in buildings with poor ventilation, poor insulation or poor heating or cooling systems are at increased risk of heat-related illnesses or cold-related emergencies. Often they might not even recognize that they are in danger of becoming ill.

Heat-Related Illness

Heat cramps, heat exhaustion and *heat stroke* are conditions caused by overexposure to heat, loss of fluids and electrolytes.

Heat Cramps

Heat cramps are the least severe of the heat-related illnesses. They often are the first signals that the body is having trouble with the heat.

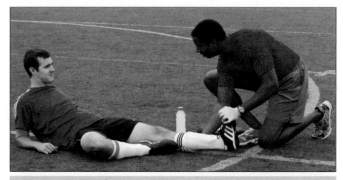

FIGURE 6-2 *Lightly stretching the muscle and gently massaging the area, along with having the person rest and giving electrolyte- and carbohydrate-containing fluids, usually is enough for the body to recover from heat cramps.*

What to Look For

Heat cramps are painful muscle spasms. They usually occur in the legs and abdomen. Think of them as a warning of a possible heat-related illness.

What to Do

To care for heat cramps, help the person move to a cool place to rest. Give an electrolyte- and carbohydrate-containing fluid such as a commercial sports drink, fruit juice or milk. Water also may be given. Lightly stretch the muscle and gently massage the area (Fig. 6-2). The person should not take salt tablets. They can worsen the situation.

When cramps stop, the person usually can start activity again if there are no other signals of illness. He or she should keep drinking plenty of fluids. Watch the person carefully for further signals of heat-related illness.

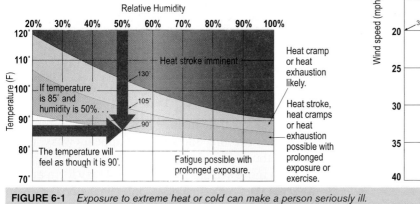

FIGURE 6-1 *Exposure to extreme heat or cold can make a person seriously ill.*

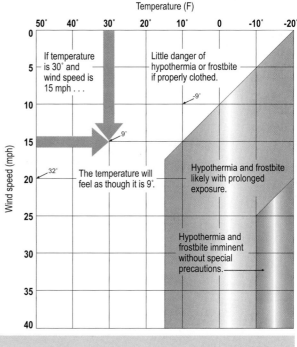

Heat Exhaustion

Heat exhaustion is a more severe condition than heat cramps. It often affects athletes, firefighters, construction workers and factory workers. It also affects those who wear heavy clothing in a hot, humid environment.

What to Look For

Signals of heat exhaustion include cool, moist, pale, ashen or flushed skin; headache; nausea; dizziness; weakness; and exhaustion.

What to Do

When a heat-related illness is recognized in its early stages, it usually can be reversed. Get the person out of the heat. Move the person to a cooler environment with circulating air. Loosen or remove as much clothing as possible and apply cool, wet cloths, such as towels or sheets, taking care to remoisten the cloths periodically (Fig. 6-3). Spraying the person with water and fanning also can help.

If the person is conscious and able to swallow, give him or her small amounts of a cool fluid such as a commercial sports drink or fruit juice to restore fluids and electrolytes. Milk or water also may be given. Do not let the conscious person drink too quickly. Give about 4 ounces of fluid every 15 minutes. Let the person rest in a comfortable position and watch carefully for changes in his or her condition. The person should not resume normal activities the same day.

If the person's condition does not improve or he or she refuses fluids, has a change in consciousness or vomits, call 9-1-1 or the local emergency number, as these are indications that the person's condition is getting worse.

Stop giving fluids and place the person on his or her side to keep the airway open. Watch for signals of breathing problems. Keep the person lying down and continue to cool the body any way you can (see What to Do Until Help Arrives).

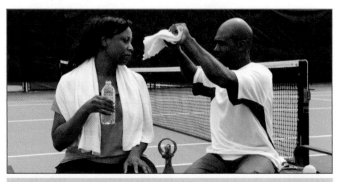

FIGURE 6-3 *When you recognize a heat-related illness, get the person out of the heat, loosen or remove clothing and apply cool, wet cloths, such as towels or sheets. Spraying the person with water and fanning also can be effective.*

Heat Stroke

Heat stroke is the least common but most severe heat-related illness. It usually occurs when people ignore the signals of heat exhaustion. Heat stroke develops when the body systems are overwhelmed by heat and begin to stop functioning. Heat stroke is a serious medical emergency.

What to Look For

Signals of heat stroke include extremely high body temperature, red skin that can be either dry or moist; changes in consciousness; rapid, weak pulse; rapid, shallow breathing; confusion; vomiting; and seizures.

When to Call 9-1-1

Call 9-1-1 or the local emergency number immediately. Heat stroke is a life-threatening emergency.

What to Do Until Help Arrives

- Preferred method: Rapidly cool the body by immersing the person up to the neck in cold water, if possible.
  OR
  Douse or spray the person with cold water.
- Sponge the person with ice water-doused towels over the entire body, frequently rotating the cold, wet towels.
- Cover with bags of ice.
- If you are not able to measure and monitor the person's temperature, apply rapid cooling methods for 20 minutes or until the person's condition improves.
- Give care according for other conditions found.

Cold-Related Emergencies

Frostbite and *hypothermia* are two types of cold-related emergencies.

Frostbite

Frostbite is the freezing of body parts exposed to the cold. Severity depends on the air temperature, length of exposure and the wind. Frostbite can result in the loss of fingers, hands, arms, toes, feet and legs.

What to Look For

The signals of frostbite include lack of feeling in the affected area, swelling and skin that appears waxy, is cold to the touch or is discolored (flushed, white, yellow or blue). In more serious cases, blisters may form and the affected part may turn black and show signs of deep tissue damage.

When to Call 9-1-1

Call 9-1-1 or the local emergency number for more serious frostbite or seek emergency medical help as soon as possible.

What to Do Until Help Arrives

To care for frostbite, handle the area gently. Remove wet clothing and jewelry, if possible, from the affected area. Never rub a frostbitten area. Rubbing causes further damage to soft tissues. Do not attempt to rewarm the frostbitten area if there is a chance that it might refreeze or if you are close to a medical facility. For minor frostbite, rapidly rewarm the affected part using skin-to-skin contact such as with a warm hand.

To care for a more serious injury, gently soak it in water not warmer than about 105° F (Fig. 6-4, A). If you do not have a thermometer, test the water temperature yourself. If the temperature is uncomfortable to your touch, it is too warm. Keep the frostbitten part in the water until normal color returns and it feels warm (20 to 30 minutes). Loosely bandage the area with a dry, sterile dressing (Fig. 6-4, B). If fingers or toes are frostbitten, place cotton or gauze between them. Do not break any blisters. Take precautions to prevent hypothermia. Monitor the person's condition, and if you see that the person is going into shock, give care accordingly. Do not give ibuprofen or other nonsteroidal anti-inflammatory drugs (NSAIDs) when caring for frostbite.

Hypothermia

In a hypothermic condition, the entire body cools because its ability to keep warm is failing. The person will die if not given the proper care.

The air temperature does not have to be below freezing for people to develop hypothermia. This is especially true if the person is wet or if it is windy. Elderly people in poorly heated homes can develop hypothermia. The homeless, the ill and young children also are at risk.

Certain conditions can more easily lead to hypothermia, including:

- Ingestion of substances that interfere with the body's ability to regulate temperature (such as alcohol, other drugs and certain medications).
- Any medical condition that impairs circulation, such as diabetes or cardiovascular disease.
- Prolonged exposure to cold, wet and/or windy conditions or wet clothing.

What to Look For

Signals of hypothermia include the following:

- Shivering
- Numbness
- Glassy stare
- Indifference
- Loss of consciousness

Shivering that stops without rewarming is a sign that the person's condition is worsening. He or she needs immediate medical care.

When to Call 9-1-1

Call 9-1-1 or the local emergency number immediately for any case of hypothermia.

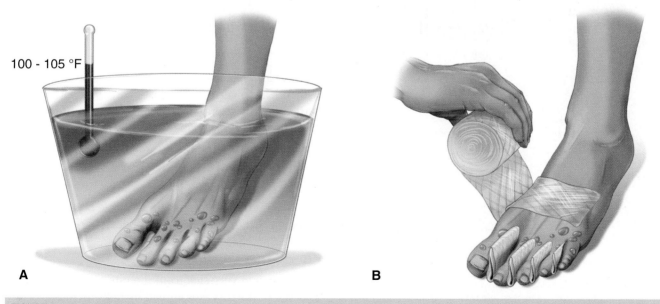

100 - 105 °F

A

B

FIGURE 6-4, A–B *To care for more serious frostbite:* **A,** *Warm the area gently by soaking the affected part in water not warmer than 105° F. Keep the frostbitten part in the water until normal color returns and it feels warm (20–30 minutes).* **B,** *Loosely bandage the area with a dry, sterile dressing.*

What to Do Until Help Arrives

To care for hypothermia, start by caring for life-threatening conditions (see below). Make the person comfortable. Gently move the person to a warm place. Remove wet clothing and dry the person. Put on dry clothing. Warm the body *gradually* by wrapping the person in blankets and plastic sheeting to hold in body heat (Fig. 6-5). Also, keep the head covered to further retain body heat.

If you are far from medical care, position the person near a heat source or apply heat pads or other heat sources to the body, such as containers filled with warm water. Carefully monitor any heat source to avoid burning the person. Keep a barrier, such as a blanket, towel or clothing, between the heat source and the person.

If the person is alert, give warm liquids that do not contain alcohol or caffeine. Alcohol can cause heat loss and caffeine can cause dehydration. Do not warm the person too quickly, such as by immersing the person in warm water. Check breathing and monitor for any changes in the person's condition and care for shock.

In cases of *severe hypothermia*, the person may be unconscious. Breathing may have slowed or stopped. The body may feel stiff because the muscles became rigid. Check for breathing for no more than 10 seconds. If the person is not breathing, perform CPR. Continue to warm the person until emergency medical services (EMS) personnel take over. Be prepared to use an automated external defibrillator (AED), if available.

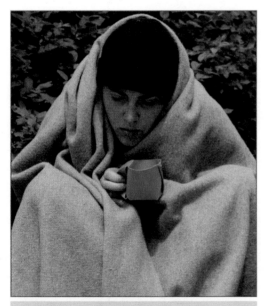

FIGURE 6-5 *For hypothermia, warm the body gradually by wrapping the person in blankets or putting on dry clothing and moving him or her to a warm place.* Courtesy of Canadian Red Cross.

Preventing Heat-Related Illnesses and Cold-Related Emergencies

In general, you can prevent illnesses caused by overexposure to extreme temperatures. To prevent heat-related illnesses and cold-related emergencies, follow these guidelines:

- Do not go outdoors during the hottest or coldest part of the day.
- Change your activity level according to the temperature.
- Take frequent breaks.
- Dress appropriately for the environment.
- Drink large amounts of fluids.

BITES AND STINGS

People are bitten and stung every day by insects, spiders, snakes, animals and marine life. Most of the time, these bites and stings do not cause serious problems. However, in rare circumstances, certain bites and stings can cause serious illness or even death in people who are sensitive to the venom.

Insect Stings

Most of the time, insect stings are harmless. If the person is allergic, an insect sting can lead to anaphylaxis, a life-threatening condition.

What to Look For

Signals of an insect sting include:

- Presence of a stinger.
- Pain.
- Swelling.
- Signals of an allergic reaction.

What to Do

If someone is stung by an insect:

- Remove any visible stinger. Scrape it away from the skin with a clean fingernail or a plastic card, such as a credit card, or use tweezers (Fig. 6-6). In the case of a bee sting, if you use tweezers, grasp the stinger, not the venom sac.
- Wash the site with soap and water.
- Cover the site and keep it clean.
- Apply a cold pack to the area to reduce pain and swelling.
- Call 9-1-1 if the person has any trouble breathing or for any other signals of anaphylaxis.

Tick-Borne Diseases

Humans can get very sick from the bite of an infected tick. Some of the diseases spread by ticks include Rocky Mountain spotted fever, *Babesia* infection, ehrlichiosis and Lyme disease.

LAYER YOUR WAY TO WARMTH

As long as seasonal changes and cold climates exist, preventing cold-related emergencies, such as hypothermia, remains important when we work or play outside.

The best way to ensure your comfort and warmth outdoors is to layer your clothing. The first layer, called the base layer, is next to your skin. The base layer helps to regulate your body temperature by moving perspiration away from your skin. This is important because if perspiration gets trapped inside your clothes, you can become chilled rapidly, which can lead to hypothermia.

Thermal underwear makes a good base layer for cold weather. The fabrics that are best at moving sweat away from the skin (also called wicking) are silk, merino wool and certain synthetics. Cotton is not a good choice because it traps moisture rather than wicking it away.

The job of the middle layer is insulation. This layer keeps you warm; it helps you retain heat by trapping air close to your body. Natural fibers, such as wool and goose down, are excellent insulators. So is synthetic fleece. Vests, jackets and tights are examples of clothing that can be worn for insulation.

The shell or outer layer protects you from wind, rain or snow. For cold weather, the shell layer should be both waterproof and "breathable." This will keep wind and water from getting inside of the other two layers while allowing perspiration to evaporate. The shell also should be roomy enough to fit easily over the other layers without restricting your movement.

One of the other advantages of layering is that you can make quick adjustments if the weather changes or you change your activity level. You can take clothes off when you become too warm and put them back on if you get cold.

In addition to layering your clothes, to stay warm in cold weather you also should wear:

- A hat.
- A scarf or knit mask that covers your face and mouth.
- Sleeves that are snug at the wrist.
- Mittens (they are warmer than gloves).
- Water-resistant boots.

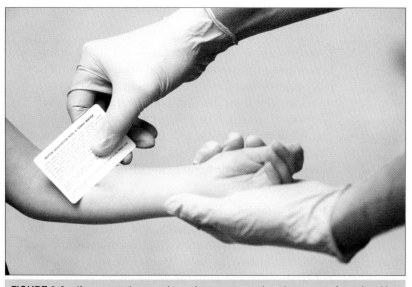

FIGURE 6-6 *If someone is stung by an insect, scrape the stinger away from the skin with a clean fingernail or a plastic card, such as a credit card.*

Rocky Mountain Spotted Fever

Rocky Mountain spotted fever is a bacterial infection spread by wood ticks in the western United States, dog ticks in the eastern United States, and other ticks in the southern United States. Rocky Mountain spotted fever occurs mostly in the spring and summer, and most cases occur in children.

What to Look For

Signals of Rocky Mountain spotted fever usually appear between 2 and 14 days after a tick bite.

Initial signals of Rocky Mountain spotted fever include the following:

- Fever
- Nausea

- Vomiting
- Muscle aches or pain
- Lack of appetite
- Severe headache

Later signals include:

- Rash: The *spotted rash* usually starts a few days after fever develops. It first appears as small spots on the wrists and ankles. It then spreads to the rest of the body. However, about one-third of persons infected with the illness do not get a rash.
- Abdominal pain.
- Joint pain.
- Diarrhea.

When to Seek Medical Care

Call a health care provider if the person develops signals of Rocky Mountain spotted fever after a tick bite. The health care provider is likely to prescribe antibiotics. In most cases, the person will recover fully. If left untreated, complications of Rocky Mountain spotted fever can be life threatening.

Babesia Infection

Babesia also called *Babesiosis* is a protozoa infection spread by deer ticks and black-legged ticks. It is more common during warm months, and most cases happen in the northeast and upper Midwest regions of the United States.

What to Look For

Many people infected with *Babesia* have no apparent symptoms. Some people may have flu-like symptoms, such as:

- Fever
- Sweats
- Chills
- Body aches and headaches
- No appetite
- Nausea
- Fatigue

Others infected with *Babesia* develop a type of anemia that can cause jaundice and dark urine. In some people, the disease can be life threatening if untreated. The elderly and persons with no spleen, a weak immune system or a serious health condition are the most susceptible.

When to Seek Medical Care

If a person develops any of the signals described above, he or she should seek medical care. Most people with signals of the disease can be treated successfully with prescription medications.

Ehrlichiosis

Most cases of infection with the bacteria *ehrlichia* in humans are caused by bites by an infected Lone Star tick, and occur mainly in the southern, eastern and south-central United States.

What to Look For

Many people with ehrlichiosis do not become ill. Some develop only mild signals that are seen 5 to 10 days after an infected tick bit the person.

Initial signals include the following:

- Fever
- Headache
- Fatigue
- Muscle aches

Other signals that may develop include the following:

- Nausea
- Vomiting
- Diarrhea
- Cough
- Joint pains
- Confusion
- Rash (in some cases)

When to Seek Medical Care

If the person becomes ill with any of the above signals described, he or she should seek medical care. Ehrlichiosis is treated with antibiotics.

Lyme Disease

Lyme disease is spreading throughout the United States. Although it is most prevalent on the east coast and the upper Midwest, cases of Lyme disease have been reported in all 50 states.

Lyme disease is spread by the deer tick and black-legged tick, which attaches itself to field mice and deer. Deer ticks are tiny and difficult to see (Fig. 6-7). They are much smaller than the common dog tick or wood tick. They can be as small as a poppy seed or the head of a pin. Adult deer ticks are only as large as a grape seed. Because of the tick's tiny size, its bite usually is painless. Many people who develop Lyme disease cannot recall having been bitten.

The tick is found around branches and in wooded and grassy areas. Like all ticks, it attaches itself to any warm-blooded animal with which it comes into direct contact, including humans. Deer ticks are active any time the temperature is above about 45° F. However, most cases of infection happen between May and late August, when ticks are most active and

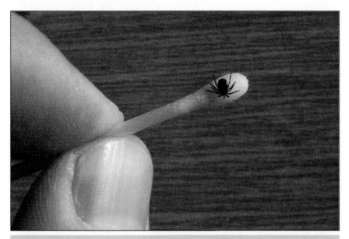

FIGURE 6-7 *Deer ticks are tiny and difficult to see.* © iStockphoto .com/Martin Pietak.

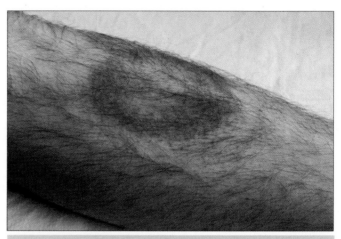

FIGURE 6-8 *A person with Lyme disease may develop a rash.* © iStockphoto.com/Heike Kampe.

people spend more time outdoors. Recent studies indicate that the tick must remain embedded in human skin for about 36 to 48 hours to transmit the disease. More information on Lyme disease may be available from your local or state health department, the American Lyme Disease Foundation (aldf.com), or the Centers for Disease Control and Prevention (CDC) (cdc.gov/features/lymedisease/).

What to Look For

The first signal of infection may appear a few days or a few weeks after a tick bite. In 80 to 90 percent of all cases of Lyme disease, a rash starts as a small red area at the site of the bite. It may spread up to 7 inches across (Fig. 6-8). In fair-skinned people, the center may be a lighter color with the outer edges red and raised. This sometimes gives the rash a bull's-eye appearance. In some individuals, the rash may appear to be solid red. In dark-skinned people, the area may look black and blue, like a bruise. The rash may or may not be warm to the touch and usually is not itchy or painful. If a rash does appear, it will do so in about 1 to 2 weeks and may last for about 3 to 5 weeks. Some people with Lyme disease never develop a rash.

Other signals of Lyme disease include fever, headache, weakness, and joint and muscle pain. These signals are similar to signals of flu and can develop slowly. They might not occur at the same time as the rash.

Lyme disease can get worse if it is not treated. Signals can include severe fatigue; fever; a stiff, aching neck; tingling or numbness in the fingers and toes; and facial paralysis.

In its advanced stages Lyme disease may cause painful arthritis; numbness in the arms, hands or legs; severe headaches; long- or short-term memory loss; confusion; dizziness; and problems

in seeing or hearing. Some of these signals could indicate problems with the brain or nervous system. Lyme disease may also cause heart problems such as an irregular or rapid heartbeat.

When to Seek Medical Care

If rash or flu-like signals develop, the person should seek medical care immediately. A health care provider usually will prescribe antibiotics to treat Lyme disease. Antibiotics work quickly and effectively if taken as soon as possible. Most people who get treated early make a full recovery. If you suspect Lyme disease, do not delay seeking treatment. Treatment time is longer and less effective when the person has been infected for a long period of time.

Preventing Tick-borne Diseases

Follow the guidelines presented in *Focus on Prevention: How to Beat Those Little Critters* in this chapter for general tips on how to prevent contact with, and bites from, ticks when you are in wooded or grassy areas.

To prevent tick-borne illnesses, always check for ticks immediately after outdoor activities. Most experts believe that the longer the tick stays attached to the skin, the greater the chances are of infection. Therefore, check for ticks at least once daily after having been outdoors. Quickly remove any ticks that you find before they become swollen with blood.

Wash all clothing. Be sure to check pets because they can carry ticks into the house, where they can then attach themselves to people or other pets. Pets also can develop signals of tick-borne diseases.

If you find a tick embedded in a person's skin, *it must be removed*. With a gloved hand, grasp the tick with fine-tipped and pointed tweezer that has a smooth inside

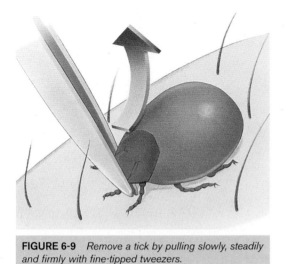

FIGURE 6-9 *Remove a tick by pulling slowly, steadily and firmly with fine-tipped tweezers.*

surface. Get as close to the skin as possible. Pull slowly, steadily and firmly with no twisting (Fig. 6-9).

■ Do not try to burn off the tick.
■ Do not apply petroleum jelly or nail polish to the tick.

Put the tick in a container or jar with rubbing alcohol to kill it. Clean the bite area with soap and water and an antiseptic. Apply an antibiotic ointment if it is available and the person has no known allergies or sensitivities to the medication. Encourage the person to seek medical advice because of the risk of contracting a tick-borne disease. If you cannot remove the tick, have the person seek advanced medical care.

Mosquito-Borne Illness: West Nile Virus

West Nile virus (WNV) is passed on to humans and other animals by mosquitoes that bite them after feeding on infected birds. Recently, WNV has been reported in some mild climate areas of North America and Europe.

WNV cannot be passed from one person to another. Also, no evidence supports that humans can acquire the disease by handling live or dead birds infected with WNV. However, it is still a good idea to use disposable gloves when handling an infected bird. Contact your local health department for instructions on reporting and disposing of the bird's body.

For most people, the risk of infection by WNV is very low. Less than 1 percent of people who are bitten by mosquitoes develop any signals of the disease. In addition, relatively few mosquitoes actually carry WNV. People who spend a lot of time outdoors are at a higher risk for catching the disease. Only about 1 in every 150 people who are infected with WNV will become seriously ill.

Preventing West Nile Virus

The easiest and best way to avoid WNV is to prevent mosquito bites. Specifically, you can:

■ Use insect repellents containing DEET (N, N-diethyl-meta-toluamide) when you are outdoors. Follow the directions on the package (see *Focus on Prevention: Repelling Those Pests*).
■ Consider staying indoors at dusk and dawn, when mosquitoes are most active. If you have to be outdoors during these times, use insect repellent and wear long sleeves and pants. Light-colored clothing can help you to see mosquitoes that land on you.
■ Make sure you have good screens on your windows and doors to keep mosquitoes out.
■ Get rid of mosquito breeding sites by emptying sources of standing water outside of the home, such as from flowerpots, buckets and barrels. Also, change the water in pet dishes and replace the water in bird baths weekly, drill drainage holes in tire swings so that water drains out and keep children's wading pools empty and on their sides when they are not being used.

For more information, visit cdc.gov/westnile or call the CDC public response hotline at (888) 246-2675 (English), (888) 246-2857 (Español) or (866) 874-2646 (TTY). Source: CDC.gov and redcross.org

What to Look For

Most people infected with WNV have no signals. Approximately 20 percent develop mild signals, such as fever and aches, which pass on their own. The risk of severe disease is higher for people 50 years and older.

People typically develop signals of WNV between 3 and 14 days after an infected mosquito bites them. Signals of WNV include the following:

■ High fever
■ Headache
■ Neck stiffness
■ Confusion
■ Coma
■ Tremors
■ Convulsions
■ Muscle weakness
■ Vision loss
■ Numbness
■ Paralysis

These signals may last several weeks. In some cases, WNV can cause fatal encephalitis, which is a swelling of the brain that leads to death.

HOW TO BEAT THOSE LITTLE CRITTERS

You can prevent bites and stings from insects, spiders, ticks or snakes by following these guidelines when you are in wooded or grassy areas:

- *Wear long-sleeved shirts and long pants.*
- *Tuck your pant legs into your socks or boots.*
- *Use a rubber band or tape to hold pants against socks so that nothing can get under clothing.*
- *Tuck your shirt into your pants.*
- *Wear light-colored clothing to make it easier to see tiny insects or ticks.*
- *When hiking in woods and fields, stay in the middle of trails. Avoid underbrush and tall grass.*
- *If you are outdoors for a long time, check yourself several times during the day. Especially check in hairy areas of the body like the back of the neck and the scalp line.*

- *Inspect yourself carefully for insects or ticks after being outdoors or have someone else do it.*
- *Avoid walking in areas where snakes are known to live.*
- *If you encounter a snake, look around for others. Turn around and walk away on the same path on which you came.*
- *Wear sturdy hiking boots.*
- *If you have pets that go outdoors, spray them with repellent made for that type of pet. Apply the repellent according to the label and check your pet for ticks often.*
- *If you will be in a grassy or wooded area for a long time or if you know that the area is highly infested with insects or ticks, consider using a repellent. Follow the directions carefully.*

When to Seek Care

If you develop signals of severe WNV illness, such as unusually severe headaches or confusion, seek medical attention immediately. Pregnant women and nursing mothers are encouraged to talk to their doctors if they develop signals that could indicate WNV. There is no specific treatment for WNV infection or a vaccine to prevent it. In more severe cases, people usually need to go to the hospital, where they will receive intravenous fluids, assistance with breathing and nursing care.

Spider Bites and Scorpion Stings

Few spiders in the United States can cause serious illness or death. However, the bites of the black widow and brown recluse spiders can, in rare cases, kill a person (Fig. 6-10, A–B). Another dangerous spider is the northwestern brown, or hobo, spider.

Widow spiders can be black, red or brown. The black widow spider is black with a reddish hourglass shape on the underside of its body and is the most venomous of the widow spiders. The brown recluse spider (also known as the violin or fiddleback spider) has a distinctive violin-shaped pattern on the back of its front body section.

These spiders prefer dark, out-of-the-way places. Examples of places where these spiders live include wood, rock and brush piles; dark garages; and attics. People often are bitten on their arms and hands when reaching into these places.

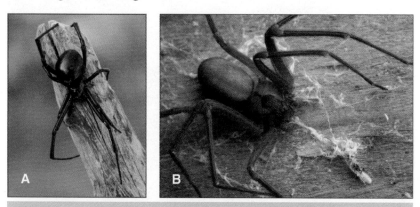

FIGURE 6-10, A–B *Bites from* **A,** *the black widow spider and* **B,** *the brown recluse spider can make a person very sick.* Fig. A © iStockphoto.com/Mark Kostich, Fig. B Image © Miles Boyer, 2010, Used under license from Shutterstock.com.

REPELLING THOSE PESTS

Insect repellent is used to keep away pests such as mosquitoes and ticks that sting and bite. DEET is the active ingredient in many insect repellents. Insect repellents that contain DEET are available in many different forms, including sprays, lotions and liquids. Using repellent with DEET is safe for most people. However, it is important to follow label directions and take proper precautions (see below).

The amount of DEET in insect repellents ranges from less than 10 percent to over 30 percent. The more DEET that a product contains, the longer it will protect from mosquito and tick bites. For example, an insect repellent containing about 24 percent DEET provides about 5 hours of protection.

Products with 10 percent DEET are as safe as products with 30 percent DEET when used properly. Precautions to follow when using products containing DEET include:

- *Apply products that contain DEET only once a day.*
- *Do not use DEET on infants under 2 months of age.*
- *Do not use a product that combines sunscreen with a DEET-containing insect repellent. Sunscreens wash off and need to be reapplied often. DEET does not wash off with water. Repeating applications may increase absorption of the chemical and cause possible toxic effects.*

Before using insect repellent, check the label carefully for the list of ingredients. If you are unsure whether the product is safe for you and your family to use, ask your health care provider. Use caution when considering insect repellents to be used by pregnant women, infants and children.

If you use a repellent, follow these general rules:

- *Keep all repellents out of the reach of children.*
- *To apply repellent to the face, first spray it on your hands and then apply it from your hands to your face. Avoid sensitive areas, such as the lips and eyes.*
- *Never use repellents on an open wound or irritated skin.*
- *Use repellents sparingly. One application will last 4 to 8 hours. Heavier or more frequent applications do not increase effectiveness.*
- *If you suspect that you are having a reaction to a repellent, wash the treated skin immediately and call your health care provider.*
- *Never put repellents on children's hands. They may put them in their eyes or mouth.*

For current information about pesticides, contact the National Pesticide Information Center at npic.orst. edu or at (800) 858-7378.

Scorpions live in dry regions such as the southwestern United States and Mexico. They live under rocks, logs and the bark of certain trees (Fig. 6-11). They are most active at night. Like spiders, only a few species of scorpions have a sting that can cause death. It is difficult to distinguish highly poisonous scorpions from nonpoisonous scorpions. Therefore, *all* scorpion stings should be treated as medical emergencies.

What to Look For

Signals of spider bites depend on the amount of poison, called *venom*, injected and the person's sensitivity to the venom. Most spider bites heal with no adverse effects or scarring. Signals of venomous spider bites can seem identical to those of other conditions and therefore can be difficult to recognize. The only way

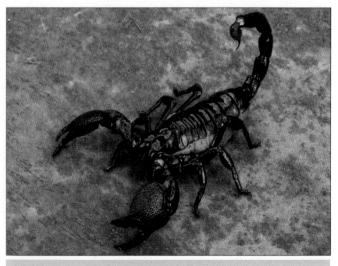

FIGURE 6-11 *A scorpion.* © iStockphoto.com/John Bell.

to be certain that a spider has bitten a person is to have witnessed it.

The bite of the black widow spider is the most painful and deadly of the widow spiders, especially in very young children and the elderly. The bite usually causes an immediate sharp pinprick pain, followed by a dull pain in the area of the bite. However, the person often does not know that he or she has been bitten until he or she starts to feel ill or notices a bite mark or swelling. Other signals of a black widow spider bite include:

- Rigid muscles in the shoulders, chest, back and abdomen.
- Restlessness.
- Anxiety.
- Dizziness.
- Headache.
- Excessive sweating.
- Weakness.
- Drooping or swelling of the eyelids.

The bite of the brown recluse spider may produce little or no pain initially. Pain in the area of the bite develops an hour or more later. A blood-filled blister forms under the surface of the skin, sometimes in a target or bull's-eye pattern. Over time, the blister increases in size and eventually ruptures, leading to tissue destruction and a black scab.

The hobo spider also can produce an open, slow-healing wound.

General signals of spider bites and scorpion stings may include:

- A mark indicating a possible bite or sting.
- Severe pain in the sting or bite area.
- A blister, lesion or swelling at the entry site.
- Nausea and vomiting.
- Stiff or painful joints.
- Chills or fever.
- Trouble breathing or swallowing or signs of anaphylaxis.
- Sweating or salivating profusely.
- Muscle aches or severe abdominal or back pain.
- Dizziness or fainting.
- Chest pain.
- Elevated heart rate.
- Infection at the site of the bite.

When to Call 9-1-1

Call 9-1-1 or the local emergency number immediately if you suspect that someone has been bitten by a black widow spider or brown recluse spider, stung by a scorpion or if the person has any other life-threatening conditions.

What to Do Until Help Arrives

If the person has been bitten by a venomous spider or stung by a scorpion:

- Wash the wound thoroughly.
- Apply an antibiotic ointment, if the person has no known allergies or sensitivities to the medication, to prevent infection.
- Bandage the wound.
- Apply an ice or cold pack to the site to reduce pain and swelling.
- Encourage the person to seek medical attention. Children and older adults may need antivenin to block the effects of the spider's venom.
- If you transport the person to a medical facility, keep the bitten area elevated and as still as possible.

Venomous Snake Bites

Snakebites kill few people in the United States. Of the estimated 7000 people bitten annually, fewer than 5 die (Fig. 6-12, A–D). Most snakebites occur near the home, not in the wild. Rattlesnakes account for most snakebites, and most of the deaths from snakebites in the United States. Most deaths occur because the bitten person has an allergic reaction, is in poor health or because too much time passes before he or she receives medical care.

What to Look For

Signals of a possibly venomous snakebite include:

- A bite mark.
- Pain.
- Swelling.

When to Call 9-1-1

If the bite is from a venomous snake such as a rattlesnake, copperhead, cottonmouth or coral snake call 9-1-1 or the local emergency number immediately.

What to Do Until Help Arrives

To care for a venomous snake bite:

- Wash the wound.
- Apply an elastic (pressure immobilization) bandage to slow the spread of venom through the lymphatic system by following these steps:

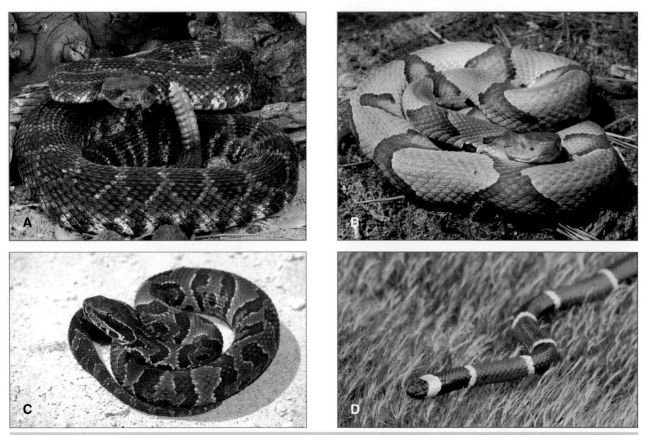

FIGURE 6-12, A–D *Venomous snakes found in the United Statics include* **A,** *rattlesnake* (Image © Audrey Snider-Bell, 2010 Used under license from Shutterstock.com). **B,** *copperhead* (© iStockphoto.com/Jake Holmes), **C,** *cottonmouth* (Image © Leighton Photography & Imaging, 2010 Used under license from Shutterstock.com), and **D,** *coral snake* (© iStockphoto.com/Mark Kostich).

○ Check for feeling, warmth and color of the limb and note changes in skin color and temperature.

○ Place the end of the bandage against the skin and use overlapping turns.

○ The wrap should cover a long body section, such as an arm or a calf, beginning at the point farthest from the heart. For a joint, such as the knee or ankle, use figure-eight turns to support the joint.

○ Check above and below the injury for feeling, warmth and color, especially fingers and toes, after you have applied an elastic roller bandage. By checking before and after bandaging, you may be able to tell if any tingling or numbness is from the elastic bandage or the injury.

○ Check the snugness of the bandaging—a finger should easily, but not loosely, pass under the bandage.

○ Keep the injured area still and *lower* than the heart. The person should walk *only* if absolutely necessary.

■ *Do not* apply ice.

■ *Do not* cut the wound.

■ *Do not* apply suction.

■ *Do not* apply a tourniquet.

■ *Do not* use electric shock, such as from a car battery.

Animal Bites

The bite of a domestic or wild animal can cause infection and soft tissue injury. The most serious possible result is rabies. Rabies is transmitted through the saliva of diseased animals such as skunks, bats, raccoons, cats, dogs, cattle and foxes.

Animals with rabies may act strangely. For example, those that are usually active at night may be active in the daytime. A wild animal that usually tries to avoid people might not run from you. Rabid animals may drool, appear to be partially paralyzed, or act aggressively or strangely quiet.

If not treated, rabies is fatal. Anyone bitten by an animal that might have rabies must get medical attention. Treatment for rabies includes a series of vaccine injections to build up immunity that will help fight the disease.

If an animal bites someone, try to get the person away from the animal without putting yourself in danger. Do not try to stop, hold or catch the animal. Do not touch a pet that may have come in contact with the animal's saliva without using or wearing some form of protection like disposable gloves.

What to Look For

Signals of an animal bite include:

- A bite mark.
- Bleeding.

When to Call 9-1-1

Call 9-1-1 or the local emergency number if the wound is bleeding seriously or you suspect the animal might have rabies.

If possible, try to remember the animal's appearance and where you last saw it. When you call 9-1-1 or the local emergency number, the call taker will direct the proper authorities, such as animal control, to the scene.

What to Do Until Help Arrives

To care for an animal bite:

- Control bleeding *first* if the wound is bleeding seriously.
- Do not clean serious wounds. The wound will be cleaned at a medical facility.
- If bleeding is minor, wash the wound with soap and water then irrigate with clean running tap water.
- Control any bleeding.
- Apply an antibiotic ointment to a minor wound, if the person has no known allergies or sensitivities to the medication, and cover the wound with a dressing.
- Watch for signals of infection.

Marine Life Stings

The stings of some forms of marine life are not only painful, but they can make you sick, and in some parts of the world, can kill you (Fig. 6-13, A–D). The side effects include allergic reactions that can cause breathing and heart problems, as well as paralysis and death. The lifeguards in your area should know the types of jellyfish that may be present.

What to Look For

Signals of marine life stings include:

- Possible puncture marks.
- Pain.
- Swelling.
- Signs of a possible allergic reaction.

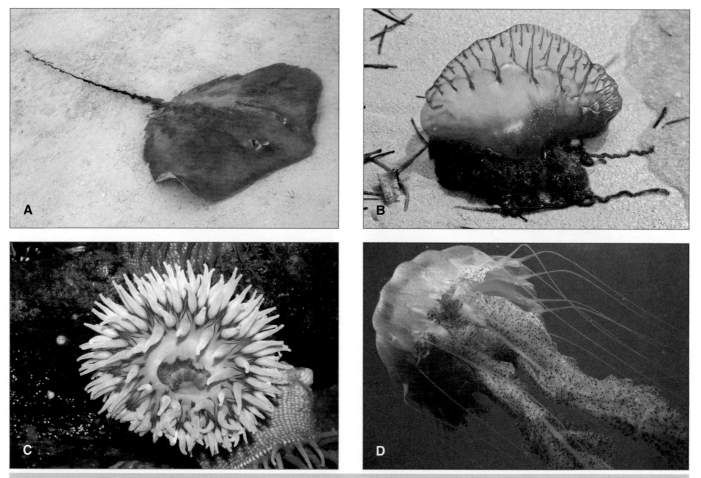

FIGURE 6-13, A–D *The painful sting of some marine animals can cause serious problems:* **A,** *stingray* (© iStockphoto.com/Dia Karanouh); **B,** *Bluebottle jellyfish/Portuguese man-of-war* (© iStockphoto.com/Mark Kostich); **C,** *sea anemone* (© iStockphoto.com/Omers); **D,** *jellyfish* (Image © Johan1900, 2010 Used under license from Shutterstock.com).

When to Call 9-1-1

Call 9-1-1 or the local emergency number if the person does not know what stung him or her, has a history of allergic reactions to marine-life stings, is stung on the face or neck, or starts to have trouble breathing.

What to Do Until Help Arrives

If you encounter someone who has a marine-life sting:

- Get a lifeguard to remove the person from the water as soon as possible. If a lifeguard is not available, use a reaching assist, if possible (see Chapter 1). Avoid touching the person with your bare hands, which could expose you to the stinging tentacles. Use gloves or a towel when removing any tentacles.

- If you know the sting is from a jellyfish, irrigate the injured part with large amounts of vinegar as soon as possible for at least 30 seconds. This can help to remove the tentacles and stop the injection of venom. Vinegar works best to offset the toxin, but a baking soda slurry also may be used if vinegar is not available.

- If the sting is known to be from a bluebottle jellyfish, also known as a Portugese man-of-war, use ocean water instead of vinegar. Vinegar triggers further envenomation.

- Do not rub the wound, apply a pressure immobilization bandage or apply fresh water or other remedies because this may increase pain.

- Once the stinging action is stopped and tentacles removed, care for pain by hot-water immersion. Have the person take a hot shower if possible for at least 20 minutes. The water temperature should be as hot as can be tolerated (non-scalding) or about 113° F if the temperature can be measured.

- If you know the sting is from a stingray, sea urchin or spiny fish, flush the wound with tap water. Ocean water also may be used. Keep the injured part still and soak the affected area in non-scalding hot water (as hot as the person can stand) for at least 20 minutes or until the pain goes away. If hot water is not available, packing the area in hot sand may have a similar effect if the sand is hot enough. Then carefully clean the wound and apply a bandage. Watch for signals of infection and check with a health care provider to determine if a tetanus shot is needed.

POISONOUS PLANTS

Every year, millions of people suffer after coming into contact with poisonous plants such as poison ivy, poison sumac and poison oak (Fig. 6-14, A–C).

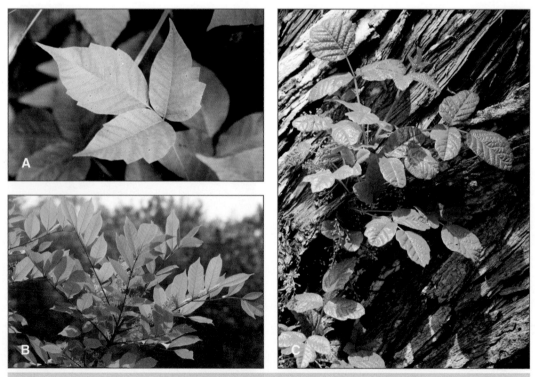

FIGURE 6-14, A–C **A,** *poison ivy* (Image © Tim Mainiero, 2010 Used under license from Shutterstock.com); **B,** *poison sumac* (Courtesy of www.poison-ivy.org); **C,** *poison oak* (Image © Dwight Smith, 2010 Used under license from Shutterstock.com).

You often can avoid or limit the irritating effects of touching or brushing against poisonous plants by following these steps:

- Remove exposed clothing and wash the exposed area thoroughly with soap and water as soon as possible after contact.
- Wash clothing exposed to plant oils since the oils can linger on fabric. Wash your hands thoroughly after handling exposed clothing. Wash your hands after touching exposed pets.
- Put a paste of baking soda and water on the area several times a day if a rash or weeping sore begins to develop. Calamine lotion and antihistamines, such as Benadryl®, may help to dry up the sores.
- See a health care provider if the condition gets worse or involves areas of the face or throat that could affect breathing. He or she may decide to give anti-inflammatory drugs, such as corticosteroids or other medications, to relieve discomfort.

LIGHTNING

Every year, lightning causes more deaths in the United States than any other weather hazard, including blizzards, hurricanes, floods, tornadoes, earthquakes and volcanic eruptions. The National Weather Service (NWS) estimates that lightning kills nearly 100 people annually and injures about 300 others.

Lightning travels at speeds of up to 300 miles per second. Anything tall—a tower, tree or person—can become a path for the electrical current. A lightning strike can throw a person through the air, burn off clothes and cause the heart to stop beating. The most severe lightning strikes carry up to 50 million volts of electricity. This is enough electricity to light 13,000 homes. Lightning can "flash" *over* a person's body or it can travel *through* blood vessels and nerves to reach the ground.

If a person survives a lightning strike, he or she may act confused. The person may describe the episode as getting hit on the head or hearing an explosion.

Prevent Lightning Injuries

What to do before a possible lightning storm:

- Pick campsites that meet safety precautions.
- Know local weather patterns, especially in summertime.
- Plan turnaround times (the amount of time you need to get back) in lightning-prone areas, based on your research, and stick to the plan.

During thunderstorms, use common sense to prevent being struck by lightning. If a thunderstorm threatens, the NWS advises people to:

- Postpone activities immediately, and not wait for rain to begin. Thunder and lightning can strike without rain.
- Watch cloud patterns and conditions for signs of an approaching storm.
- Designate safe locations and move or evacuate to a safe location at the first sound of thunder. Every 5 seconds between the flash of lightning and the sound of thunder equals 1 mile of distance.
- Where possible, quickly find shelter in a substantial building (not a carport, open garage or covered patio), or in a fully enclosed metal vehicle, such as a hardtop car (not a convertible), truck or van, with the windows completely shut.
- Use the *30-30 rule* where visibility is good and there is nothing obstructing your view of the thunderstorm. When you see lightning, count the time until you hear thunder. If that time is 30 seconds or less, the thunderstorm is within 6 miles. Seek shelter immediately. The threat of lightning continues for a much longer period than most people realize. Wait *at least 30 minutes* after the last clap of thunder before leaving shelter. If inside during a storm, keep away from windows. Injuries may occur from flying debris or glass if a window breaks.
- Stay away from plumbing, electrical equipment and wiring during a thunderstorm.
- Do *not* use a corded telephone or radio transmitter except for emergencies.
- If there is a tornado alert, go to the basement of the lowest interior level of a building.

In a lightning storm, reach safety by following these guidelines:

- Move downhill.
- Do not stay in a meadow or any other wide-open space.
- Seek uniform cover, such as low rolling hills or trees of about the same size.
- If you are boating or swimming, get to land and move away from the shore.
- Avoid all of the following:
  - Metal
  - Anything connected to electrical power
  - High places and high objects such as tall trees
  - Open places
  - Damp, shallow caves and tunnels
  - Overhangs
  - Flood zones

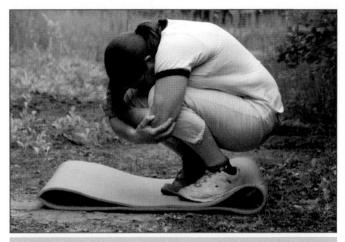

FIGURE 6-15 *If lightning strikes and you cannot get inside, squat or sit in a tight body position, preferably on insulating material such as a sleeping pad or life jacket.* Courtesy of the Canadian Red Cross.

○ Places obviously struck by lightning in the past
○ Long conductors, such as fences

If lightning is striking nearby when people are outside, they should assume a safe position:

- Squat or sit in a tight body position on insulating material such as a sleeping pad or a life jacket (Fig. 6-15).
- Take off any metal-framed packs and toss hiking poles away from the group.
- Do not lie down; instead, try to make as little contact with the ground as possible.
- If you feel your hair stand on end or your skin get tingly, cover your ears with your hands, close your eyes and get your head close to your knees.
- Avoid squatting or sitting close to other people. Maintain a minimum distance of at least 15 feet between people. Keep everyone in sight if possible.

Lightning Injuries

Lightning injuries are serious and can be fatal. Being struck by lightning can cause cardiac and pulmonary arrest, neurological problems, blindness, deafness, burns, bone fractures, loss of hearing, eyesight and trauma.

What to Look For

When checking a person struck by lightning, look the person over from head to toe in the front and back for any of the following signals:

- Unconsciousness
- Dazed, confused behavior
- Trouble breathing
- No breathing
- Burn marks on the skin or other open wounds
- Muscle, bone or joint injuries such as fractures or dislocations

When to Call 9-1-1

Call **9-1-1** immediately if a person is struck by lightning.

Even if the person seems to have recovered soon after the incident, advanced medical care still is necessary because serious problems can develop later.

What to Do Until Help Arrives

- Immediately perform CPR if needed.
- Give care for any injuries as needed including care for thermal burns.
- Be ready to care for other conditions, such as hypothermia in a wet, injured person.

PUTTING IT ALL TOGETHER

Outdoor activities in all kinds of weather are healthy and fun, but environmental emergencies can occur. Children and adults become seriously injured, and even die, from heat stroke, hypothermia, snakebites and lightning strikes.

The good news is that you can prevent environmental emergencies most of the time. Be prepared for all kinds of weather and situations before you head out to hike, swim, ski or camp. Know how to dress appropriately, what precautions to take and what to do if a situation becomes uncertain.

Even with excellent preparation, emergencies still happen. Know the signals—especially the early ones—of environmentally caused illnesses. This will allow you to make quick decisions for yourself or others. Quick decisions about when to call 9-1-1 and when to seek medical care can mean the difference between life and death in an environmental emergency!

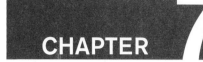

Soft Tissue Injuries

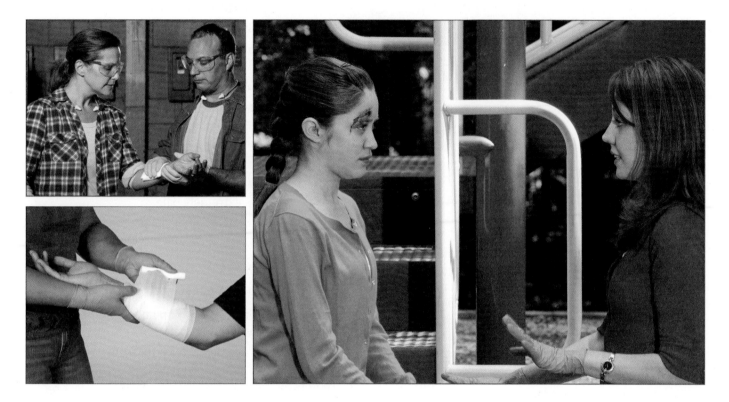

Soft tissue injuries happen to children and adults of all ages. They can be minor, serious or life threatening. Examples of minor soft tissue injuries include scrapes, bruises and mild sunburns. Examples of serious soft tissue injuries include large cuts that require stitches and partial-thickness burns. Life-threatening soft tissue injuries include stab wounds to the abdomen, lacerations that cause serious bleeding and full-thickness burns.

This chapter discusses the signals of soft tissue injuries, including closed wounds, open wounds and burns. You will read about the differences between major wounds and minor wounds and between different types of burns. In addition, you will learn when to call 9-1-1 or the local emergency number and how to give care.

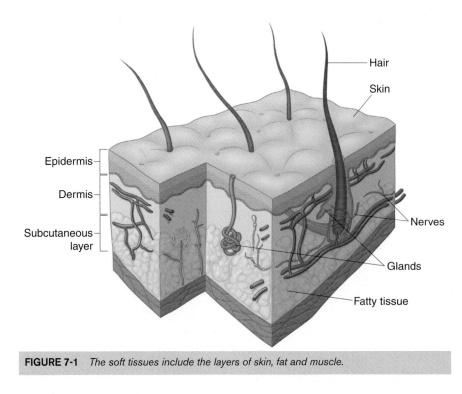

FIGURE 7-1 *The soft tissues include the layers of skin, fat and muscle.*

into the surrounding tissues, causing the area to swell and change color.

A more serious closed wound can be caused by a violent force hitting the body. This type of force can injure larger blood vessels and deeper layers of muscle tissue, which may result in heavy bleeding beneath the skin and damage to internal organs.

What to Look For

Signals of internal bleeding include:

- Tender, swollen, bruised or hard areas of the body, such as the abdomen.
- Rapid, weak pulse.
- Skin that feels cool or moist or looks pale or bluish.
- Vomiting blood or coughing up blood.
- Excessive thirst.
- An injured extremity that is blue or extremely pale.
- Altered mental state, such as the person becoming confused, faint, drowsy or unconscious.

When to Call 9-1-1

Call 9-1-1 or the local emergency number if:

- A person complains of severe pain or cannot move a body part without pain.
- You think the force that caused the injury was great enough to cause serious damage.
- An injured extremity is blue or extremely pale.
- The person's abdomen is tender and distended.
- The person is vomiting blood or coughing up blood.
- The person shows signals of shock or becomes confused, drowsy or unconscious.

WOUNDS

Soft tissues are the layers of skin and the fat and muscle beneath the skin's outer layer (Fig. 7-1). An injury to the soft tissue commonly is called a *wound*. Any time the soft tissue is damaged or torn, the body is threatened. Injuries may damage the soft tissue at or near the skin's surface or deep in the body. Severe bleeding can occur at the skin's surface or beneath, where it is harder to detect. Germs can enter the body through the wound and cause infection.

Wounds usually are classified as either closed or open. In a *closed wound*, the skin's surface is not broken; therefore, tissue damage and any bleeding occur below the surface. In an *open wound*, the skin's surface is broken, and blood may come through the tear in the skin.

Fortunately, most of the bleeding you will encounter will not be serious. In most cases it usually stops by itself within a few minutes with minimal intervention. The trauma may cause a blood vessel to tear causing bleeding, but the blood at the wound site usually clots quickly and stops flowing. Sometimes, however, the damaged blood vessel is too large or the pressure in the blood vessel is too great for the blood to clot, then bleeding can be life threatening. This can happen with both closed and open wounds.

Closed Wounds

The simplest closed wound is a bruise. A bruise develops when the body is bumped or hit, such as when you bump your leg on a table or chair (Fig. 7-2). The force of the blow to the body damages the soft tissue layers beneath the skin. This causes internal bleeding. Blood and other fluids seep

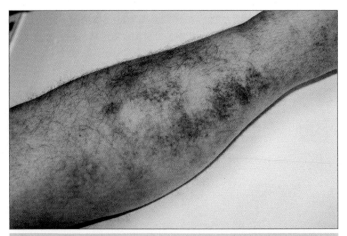

FIGURE 7-2 *The simplest closed wound is a bruise, which develops when the body is bumped or hit.* Courtesy of Ted Crites.

What to Do Until Help Arrives

Many closed wounds, like bruises, do not require special medical care. To care for a closed wound, you can apply an ice pack to the area to decrease bleeding beneath the skin.

Applying cold also can be effective in helping to control both pain and swelling (Fig. 7-3). Fill a plastic bag with ice and water or wrap ice in a wet cloth and apply it to the injured area for periods of about 20 minutes. Place a thin barrier between the ice and bare skin. Remove the ice and wait for 20 minutes before reapplying. If the person is not able to tolerate a 20–minute application, apply the ice pack for periods of 10 minutes on and off. Elevating the injured part may help to reduce swelling; however, *do not* elevate the injured part if it causes more pain.

Do not assume that all closed wounds are minor injuries. Take the time to find out whether more serious injuries could be present.

With all closed wounds, help the person to rest in the most comfortable position possible. In addition, keep the person from getting chilled or overheated. It also is helpful to comfort and reassure the person. Be sure that a person with an injured lower extremity does not bear weight on it until advised to do so by a medical professional.

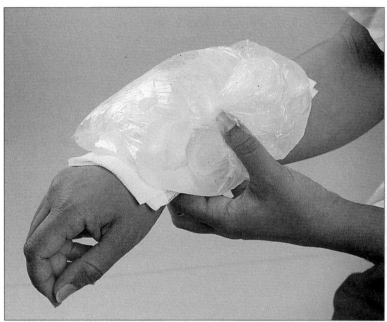

FIGURE 7-3 *Apply ice to a closed wound to help control pain and swelling.*

Open Wounds

In an open wound, the break in the skin can be as minor as a scrape of the surface layers or as severe as a deep penetration. The amount of bleeding depends on the location and severity of the injury.

The four main types of open soft tissue wounds are abrasions, lacerations, avulsions and punctures.

Abrasions

Abrasions are the most common type of open wound (Fig. 7-4). They usually are caused by something rubbing roughly against the skin. Abrasions do not bleed much. Any bleeding that occurs comes from *capillaries* (tiny blood vessels). Dirt and germs frequently have been rubbed into this type of wound, which is why it is important to clean and irrigate an abrasion thoroughly with soap and water to prevent infection.

Other terms for an abrasion include a scrape, a rug burn, a road rash or a strawberry. Abrasions usually are painful because scraping of the outer skin layers exposes sensitive nerve endings.

Lacerations

A *laceration* is a cut in the skin, which commonly is caused by a sharp object, such as a knife, scissors or broken glass (Fig. 7-5). A laceration also can occur when a blunt force splits the skin. Deep lacerations may cut layers of fat and muscle, damaging both nerves and blood vessels. Bleeding may be heavy or there may be none at all. Lacerations are not always painful because damaged nerves cannot send pain signals to the brain. Infection can easily occur with lacerations if proper care is not given.

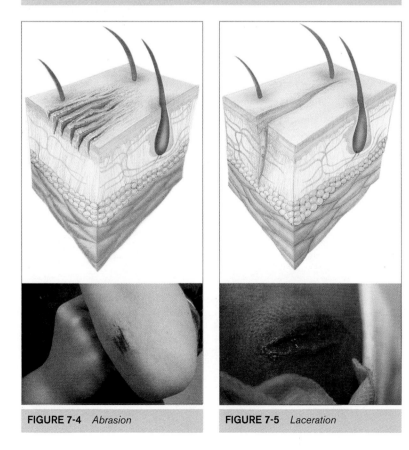

FIGURE 7-4 *Abrasion*

FIGURE 7-5 *Laceration*

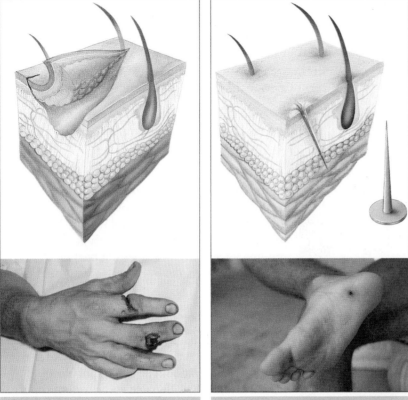

FIGURE 7-6 *Avulsion*   **FIGURE 7-7** *Puncture*

What to Do Until Help Arrives

Give general care for all open wounds. Specific care depends on whether the person has a minor or a major open wound.

General Care for Open Wounds

General care for open wounds includes controlling bleeding, preventing infection and using dressings and bandages.

Preventing Infection

When the skin is broken, the best initial defense against infection is to clean the area. For minor wounds, after controlling any bleeding, wash the area with soap and water and, if possible, irrigate with large amounts of fresh running water to remove debris and germs. You should not wash more serious wounds that require medical attention because they involve more extensive tissue damage or bleeding and it is more important to control the bleeding.

Sometimes even the best care for a soft tissue injury is not enough to prevent infection. You usually will be able to recognize the early signals of infection. The area around the wound becomes swollen and red (Fig. 7-8). The area may feel warm or throb with pain. Some wounds discharge pus. Serious infections may cause a person to develop a fever and feel ill. Red streaks may develop that progress from the wound toward the heart. If this happens, the infected person should seek immediate professional medical attention.

If you see any signals of infection, keep the area clean, soak it in clean, warm water and apply an antibiotic ointment if the person has no known allergies or sensitivities to the medication. Change coverings over the wound daily.

Avulsions

An *avulsion* is a serious soft tissue injury. It happens when a portion of the skin, and sometimes other soft tissue, is partially or completely torn away (Fig. 7-6). This type of injury often damages deeper tissues, causing significant bleeding. Sometimes a violent force may completely tear away a body part, including bone, such as a finger. This is known as an *amputation*. With amputations, sometimes bleeding is easier to control because the tissues close around the vessels at the injury site. If there is a violent tearing, twisting or crushing of the extremity, the bleeding may be hard to control.

Punctures

Punctures usually occur when a pointed object, such as a nail, pierces the skin (Fig. 7-7). A gunshot wound is a puncture wound. Puncture wounds do not bleed much unless a blood vessel has been injured. However, an object that goes into the soft tissues beneath the skin can carry germs deep into the body. These germs can cause infections—sometimes serious ones. If the object remains in the wound, it is called an *embedded object*.

When to Call 9-1-1

Call 9-1-1 or the local emergency number immediately for any major open or closed wound.

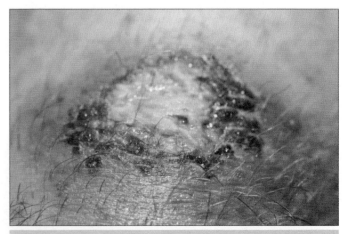

FIGURE 7-8 *The area around an infected wound becomes swollen and red.* Image © Fedor Kondratenko, 2010 Used under license from Shutterstock.com.

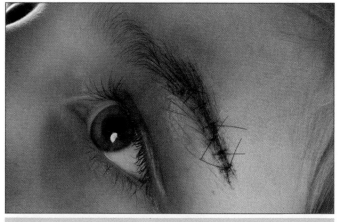

FIGURE 7-9 *Wounds to the face could cause scarring and therefore often require stitches.* © iStockphoto.com/Angie Kohler.

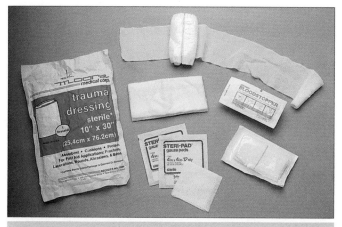

FIGURE 7-10 *Dressings are placed directly on the wound to absorb blood and prevent infection.*

Determining if the Person Needs Stitches

It can be difficult to judge when a wound requires stitches. One rule of thumb is that a health care provider will need to stitch a wound if the edges of skin do not fall together, the laceration involves the face or when any wound is over ½ inch long (Fig. 7-9).

Stitches speed the healing process, lessen the chances of infection and minimize scarring. They should be placed within the first few hours after the injury. The following major injuries often require stitches:

- Bleeding from an artery or uncontrolled bleeding.
- Wounds that show muscle or bone, involve joints, gape widely, or involve hands or feet.
- Wounds from large or deeply embedded objects.
- Wounds from human or animal bites.
- Wounds that, if left unstitched, could leave conspicuous scars, such as those on the face.

Using Dressings and Bandages

All open wounds need some type of covering to help control bleeding and prevent infection. These coverings commonly are referred to as dressings and bandages, and there are many types.

Dressings are pads placed directly on the wound to absorb blood and other fluids and to prevent infection. To minimize the chance of infection, dressings should be sterile. Most dressings are porous, allowing air to circulate to the wound to promote healing. Standard dressings include varying sizes of cotton gauze, commonly ranging from 2 to 4 inches square (Fig. 7-10). Larger dressings are used to cover very large wounds and multiple wounds in one body area. Some dressings have nonstick surfaces to prevent them from sticking to the wound.

An *occlusive dressing* is a bandage or dressing that closes a wound or damaged area of the body and

FOCUS ON PREVENTION

TETANUS

Tetanus *is a severe infection that can result from a puncture or a deep cut. Tetanus is a disease caused by bacteria. These bacteria produce a powerful poison in the body. The poison enters the nervous system and can cause muscle paralysis. Once tetanus reaches the nervous system, its effects are highly dangerous and can be fatal. Fortunately, tetanus often can be successfully treated with medicines called* antitoxins.

One way to prevent tetanus is through immunizations. All of us need to have a shot to protect against tetanus. We also need a booster shot at least every 10 years. Check with your health care provider to learn whether you need a booster shot if either of the following happens:

- *Your skin is punctured or cut by an object that could carry infection, such as a rusty nail.*
- *You are bitten by an animal.*

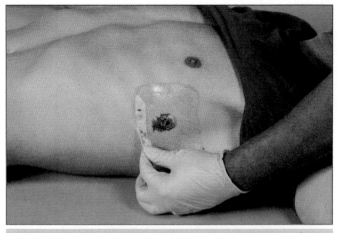

FIGURE 7-11 *Occlusive dressings are designed to close a wound or damaged area of the body and prevent it from being exposed to the air or water.*

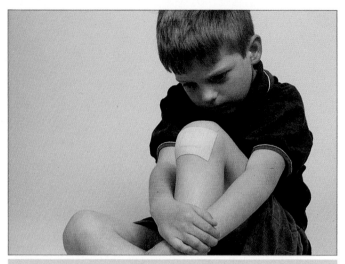

FIGURE 7-13 *Adhesive compress*

prevents it from being exposed to the air or water (Fig. 7-11). By preventing exposure to the air, occlusive dressings help to prevent infection. Occlusive dressings help to keep in place medications that have been applied to the affected area. They also help to keep in heat, body fluids and moisture. Occlusive dressings are manufactured but can be improvised. An example of an improvised occlusive dressing is plastic wrap secured with medical tape. This type of dressing can be used for certain chest and abdominal injuries.

A *bandage* is any material that is used to wrap or cover any part of the body. Bandages are used to hold dressings in place, to apply pressure to control bleeding, to protect a wound from dirt and infection, and to provide support to an injured limb or body part (Fig. 7-12). Any bandage applied snugly to create pressure on a wound or an injury is called a *pressure bandage*.

You can purchase many different types of bandages, including:

- *Adhesive compresses*, which are available in assorted sizes and consist of a small pad of nonstick gauze on a strip of adhesive tape that is applied directly to minor wounds (Fig. 7-13).
- *Bandage compresses*, which are thick gauze dressings attached to a bandage that is tied in place. Bandage compresses are specially designed to help control severe bleeding and usually come in sterile packages.
- *Roller bandages*, which are usually made of gauze or gauze-like material (Fig. 7-14). Roller bandages are available in assorted widths from ½ to 12 inches (1.3–30.5 cm) and in lengths from 5 to 10 yards. A narrow bandage would be used to wrap a hand or wrist. A medium-width bandage would be used

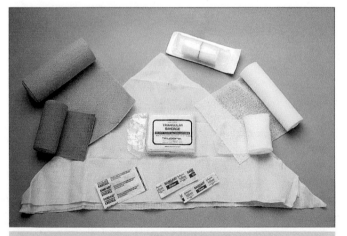

FIGURE 7-12 *Bandages are used to hold dressings in place, control bleeding, protect wounds and provide support to an injured limb or body part.*

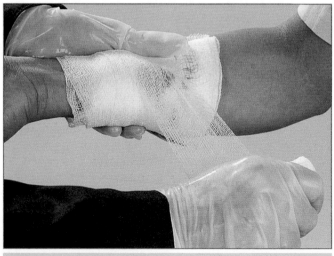

FIGURE 7-14 *Roller bandage*

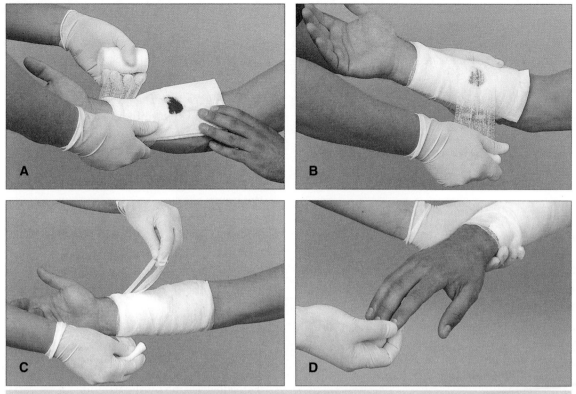

FIGURE 7-15, A–D   *To apply a roller bandage:* **A,** *Start by securing the bandage in place.* **B,** *Use overlapping turns to cover the dressing completely.* **C,** *Tie or tape the bandage in place.* **D,** *Check the fingers or toes for feeling, warmth and color.*

for an arm or ankle. A wide bandage would be used to wrap a leg. A roller bandage generally is wrapped around the body part. It can be tied or taped in place. A roller bandage also may be used to hold a dressing in place, secure a splint or control external bleeding.

Follow these general guidelines when applying a roller bandage:

- Check for feeling, warmth and color of the area below the injury site, especially fingers and toes, before and after applying the bandage.

- Elevate the injured body part only if you do not suspect that a bone has been broken and if doing so does not cause more pain.

- Secure the end of the bandage in place with a turn of the bandage. Wrap the bandage around the body part until the dressing is completely covered and the bandage extends several inches beyond the dressing. Tie or tape the bandage in place (Fig. 7-15, A–C).

- Do not cover fingers or toes. By keeping these parts uncovered, you will be able to see if the bandage is too tight (Fig. 7-15, D). If fingers or toes become cold or begin to turn pale, blue or ashen, the bandage is too tight and should be loosened slightly.

- Apply additional dressings and another bandage if blood soaks through the first bandage. Do not remove the blood-soaked bandages and dressings. Disturbing them may disrupt the formation of a clot and restart the bleeding.

Elastic roller bandages, sometimes called elastic wraps, are designed to keep continuous pressure on a body part (Fig. 7-16). Elastic bandages are available in 2-, 3-, 4- and 6-inch widths. As with roller bandages, the

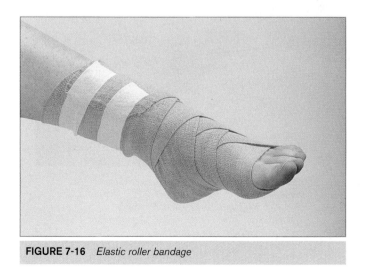

FIGURE 7-16   *Elastic roller bandage*

first step in using an elastic bandage is to select the correct size of the bandage: a narrow bandage is used to wrap a hand or wrist; a medium-width bandage is used for an arm or ankle and a wide bandage is used to wrap a leg.

When properly applied, an elastic bandage may control swelling or support an injured limb, as in the care for a venomous snakebite. However, an improperly applied elastic bandage can restrict blood flow, which is not only painful but also can cause tissue damage if not corrected.

To apply an elastic roller bandage:

- Check the circulation of the limb beyond where you will be placing the bandage by checking for feeling, warmth and color.
- Place the end of the bandage against the skin and use overlapping turns (Fig. 7-17, A).
- Gently stretch the bandage as you continue wrapping (Fig. 7-17, B). The wrap should cover a long body section, like an arm or a calf, beginning at the point farthest from the heart. For a joint like

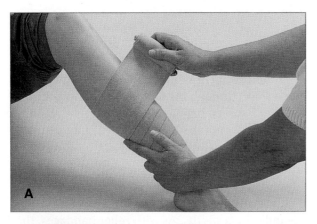

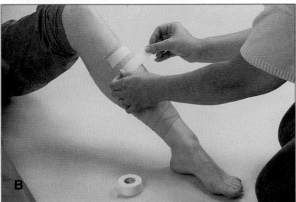

FIGURE 7-17, A–B A, To apply an elastic bandage: Place the bandage against the skin and use overlapping turns. B, Gently stretch the bandage as you continue wrapping. The wrap should cover a long body section, like an arm or a calf, beginning at the point farthest from the heart.

a knee or an ankle, use figure-eight turns to support the joint.

- Check the snugness of the bandaging—a finger should easily, but not loosely, pass under the bandage.
- Always check the area above and below the injury site for feeling, warmth and color, especially fingers and toes, after you have applied an elastic roller bandage. By checking both before and after bandaging, you will be able to tell if any tingling or numbness is from the bandaging or the injury.

Specific Care Guidelines for Minor Open Wounds

In minor open wounds, such as abrasions, there is only a small amount of damage and minimal bleeding.

To care for a minor open wound, follow these general guidelines:

- Use a barrier between your hand and the wound. If readily available, put on disposable gloves and place a sterile dressing on the wound.
- Apply direct pressure for a few minutes to control any bleeding.
- Wash the wound thoroughly with soap and water. If possible, irrigate an abrasion for about 5 minutes with clean, warm, running tap water.
- Apply an antibiotic ointment to a minor wound if the person has no known allergies or sensitivities to the medication.
- Cover the wound with a sterile dressing and a bandage or with an adhesive bandage to keep the wound moist and prevent drying.

Specific Care Guidelines for Major Open Wounds

A major open wound has serious tissue damage and severe bleeding. To care for a major open wound, you must act at once. Follow these steps:

- Put on disposable gloves. If you suspect that blood might splatter, you may need to wear eye and face protection.
- Control bleeding by:
  ○ Covering the wound with a dressing and firmly pressing against the wound with a gloved hand until the bleeding stops.
  ○ Applying a pressure bandage over the dressing to maintain pressure on the wound and to hold the dressing in place. If blood soaks through the bandage, do not remove the blood-soaked bandages. Instead, add more

dressings and bandages and apply additional direct pressure.

- Continue to monitor the person's condition. Observe the person closely for signals that may indicate that the person's condition is worsening, such as faster or slower breathing, changes in skin color and restlessness.
- Care for shock. Keep the person from getting chilled or overheated.
- Have the person rest comfortably and provide reassurance.
- Wash your hands immediately after giving care, even if you wore gloves.

Using Tourniquets When Help Is Delayed

A *tourniquet* is a tight band placed around an arm or leg to constrict blood vessels in order to stop blood flow to a wound. Because of the potential for adverse effects, a tourniquet should be used *only as a last resort* in cases of delayed care or situations where response from emergency medical services (EMS) is delayed, when direct pressure does not stop the bleeding or you are not able to apply direct pressure.

For example, a tourniquet may be appropriate if you cannot reach the wound because of entrapment, there are multiple injuries or the size of the wound prohibits application of direct pressure. In most areas, application of a tourniquet is considered to be a skill at the emergency medical technician (EMT) level or higher and requires proper training. There are several types of manufactured tourniquets available and are preferred over makeshift (improvised) devices. For a manufactured tourniquet, always follow the manufacturer's instructions.

In general, the tourniquet is applied around the wounded extremity, just above the wound. The tag end of the strap is routed through the buckle, and the strap is pulled tightly, which secures the tourniquet in place. The rod (windlass) then is twisted to tighten the tourniquet until the bright-red bleeding stops. The rod then is secured in place (Fig. 7-18, A–B). The tourniquet should *not* be removed in the prehospital setting once it is applied. The time that the tourniquet was applied should be noted and recorded and then given to EMS personnel.

Blood pressure cuffs sometimes are used as a tourniquet to slow the flow of blood in an upper extremity. Another technique is to use a bandage that is 4 inches wide and six to eight layers deep. Always follow local protocols when the use of a tourniquet is considered.

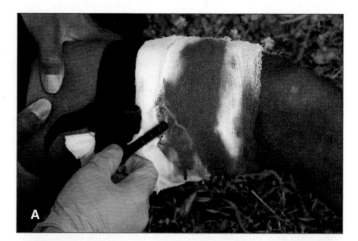
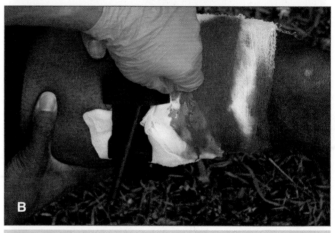

FIGURE 7-18, A–B *When applying a tourniquet:* **A,** *Twist the rod to tighten until bright-red bleeding stops.* **B,** *Secure it in place.*

Hemostatic Agents

Hemostatic agents generally are substances that speed clot formation by absorbing the excess moisture caused by the bleeding. Hemostatic agents are found in a variety of forms, including treated sponge or gauze pads and powder or granular forms. The powder or granular forms are poured directly on the bleeding vessel, then other hemostatic agents, such as gauze pads, are used in conjunction with direct pressure.

Over-the-counter versions of hemostatic bandages are available in addition to hemostatic agents intended for use by professional rescuers. Some are more effective than others. However, because some types present a risk of further injury or tissue damage, the routine use of hemostatic agents in first aid settings is not recommended.

BURNS

Burns are a special kind of soft tissue injury. Like other types of soft tissue injury, burns can damage the top layer of skin or the skin and the layers of fat, muscle and bone beneath.

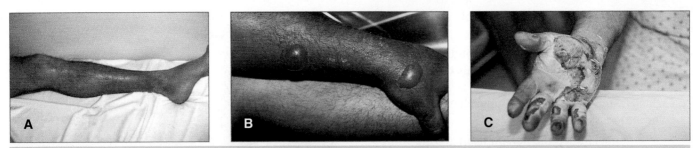

FIGURE 7-19, A–C *The three classifications of burns are* **A,** *superficial burns,* **B,** *partial-thickness burns and* **C,** *full-thickness burns.* Courtesy of Alan Dimick, M.D., Professor of Surgery, Former Director of UAB Burn Center.

Burns are classified by their depth. The deeper the burn, the more severe it is. The three classifications of burns are as follows: superficial (sometimes referred to as first degree) (Fig. 7-19, A), partial thickness (sometimes referred to as second degree) (Fig. 7-19, B) and full thickness (sometimes referred to as third degree) (Fig. 7-19, C). Burns also are classified by their source: heat (thermal), chemical, electrical and radiation (such as from the sun).

A *critical burn* requires immediate medical attention. These burns are potentially life threatening, disfiguring and disabling. Unfortunately, it often is difficult to tell if a burn is critical. Even superficial burns can be critical if they affect a large area or certain body parts. You cannot judge a burn's severity by the person's level of pain because nerve endings may be destroyed.

Be aware that burns to a child or an infant could be caused by child abuse. Burns that are done intentionally to a child often leave an injury that cannot be hidden. One example is a sharp line dividing the burned and unburned skin such as from scalding water in a tub. If you think you have reasonable cause to believe that abuse has occurred, report your suspicions to the appropriate community or state agency. For more information on child abuse, see Chapter 9.

What to Look For

Signals of burns depend on whether the burn is superficial, partial thickness or full thickness.

- *Superficial burns:*
  - ○ Involve only the top layer of skin.
  - ○ Cause skin to become red and dry, usually painful and the area may swell.
  - ○ Usually heal within a week without permanent scarring.
- *Partial-thickness burns:*
  - ○ Involve the top layers of skin.
  - ○ Cause skin to become red; usually painful; have blisters that may open and weep clear fluid, making the skin appear wet; may appear mottled; and often swells.
  - ○ Usually heal in 3 to 4 weeks and may scar.
- *Full-thickness burns:*
  - ○ May destroy all layers of skin and some or all of the underlying structures—fat, muscles, bones and nerves.
  - ○ The skin may be brown or black (charred), with the tissue underneath sometimes appearing white, and can either be extremely painful or relatively painless (if the burn destroys nerve endings).
  - ○ Healing may require medical assistance; scarring is likely.

When to Call 9-1-1

You should always call 9-1-1 or the local emergency number if the burned person has:

- Trouble breathing.
- Burns covering more than one body part or a large surface area.
- Suspected burns to the airway. Burns to the mouth and nose may be a sign of this.
- Burns to the head, neck, hands, feet or genitals.
- A full-thickness burn and is younger than 5 years or older than 60 years.
- A burn caused by chemicals, explosions or electricity.

What to Do Until Help Arrives

Care given for burns depends on the type of burn.

Heat (Thermal) Burns

Follow these basic steps when caring for a *heat* burn:

- Check the scene for safety.
- Stop the burning by removing the person from the source of the burn.
- Check for life-threatening conditions.

- As soon as possible, cool the burn with large amounts of cold running water, at least until pain is relieved (Fig. 7-20, A).
- Cover the burn loosely with a sterile dressing (Fig. 7-20, B).
- Take steps to minimize shock. Keep the person from getting chilled or overheated.
- Comfort and reassure the person.
- *Do not* apply ice or ice water to any burn. Ice and ice water can cause the body to lose heat rapidly and further damages body tissues.
- *Do not* touch a burn with anything except a clean covering.
- *Do not* remove pieces of clothing that stick to the burned area.
- *Do not* try to clean a severe burn.
- *Do not* break blisters.
- *Do not* use any kind of ointment on a severe burn.

When a person suffers a burn, he or she is less able to regulate body temperature. As a result, a person who has been burned tends to become chilled. To help maintain body temperature and prevent hypothermia, keep the person warm and away from drafts. Remember that cooling a burn over a large area of the body can bring on hypothermia. Be aware of this risk and look for signals of hypothermia. If possible, monitor the person's core body temperature when cooling a burn that covers a large area.

Chemical Burns

When caring for *chemical burns* it is important to remember that the chemical will continue to burn as long as it is on the skin. You must remove the chemical from the skin as quickly as possible. To do so, follow these steps:

- If the burn was caused by dry chemicals, brush off the chemicals using gloved hands or a towel and remove any contaminated clothing before flushing with tap water (under pressure). Be careful not to get the chemical on yourself or on a different area of the person's skin.
- Flush the burn with large amounts of cool running water. Continue flushing the burn for at least 20 minutes or until EMS personnel take over.
- If an eye is burned by a chemical, flush the affected eye with water until EMS personnel take over. Tilt the head so that the affected eye is lower than the unaffected eye as you flush (Fig. 7-21).
- If possible, have the person remove contaminated clothes to prevent further contamination while you continue to flush the area.

Be aware that chemicals can be inhaled, potentially damaging the airway or lungs.

Electrical Burns

If you encounter a person with an *electrical burn*, you should:

- Never go near the person until you are sure he or she is not still in contact with the power source.
- Turn off the power at its source and care for any life-threatening conditions.
- Call 9-1-1 or the local emergency number. Any person who has suffered an electrical shock needs to be evaluated by a medical professional to determine the extent of injury.

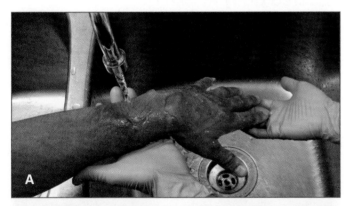

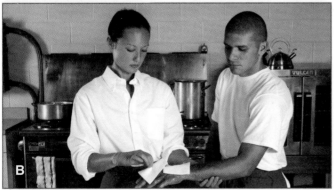

FIGURE 7-20 A–B A, *Cool a thermal burn with large amounts of cold running water until the pain is relieved.* B, *Cover a thermal burn loosely with a sterile dressing.*

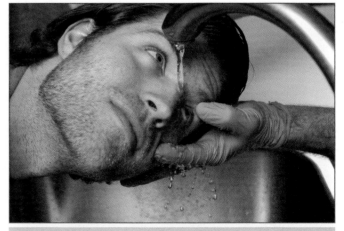

FIGURE 7-21 *If an eye is burned by a chemical, flush the affected eye with water until EMS personnel take over.*

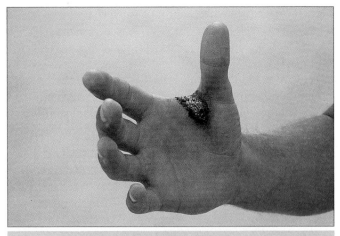

FIGURE 7-22 *For an electrical burn, look for entry and exit wounds and give the appropriate care.*

- Be aware that electrocution can cause cardiac and respiratory emergencies. Therefore, be prepared to perform CPR or use an automated external defibrillator (AED).
- Care for shock and thermal burns.
- Look for entry and exit wounds and give the appropriate care (Fig. 7-22).
- Remember that anyone suffering from electric shock requires advanced medical care.

Radiation Burns

Care for a *radiation (sun) burn* as you would for any thermal burn (Fig. 7-23). Always cool the burn and protect the area from further damage by keeping the person away from the source of the burn.

Preventing Burns

- Heat burns can be prevented by following safety practices that prevent fire and by being careful around sources of heat.

- Chemical burns can be prevented by following safety practices around all chemicals and by following manufacturers' guidelines when handling chemicals.
- Electrical burns can be prevented by following safety practices around electrical lines and equipment and by leaving outdoor areas when lightning could strike.
- Sunburn can be prevented by wearing appropriate clothing and using sunscreen. Sunscreen should have a sun protection factor (SPF) of at least 15.

SPECIAL SITUATIONS

Certain types of wounds need special attention or care. These types of situations include crush injury; severed body parts (amputations); impaled objects; and injury to the mouth, nose, lip, tooth, chest and abdomen.

Crush Injuries

A crush injury is caused by strong pressure against a body part, often a limb. It may result in serious damage to underlying tissue, causing bruising, bleeding, lacerations, fractures, shock and internal injuries. Call 9-1-1 or the local emergency number for any serious or life-threatening condition. Care for specific injuries found and assume that internal injuries are present. Also care for shock.

Severed Body Parts

If part of the body has been torn or cut off, call 9-1-1 or the local emergency number, then try to find the part and wrap it in sterile gauze or any clean material, such as a washcloth. Put the wrapped part in a plastic bag and seal the bag. Keep the part cold and bag cool by placing it in a larger bag or container of an ice and water slurry, *not* on ice alone and *not* on dry ice, if possible, but do not freeze (Fig. 7-24). Be sure the part is taken to the hospital with the person. Doctors may be able to reattach it.

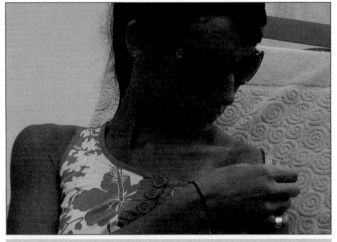

FIGURE 7-23 *Care for sunburn as you would for any thermal burn.*

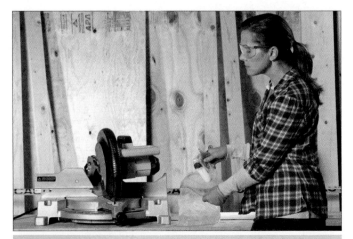

FIGURE 7-24 *Wrap a severed body part in sterile gauze, put it in a plastic bag and put the bag on ice.*

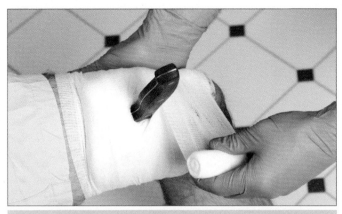
FIGURE 7-25 *Place several dressings around an embedded object to keep it from moving. Bandage the dressings in place around the object.*

Embedded Objects

If an object, such as a knife or a piece of glass or metal, is embedded in a wound, do not remove it. Place several dressings around it to keep it from moving (Fig. 7-25). Bandage the dressings in place around the object.

If it is only a splinter in the surface of the skin, it can be removed with tweezers. After removing the splinter from the skin, wash the area with soap and water, rinsing the area with tap water for about 5 minutes. After drying the area, apply an antibiotic ointment to the area if the person has no known allergies or sensitivities to the medication and then cover it to keep it clean. If the splinter is in the eye, do not attempt to remove it. Call 9-1-1 or the local emergency number.

Nose Injuries

Nose injuries usually are caused by a blow from a blunt object, often resulting in a nosebleed. High blood pressure or changes in altitude also can cause nosebleeds. In most cases, you can control bleeding by having the person sit with the head slightly forward while pinching the nostrils together for about 10 minutes (Fig. 7-26). If pinching the nostrils does not control the bleeding, other methods include applying an ice pack to the bridge of the nose or putting pressure on the upper lip just beneath the nose. Remember, ice should not be applied directly to the skin since it can damage the skin tissue. Place a cloth between the ice and the skin. Seek medical attention if the bleeding persists or recurs or if the person says that it is caused by high blood pressure.

Mouth Injuries

With mouth injuries, you must make sure the person is able to breathe. Injuries to the mouth may cause breathing problems if blood or loose teeth block the airway.

If the person is bleeding from the mouth and you do not suspect a serious head, neck or spinal injury, place the person in a seated position leaning slightly forward. This will allow any blood to drain from the mouth. If this position is not possible, place the person on his or her side.

Lip Injuries

For injuries that penetrate the lip, place a rolled dressing between the lip and the gum. You can place another dressing on the outer surface of the lip. If the tongue is bleeding, apply a dressing and direct pressure. Applying cold to the lips or tongue can help to reduce swelling and ease pain.

Tooth Injuries

If a person's tooth is knocked out, control the bleeding and save the tooth so it may possibly be reinserted. When the fibers and tissues are torn from the socket, it is important for the person to seek dental or emergency care as soon as possible after the injury. Generally, the sooner the tooth is replaced, the better the chance is that it will survive.

If the person is conscious and able to cooperate, rinse out the mouth with cold tap water if available. You can control the bleeding by placing a rolled sterile dressing into the space left by the missing tooth (Fig. 7-27). Have

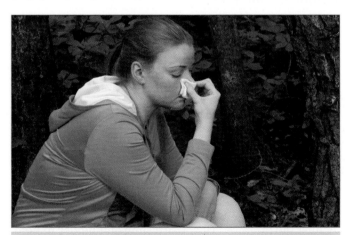
FIGURE 7-26 *To control a nosebleed, have the person lean forward and pinch the nostrils together until bleeding stops (about 10 minutes).*

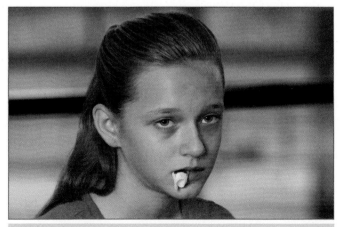
FIGURE 7-27 *You can control the bleeding by placing a rolled sterile dressing and inserting it into the space left by the missing tooth.*

the person gently bite down to maintain pressure. To save the tooth, place it in milk, if possible, or cool water if milk is not available. Be careful to pick up the tooth only by the crown (white part) rather than by the root.

Chest Injuries

The chest is the upper part of the trunk. It is shaped by 12 pairs of ribs. Ten of the pairs attach to the *sternum* (breastbone) in front and to the spine in back. Two pairs, the *floating ribs*, attach only to the spine. The *rib cage*, formed by the ribs, the sternum and the spine, protects vital organs, such as the heart, major blood vessels and the lungs. Also in the chest are the esophagus, trachea and muscles used for respiration.

Chest injuries are a leading cause of trauma deaths each year. Injuries to the chest may result from a wide variety of causes, such as motor vehicle crashes, falls, sports mishaps and crushing or penetrating forces. Chest injuries may involve the bones that form the chest cavity or the organs or other structures in the cavity itself.

Chest wounds may be either closed or open. A *closed chest wound* does not break the skin. Closed chest wounds generally are caused by blunt objects, such as steering wheels. *Open chest wounds* occur when an object, such as a knife or bullet, penetrates the chest wall. Fractured ribs may break through the skin to cause an open chest injury.

Rib fractures usually are caused by direct force to the chest.

Puncture wounds to the chest range from minor to life threatening. Stab and gunshot wounds are examples of puncture injuries. The penetrating object can injure any structure or organ within the chest, including the lungs. A puncture injury can allow air to enter the chest through the wound. Air in the chest cavity does not allow the lungs to function normally.

Puncture wounds cause varying degrees of internal and external bleeding. A puncture wound to the chest is a life-threatening injury. If the injury penetrates the rib cage, air can pass freely in and out of the chest cavity and the person cannot breathe normally. With each breath the person takes, you will hear a sucking sound coming from the wound. This sound is the primary signal of a penetrating chest injury called a *sucking chest wound* (Fig. 7-28). Without proper care, the person's condition will worsen. The affected lung or lungs will fail to function, and breathing will become more difficult.

What to Look For

Signals of a serious chest injury include:

- Trouble breathing.
- Severe pain at the site of the injury.

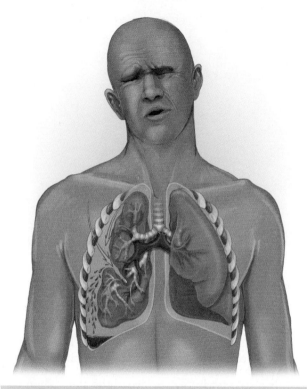

FIGURE 7-28 *If the injury penetrates the rib cage, air can pass freely in and out of the chest cavity and the person cannot breathe normally.*

- Flushed, pale, ashen or bluish skin.
- Obvious deformity, such as that caused by a fracture.
- Coughing up blood (may be bright red or dark, like coffee grounds).
- Bruising at the site of a blunt injury, such as that caused by a seat belt.
- A "sucking" noise or distinct sound when the person breathes.

When to Call 9-1-1

Call 9-1-1 or the local emergency number for any open or closed chest wound, especially if the person has a puncture wound to the chest. Also call if the person has trouble breathing or a sucking chest wound, or if you suspect rib fractures.

What to Do Until Help Arrives

Care for a chest injury depends on the type of injury.

Caring for Rib Fractures

Although painful, a simple rib fracture is rarely life threatening. Give the person a blanket or pillow to hold against the fractured ribs. Use a sling and binder to hold the person's arm against the injured side of the chest. Monitor breathing.

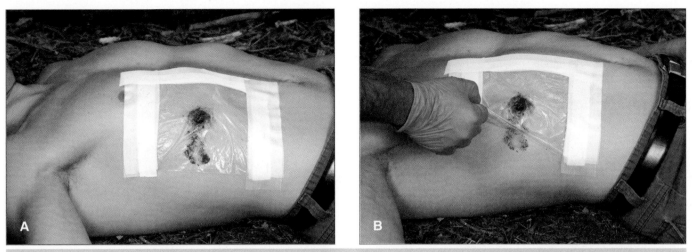

FIGURE 7-29, A–B **A,** *An occlusive dressing helps keep air from entering a chest wound when the person inhales.* **B,** *Having an open corner allows air to escape when the person exhales.*

Caring for a Sucking Chest Wound

To care for a sucking chest wound, cover the wound with a large occlusive dressing (Fig. 7-29, A–B). A piece of plastic wrap, or a plastic bag folded several times and placed over the wound, makes an effective occlusive dressing. Tape the dressing in place except for one side or corner, which should remain loose. A taped-down dressing keeps air from entering the wound when the person inhales, and having an open corner allows air to escape when the person exhales. If these materials are not available to use as dressings, use a folded cloth. Take steps to minimize shock. Monitor the person's breathing.

Abdominal Injury

Like a chest injury, an injury to the abdomen may be either open or closed. Injuries to the abdomen can be very painful. Even with a closed wound, the rupture of an organ can cause serious internal bleeding, resulting in shock. It is especially difficult to determine if a person has an internal abdominal injury if he or she is unconscious.

Always suspect an abdominal injury in a person who has multiple injuries.

What to Look For

Signals of serious abdominal injury include:

■ Severe pain.
■ Bruising.
■ External bleeding.
■ Nausea.
■ Vomiting (sometimes blood).
■ Weakness.
■ Thirst.
■ Pain, tenderness or a tight feeling in the abdomen.

■ Organs protruding from the abdomen.
■ Rigid abdominal muscles.
■ Other signals of shock.

When to Call 9-1-1

Call 9-1-1 or the local emergency number for any serious abdominal injury.

What to Do Until Help Arrives

With a severe open injury, abdominal organs sometimes protrude through the wound (Fig. 7-30, A).

To care for an *open wound to the abdomen*, follow these steps:

1. Put on disposable gloves or use another barrier.
2. Carefully position the person on his or her back with the knees bent, if that position does not cause pain.
3. Do not apply direct pressure.
4. Do not push any protruding organs back into the open wound.
5. Remove clothing from around the wound (Fig. 7-30, B).
6. Apply moist, sterile dressings loosely over the wound (clean, warm tap water can be used) (Fig. 7-30, C).
7. Cover dressings loosely with plastic wrap, if available (Fig. 7-30, D).

To care for a *closed wound to the abdomen*:

■ While keeping the injured area still, apply cold to the affected area to control pain and swelling.
■ Carefully position the person on his or her back with the knees bent, if that position does not cause pain.
■ Keep the person from getting chilled or overheated.

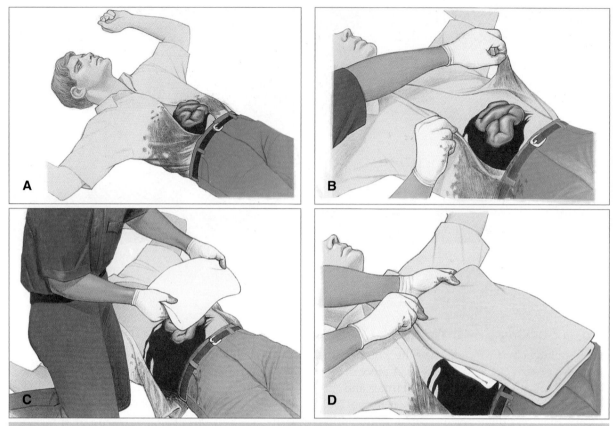

FIGURE 7-30, A–D **A,** *Wounds to the abdomen can cause the organs to protrude.* **B,** *Carefully remove clothing from around the wound.* **C,** *Cover the organs loosely with a moist, sterile dressing.* **D,** *Cover the dressings loosely with plastic wrap, if available.*

PUTTING IT ALL TOGETHER

For minor soft tissue injuries like scrapes, bruises and sunburns, it is important to give quick care and take steps to prevent infection. If you do this, these types of wounds and burns usually heal quickly and completely.

Serious and life-threatening soft tissue injuries are emergencies.

Call 9-1-1 or the local emergency number and give immediate care. These are crucial steps for any serious wound or burn.

CONTROLLING EXTERNAL BLEEDING

AFTER CHECKING THE SCENE AND THE INJURED OR ILL PERSON:

1 COVER THE WOUND

Cover the wound with a sterile dressing.

2 APPLY DIRECT PRESSURE

Apply pressure until bleeding stops.

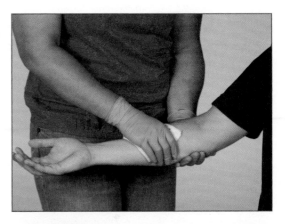

3 COVER DRESSING WITH BANDAGE

Check for circulation beyond the injury
(check for feeling, warmth and color).

4 APPLY MORE PRESSURE AND CALL 9-1-1

If bleeding does not stop:

- Apply more dressings and bandages and continue to apply additional pressure.
- Take steps to minimize shock.
- **CALL** 9-1-1 if not already done.

TIP: *Wash hands with soap and water after giving care.*

USING A MANUFACTURED TOURNIQUET

NOTE: *Always follow standard precautions and follow manufacturer's instructions when applying a tourniquet. Call 9-1-1 or the local emergency number.*

1 POSITION THE TOURNIQUET

Place the tourniquet around the limb, approximately **2** inches (about two finger widths) above the wound but not over a joint.

2 PULL STRAP THROUGH BUCKLE

- Route the tag end of the strap through the buckle, if necessary.
- Pull the strap tightly and secure it in place.

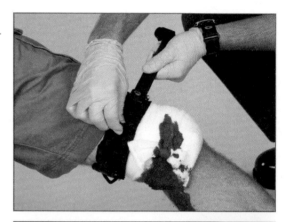

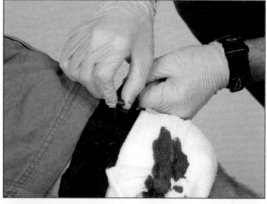

3 TWIST THE ROD

Tighten the tourniquet by twisting the rod until the flow of bleeding stops and secure the rod in place. *Do not* cover the tourniquet with clothing.

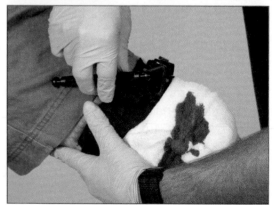

4 RECORD TIME

Note and record the time that you applied the tourniquet and give this information to EMS personnel.

CHAPTER 8

Injuries to Muscles, Bones and Joints

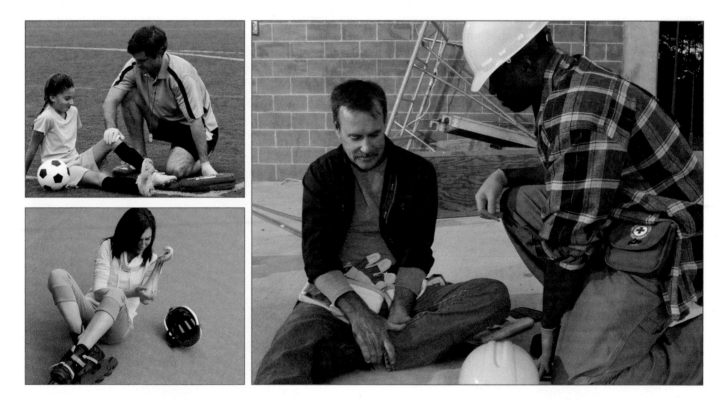

Injuries to muscles, bones and joints happen to people of all ages at home, work and play. A person may fall while walking in the park and bruise the muscles of a leg. Equipment may fall on a worker and break bones. A skier may fall and twist a leg, tearing muscles in the process.

These injuries are painful and make life difficult, but they seldom are life threatening. However, if they are not recognized and care is not given, they can cause serious problems. In the rare case of a head, neck or spinal injury, lifelong disability, or even death, can result if immediate care is not given.

This chapter discusses the signals of muscle, bone and joint injuries and how to give care for these injuries. In addition, you will read about how to recognize head, neck and spinal injuries, and how to give immediate, potentially life-saving care in these situations.

BACKGROUND

The body's skeleton is made up of bones, muscles, and the tendons and ligaments that connect them. They give the body shape and stability. Bones and muscles give the body shape and mobility. Tendons and ligaments connect to muscle and bones, giving support. They all work together to allow the body to move.

Muscles

Muscles are soft tissues. The body has over 600 muscles, most of which are attached to bones by strong tissues called *tendons* (Fig. 8-1). Unlike other soft tissues, muscles are able to shorten and lengthen—contract and relax. This contracting and relaxing enables the body to move. The brain directs the muscles to move through the spinal cord, a pathway of nerves in the spine. Tiny jolts of electricity called *electrical impulses* travel through the nerves to the muscles. They cause the muscles to contract. When the muscles contract, they pull at the bones, causing motion at a joint.

Injuries to the brain, spinal cord or nerves can affect muscle control. When nerves lose control of muscles, it is called *paralysis*. When a muscle is injured, a nearby muscle often takes over for the injured one.

Bones

Approximately 200 bones in various sizes and shapes form the *skeleton* (Fig. 8-2). The skeleton protects many of the organs inside the body. Bones are hard and dense. Because they are strong and rigid, they are not injured easily. Bones have a rich supply of blood and nerves. Bone injuries can bleed and usually are painful. If care is not given for the injury, the bleeding can become life threatening. Children have more flexible bones than adults; their bones break less easily. But if a child sustains a fracture to a *growth plate* (areas of developing cartilage near the ends of long bones), it can affect future bone growth. Bones weaken with age. Older adults have more brittle bones. Sometimes they break surprisingly easily. This gradual weakening of bones is called *osteoporosis*.

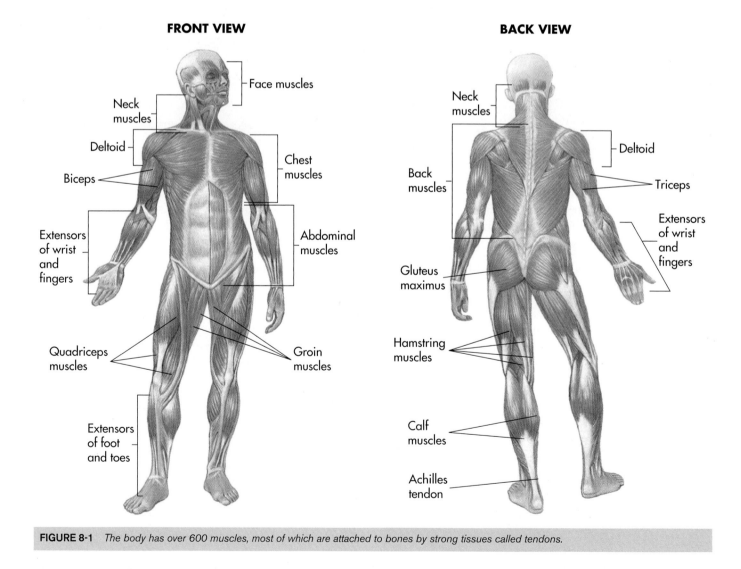

FRONT VIEW

BACK VIEW

FIGURE 8-1 *The body has over 600 muscles, most of which are attached to bones by strong tissues called tendons.*

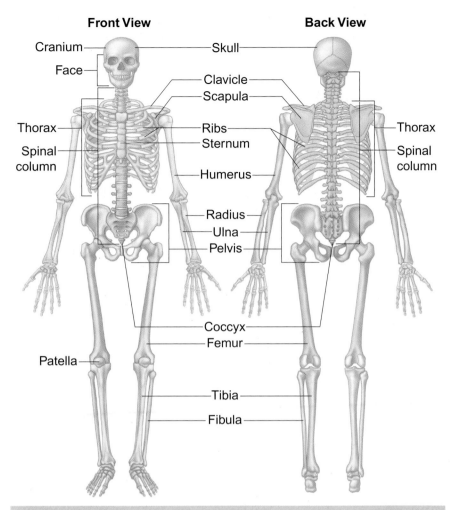

Front View

Cranium — Skull
Face
Clavicle
Scapula
Thorax — Ribs
Sternum
Spinal column
Humerus

Radius
Ulna
Pelvis

Patella

Coccyx
Femur

Tibia
Fibula

Back View

Skull
Thorax
Spinal column

FIGURE 8-2 *Approximately 200 bones in various sizes and shapes form the skeleton. The skeleton protects many of the organs inside of the body.*

Joints

The ends of two or more bones coming together at one place form a *joint* (Fig. 8-3). Strong, tough bands called *ligaments* hold the bones at a joint together. All joints have a normal range of movement in which they can move freely, without too much stress or strain. When joints are forced beyond this range, ligaments stretch and tear.

TYPES OF INJURIES

The four basic types of injuries to muscles, bones and joints are fractures, dislocations, sprains and strains. They occur in a variety of ways.

Fractures

A *fracture* is a complete break, a chip or a crack in a bone (Fig. 8-4). A fall, a blow or sometimes even a twisting movement can cause a fracture. Fractures are open or closed. An *open fracture* involves an open wound. It occurs when the end of a bone tears through the skin. An object that goes into the skin and breaks the bone, such as a bullet, also can cause an open fracture. In a *closed fracture* the skin is not broken.

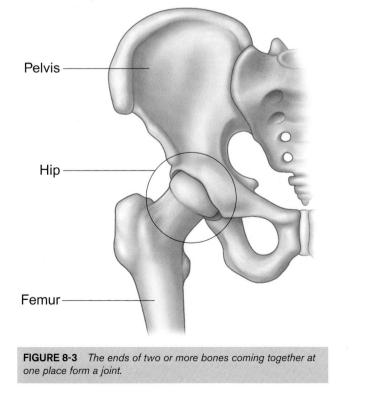

Pelvis

Hip

Femur

FIGURE 8-3 *The ends of two or more bones coming together at one place form a joint.*

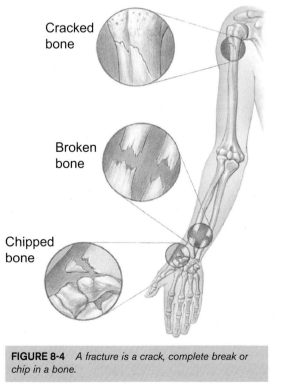

Cracked bone

Broken bone

Chipped bone

FIGURE 8-4 *A fracture is a crack, complete break or chip in a bone.*

THE BREAKING POINT

Osteoporosis is a disease that causes the bones to fracture easily. Approximately 10 million Americans have osteoporosis, and 80 percent of these are women. In 2005, some 2 million spine, hip, wrist and other fractures occurred in the United States because of osteoporosis. People usually have osteoporosis for decades before they experience signals. People do not usually become aware they have this "silent" disease until after the age of 60 years.

The disease is caused by a decrease in calcium content of the bones. Normal bones are hard, dense tissues that endure great stresses. Calcium is a key to bone growth, development and repair. When the calcium content of bones decreases, bones become frail and less dense. They are less able to repair the normal damage they incur. This leaves bones, especially hip, back and wrist, more prone to fractures. These fractures may occur with only a little force. Some even occur without force. The person may be taking a walk or washing dishes when the fracture occurs.

Risk Factors

The risk of an American woman suffering a hip fracture alone is equal to her combined risk of breast, uterine and ovarian cancer. Some risk factors for osteoporosis cannot be changed, including:

- *Being female.*
- *Having ancestors from northern Europe, the British Isles, Japan or China.*
- *Being of an advanced age.*
- *Having a family history of the disease.*
- *Having a small, thin body frame.*
- *Reaching menopause.*

However, other risk factors can be changed; there are steps that a person can take to lower the risk of developing osteoporosis. These involve lifestyle choices, including improving diet and exercise, reducing alcohol consumption and stopping smoking.

Preventing Osteoporosis

Osteoporosis can begin as early as 30 years of age. Building strong bones before age 35 years is the key to preventing osteoporosis. To help prevent osteoporosis, take the following steps:

- **Eat a Well-Balanced Diet.** *A diet rich in calcium, vitamins and minerals and low in salt is essential for bone health. Limiting caffeine intake and avoiding a high protein diet also are important for bone health.*

  As a person ages, the amount of calcium absorbed from the diet declines, making it more important to have an adequate calcium intake. Calcium is necessary to bone building and maintenance. Three to four daily servings of low-fat dairy products should provide enough calcium for good bone health.

  Vitamin D also is necessary because it helps the body to absorb the calcium to strengthen bones. Exposure to sunshine enables the body to make vitamin D. People who do not receive adequate exposure to the sun need to eat foods that contain vitamin D. The best sources are vitamin-fortified milk and fatty fish, such as tuna, salmon and eel. When exposing yourself to the sun, however, you should not risk a burn or deep tan because both increase the risk of skin cancer.

- **Take Vitamins and Supplements if Necessary.** *People who do not take in adequate calcium may be able to make up for the loss by taking calcium supplements. Some are combined with vitamin D. Before taking a calcium supplement, consult your health care provider. Many highly advertised calcium supplements are ineffective because they do not dissolve in the gastrointestinal tract and cannot be absorbed. An insufficient intake of phosphorous, magnesium, and vitamins K, B_6 and B_{12} also can increase your risk for osteoporosis. To ensure that you are getting enough of these vitamins and minerals, talk to your health care provider about taking a daily multivitamin.*

- **Exercise.** *Exercise also is necessary to building strong bones. Weight-bearing exercise increases bone density and the activity of bone-building cells. Regular exercise may reduce the rate of bone loss by promoting new bone formation. It also may stimulate the*

(Continued)

skeletal system to repair itself. An effective exercise program, such as aerobics, jogging or walking, involves the weight-bearing bones and muscles of the legs.

- **Stop Smoking.** *Smoking is bad for your bone health since it can block your body's ability to absorb calcium. The chemicals in cigarettes are bad for bone cells. Also, in women, smoking can block the bone-protective effects of the*

hormone estrogen, which can affect bone density.

- **Avoid Too Much Alcohol.** *Alcohol intake should be limited to two drinks a day. Drinking more than this on a regular basis can reduce bone formation. Too much alcohol also can reduce calcium levels in the body.*

If you have questions about your health and osteoporosis, consult your health care provider.

Closed fractures are more common, but open fractures are more dangerous because they carry a risk of infection and severe bleeding. In general, fractures are life threatening only if they involve breaks in large bones such as the thigh, sever an artery or affect breathing. Since you cannot always tell if a person has a fracture, you should consider the cause of the injury. A fall from a significant height or a motor vehicle crash could signal a possible fracture.

Dislocations

Dislocations usually are more obvious than fractures. A *dislocation* is the movement of a bone at a joint away from its normal position (Fig. 8-5). This movement

usually is caused by a violent force tearing the ligaments that hold the bones in place. When a bone is moved out of place, the joint no longer functions. The displaced end of the bone often forms a bump, a ridge or a hollow that does not normally exist.

Sprains

A *sprain* is the tearing of ligaments at a joint (Fig. 8-6). Mild sprains may swell but usually heal quickly. The person might not feel much pain and is active again soon. If a person ignores the signals of swelling and pain and becomes active too soon, the joint will not heal properly and will remain weak. There is a good chance that it will become reinjured, only this time more severely. A severe sprain also can involve a fracture or dislocation of the bones at the joint. The joints most easily injured are at the ankle, knee, wrist and fingers.

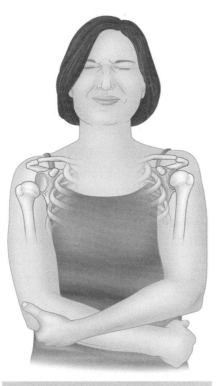

FIGURE 8-5 *A dislocation is the movement of a bone at a joint away from its normal position.*

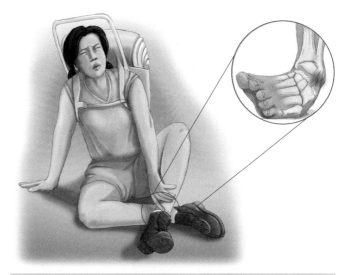

FIGURE 8-6 *A sprain is the tearing of ligaments at a joint.*

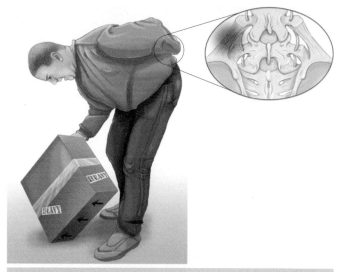

FIGURE 8-7 *A strain is a stretching and tearing of muscles or tendons.*

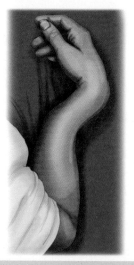

FIGURE 8-8 *A severely injured bone or joint may appear to be deformed.*

Strains

A *strain* is a stretching and tearing of muscles or tendons (Fig. 8-7). Strains often are caused by lifting something heavy or working a muscle too hard. They usually involve the muscles in the neck, back, thigh or the back of the lower leg. Some strains can reoccur, especially in the neck and back.

What to Look For

Always suspect a *severe injury* when any of the following signals are present:

- There is pain. One of the most common signals in any muscle, bone or joint injury is pain. The injured area may be very painful to touch and move.
- There is significant bruising and swelling. The area may be swollen and red or bruised.
- There is significant deformity. The area may be twisted or strangely bent (Fig. 8-8). It may have abnormal lumps, ridges and hollows.
- The person is unable to use the affected part normally.
- There are bone fragments sticking out of a wound.
- The person feels bones grating or the person felt or heard a snap or pop at the time of injury.
- The injured area is cold, numb and tingly.
- The cause of the injury suggests that it may be severe.

It can be difficult to tell if an injury is to a muscle, bone or joint. Sometimes an x-ray, computer assisted tomography (CAT) scan or magnetic resonance imaging (MRI) is needed to determine the extent of the injury.

When to Call 9-1-1

Call 9-1-1 or the local emergency number for the following situations:

- There is obvious deformity.

- There is moderate or severe swelling and discoloration.
- Bones sound or feel like they are rubbing together.
- A snap or pop was heard or felt at the time of the injury.
- There is a fracture with an open wound at, or bone piercing through, the injury site.
- The injured person cannot move or use the affected part normally.
- The injured area is cold and numb.
- The injury involves the head, neck or spine.
- The injured person has trouble breathing.
- The cause of the injury suggests that the injury may be severe.
- It is not possible to safely or comfortably move the person to a vehicle for transport to a hospital.

What to Do Until Help Arrives

General care for injuries to muscles, bone and joints includes following the mnemonic RICE:

- **R**est—Do not move or straighten the injured area.
- **I**mmobilize—Stabilize the injured area in the position it was found. Splint the injured part only if the person must be moved or transported to receive medical care and it does not cause more pain (see Splinting an Injury). Minimizing movement can prevent further injury.
- **C**old—Fill a plastic bag with ice and water or wrap ice with a damp cloth and apply ice to the injured area for periods of about 20 minutes (Fig. 8-9). Place a thin barrier between the ice and bare skin. If 20-minute icing cannot be tolerated, apply ice for periods of 10 minutes. If continued icing is needed, remove the pack for 20 minutes, and then replace it. Cold reduces internal bleeding, pain and swelling. Do *not* apply heat as there is no evidence that applying heat helps muscle, bone or joint injuries.

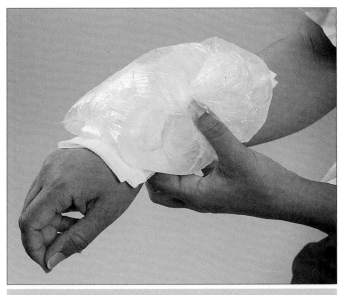

FIGURE 8-9 *Applying ice can help to control swelling and reduce pain.*

■ **Elevate**—Elevate the injured part only if it *does not* cause more pain. Elevating the injured part may help reduce swelling.

Some injuries, such as a broken finger, may not require you to call 9-1-1 or the local emergency number, yet they still need medical attention. When transporting the person to a medical facility, have someone else drive. This way you can keep an eye on the person and give care if needed. Injuries to the pelvis, hip or thigh can be life threatening. A person with such an injury should not be moved unnecessarily. Minimizing movement until EMS personnel take over can help to prevent the injury from becoming worse.

Splinting an Injury

Splinting is a method of immobilizing an injured part to minimize movement and prevent further injury and should be used *only* if you have to move or transport the person to seek medical attention *and* if it does not cause more pain. Splint an injury in the position in which you find it. For fractures, splint the *joints* above and below the site of the injury. For sprains or joint injuries, splint the *bones* above and below the site of the injury. If you are not sure if the injury is a fracture or a sprain, splint both the bones and joints above and below the point of injury. Splinting materials should be soft or padded for comfort. Check for circulation (feeling, warmth and color) before and after splinting to make sure that the splint is not too tight.

There are many methods of splinting, including:

■ Anatomic splints. The person's body is the splint. For example, you can splint an arm to the chest or an injured leg to the uninjured leg (Fig. 8-10).
■ Soft splints. Soft materials, such as a folded blanket, towel, pillow or folded triangular bandage, can be

used for the splint (Fig. 8-11). A sling is a specific kind of soft splint that uses a triangular bandage tied to support an injured arm, wrist or hand.
■ Rigid splints. Padded boards, folded magazines or newspapers, or padded metal strips that do not have any sharp edges can serve as splints (Fig. 8-12).
■ The ground. An injured leg stretched out on the ground is supported by the ground.

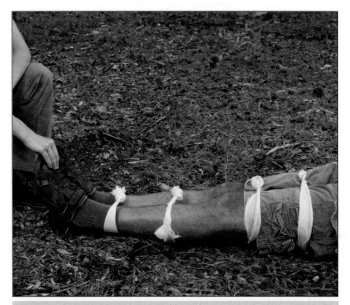

FIGURE 8-10 *An anatomic splint uses a part of the body as the splint.*

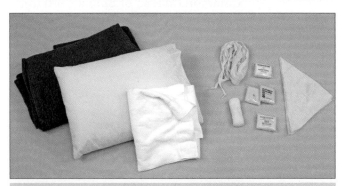

FIGURE 8-11 *Folded blankets, towels, pillows or a triangular bandage tied as a sling can be used as soft splints.*

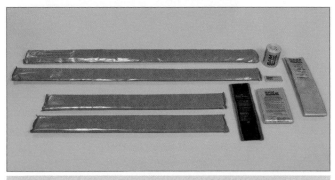

FIGURE 8-12 *Commercially made rigid splints are available (shown), but many items, such as padded boards or folded newspapers, can be used.*

After you have splinted the injury, apply ice to the injured area. Keep the person from getting chilled or overheated and be reassuring.

Head, Neck and Spinal Injuries

Although head, neck and spinal injuries make up only a small fraction of all injuries, these injuries may be life threatening or cause permanent life-altering damage. Each year, approximately 12,000 Americans suffer a spinal cord injury. Most are male victims with an average age of about 40 years. The leading causes of spinal cord injuries are motor vehicle crashes, followed by falls, violence and sports (Fig. 8-13).

Injuries to the head, neck or spine can cause paralysis, speech or memory problems or other disabling conditions. These injuries can damage bone and soft tissue, including the brain and spinal cord. Since generally only x-rays, CAT scans or MRIs can show the severity of a head, neck or spinal injury, you should always care for such injuries as if they were serious.

An injury to the brain can cause bleeding inside the skull (Fig. 8-14). The blood can build up and cause pressure, resulting in more damage. The first and most important signal of brain injury is a change in the person's level of consciousness. He or she may be dizzy or confused or may become unconscious.

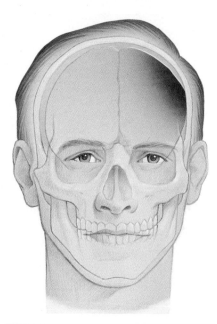

FIGURE 8-14 *Injuries to the head can rupture blood vessels in the brain. Pressure builds within the skull as blood accumulates, causing brain injury.*

The spine is a strong, flexible column of small bones that support the head and trunk (Fig. 8-15, A–C). The spinal cord runs through the circular openings of the small bones called the *vertebrae*. The vertebrae are separated from each other by cushions of cartilage called *disks*. Nerves originating in the brain form branches extending to various parts of the body through openings in the vertebrae. Injuries to the spine can fracture vertebrae and tear ligaments. In some cases, the vertebrae can shift and cut or squeeze the spinal cord. This can paralyze the person or be life threatening.

What to Look For

When you encounter an injured person, try to determine if there is a head, neck or spinal injury. Think about whether the forces involved were great enough to cause one of these injuries. Someone may have fallen from a significant height or struck his or her head while diving. He or she might have been in a motor vehicle crash and had not been wearing a safety belt. Maybe the person was thrown from the vehicle. Perhaps the person was struck by lightning, or maybe a bullet that pierced his or her back struck the spine. Always suspect

Common Causes of Spinal Cord Injury

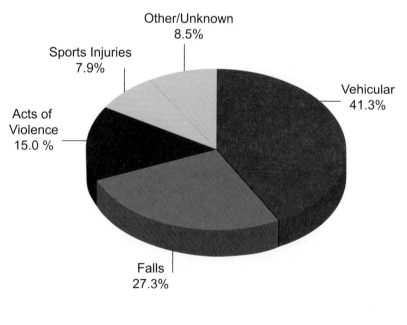

- Other/Unknown 8.5%
- Sports Injuries 7.9%
- Acts of Violence 15.0 %
- Vehicular 41.3%
- Falls 27.3%

Source: National Spinal Cord Injury Statistical Center 2010

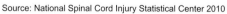

FIGURE 8-13 *The leading causes of spinal cord injuries are motor vehicle crashes, followed by falls, violence and sports.*

A

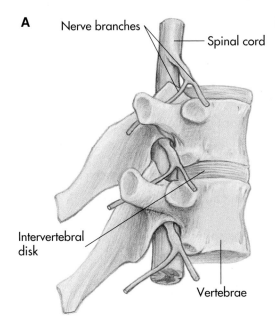

Nerve branches

Spinal cord

Intervertebral disk

Vertebrae

a head, neck or spinal injury if a person is unconscious and/or if his or her safety helmet is broken.

You also should suspect a head, neck or spinal injury if the injured person:

- Was involved in a motor vehicle crash or subjected to another significant force.
- Was injured as a result of a fall from greater than a standing height.
- Is wearing a safety helmet that is broken.
- Complains of neck or back pain.
- Has tingling or weakness in the extremities.
- Is not fully alert.
- Appears to be intoxicated.
- Appears to be frail or older than 65 years.
- Is a child younger than 3 years with evidence of a head or neck injury.

When to Call 9-1-1

If you think a person has a head, neck or spinal injury, call 9-1-1 or the local emergency number.

What to Do Until Help Arrives

While you are waiting for emergency medical services (EMS) personnel to arrive, the best care you can give is to minimize movement of the person's head, neck and spine. As long as the person is breathing normally, support the head and neck in the position

B

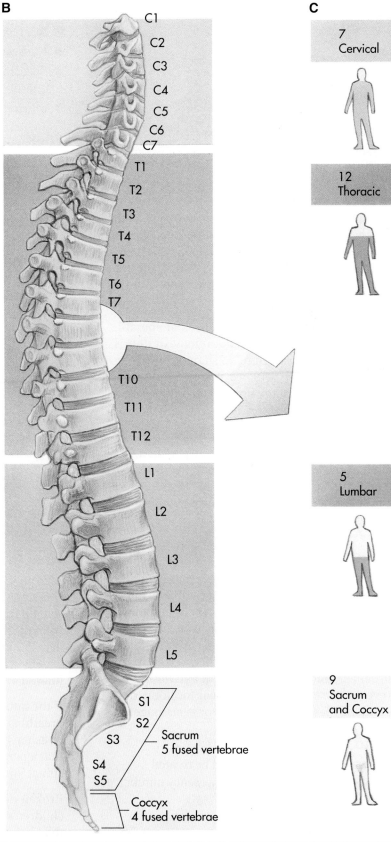

C1
C2
C3
C4
C5
C6
C7

T1
T2
T3
T4
T5
T6
T7

T10
T11
T12

L1
L2
L3
L4
L5

S1
S2
S3
Sacrum
5 fused vertebrae
S4
S5

Coccyx
4 fused vertebrae

C

7
Cervical

12
Thoracic

5
Lumbar

9
Sacrum and Coccyx

FIGURE 8-15, A–C   A, *Vertebrae are separated by cushions of cartilage called disks.* **B,** *The spine is divided into five regions.* **C,** *Traumatic injury to a region of the spine can paralyze specific body parts.*

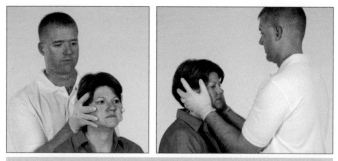

FIGURE 8-16 *Place your hands on both sides of the person's head and support it in the position in which you found it until EMS personnel take over.*

found. Do this by placing your hands on both sides of the person's head in the position in which you found it. Support the person's head in that position until EMS personnel take over supporting the person's head (Fig. 8-16). If the head is sharply turned to one side, do not move it. Support the head and neck in the position found.

If a person with a suspected head, neck or spinal injury is wearing a helmet, do not remove it unless you are specifically trained to do so *and* it is necessary to assess or access the person's airway. Minimize movement using the same manual technique you would use if the person were not wearing headgear.

The person may become confused, drowsy or unconscious. Breathing may stop. The person may be bleeding. If the person is unconscious, keep the airway open and check breathing. You should take steps to control severe bleeding and keep the person from getting chilled or overheated.

Concussion

A concussion is a type of brain injury that involves a temporary loss of brain function resulting from a blow to the head. A person with a concussion may not always lose consciousness. The effects of a concussion can appear immediately or very soon after the blow to the head and include sleep, mood and cognitive disturbances, and sensitivity to light and noise. However, some effects do not appear for hours or even days and may last for several days or even longer.

When to Call 9-1-1

Every suspected concussion should be treated seriously—call 9-1-1 or the local emergency number.

What to Look For

Signals of a concussion include:

- Confusion, which may last from moments to several minutes.
- Headache.
- Repeated questioning about what happened.

- Temporary memory loss, especially for periods immediately before and after the injury.
- Brief loss of consciousness.
- Nausea and vomiting.
- Speech problems (patient is unable to answer questions or obey simple commands).
- Blurred vision or light sensitivity.

What to Do Until Help Arrives

To care for a person with a suspected concussion:

- Support the head and neck in the position in which you found it.
- Maintain an open airway.
- Control any bleeding and apply dressings to any open wounds.
- Do not apply direct pressure if there are any signs of an obvious skull fracture.
- If there is clear fluid leaking from the ears or a wound in the scalp, cover the area loosely with a sterile gauze dressing.
- Monitor the person for any changes in condition.
- Try to calm and reassure the person. Encourage the person to talk with you; it may prevent loss of consciousness.

Chest Injuries

Injuries to the chest may be caused by falls, sports mishaps or crushing or penetrating forces. Chest injuries range from a simple broken rib to serious life-threatening injuries.

What to Look For

Although painful, a simple broken rib rarely is life threatening. A person with a broken rib generally remains calm. However, a person with a broken rib will take small, shallow breaths because normal or deep breathing is uncomfortable or painful. The person usually will attempt to ease the pain by supporting the injured area with a hand or arm.

If the injury is serious, the person will have trouble breathing. The person's skin may appear flushed, pale or ashen and he or she may cough up blood. Remember that a person with a serious chest injury also may have a spinal injury.

Broken ribs are less common in children because children's ribs are more flexible and tend to bend rather than break. However, the forces that can cause a broken rib in adults can severely bruise the lung tissue of children, which can be a life-threatening injury. Look for signals, such as what caused the injury, bruising on the chest and trouble breathing, to determine if a child has potential chest injury.

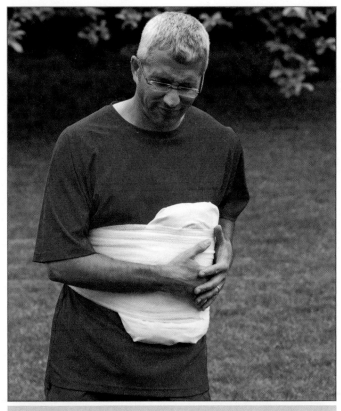

FIGURE 8-17 *Use an object, such as a pillow or rolled blanket, to support and immobilize the injured area.*

cause severe internal bleeding. Signals of a pelvic injury include the following:

- Severe pain.
- Bruising.
- Possible external bleeding.
- Nausea.
- Vomiting (which may include blood).
- Weakness.
- Thirst.
- Tenderness or a tight feeling in the abdomen.
- Possible loss of sensation in the legs or inability to move the legs.

Be alert for the signals of shock, which could indicate internal bleeding and/or blood loss. Signals of shock include:

- Nausea and vomiting
- Restlessness or irritability.
- Altered level of consciousness.
- Pale, ashen or grayish, cool, moist skin.
- Rapid breathing and pulse.

When to Call 9-1-1

If you think that the injury is serious, involves trouble breathing or the spine also has been injured, do not move the person and call 9-1-1 or the local emergency number. If the person is standing, do not have the person lie down. Continue to watch the person and minimize movement until EMS personnel take over.

What to Do Until Help Arrives

If you suspect injured or broken ribs, have the person rest in a position that will make breathing easier. Binding the person's upper arm to the chest on the injured side will help to support the injured area and make breathing more comfortable. You can use an object, such as a pillow or rolled blanket, to support and immobilize the area (Fig. 8-17). Monitor breathing and skin condition, and take steps to minimize shock.

Pelvic Injuries

The large, heavy bones of the hip make up the *pelvis*. Like the chest, injury to the pelvic bones can range from simple to life threatening.

What to Look For

An injury to the pelvis may be serious or life threatening because of the risk of damage to major arteries or internal organs. Fractures of bones in this area may

When to Call 9-1-1

Call 9-1-1 or the local emergency number if you suspect a pelvic injury.

What to Do Until Help Arrives

Because an injury to the pelvis also can involve injury to the lower spine, it is best not to move the person. If possible, try to keep the person lying flat. Watch for signals of internal bleeding and take steps to minimize shock until EMS personnel take over.

PUTTING IT ALL TOGETHER

Most of the time, injuries to muscles, bones and joints are painful but not life threatening. Be prepared to recognize signals of these types of injuries. The general care for a muscle, bone or joint injury is to minimize movement of the injured area, follow the RICE mnemonic and make sure that the person gets medical care in a timely manner.

Although head, neck and spinal injuries make up only a small fraction of all injuries, these injuries may be life threatening or cause permanent life-altering damage. Recognizing signals of these types of injuries, calling 9-1-1 or the local emergency number and knowing how to give proper care could save a life or prevent further injury.

APPLYING AN ANATOMIC SPLINT

AFTER CHECKING THE SCENE AND THE INJURED PERSON:

1 GET CONSENT

2 SUPPORT INJURED PART

Support both above and below the site of the injury.

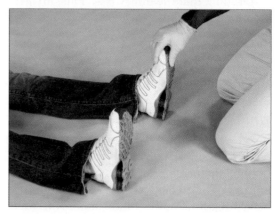

3 CHECK CIRCULATION

Check for feeling, warmth and color
beyond the injury.

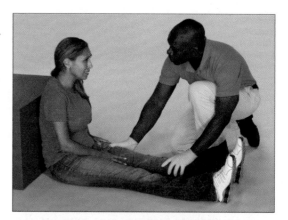

4 POSITION BANDAGES

Place several folded triangular bandages
above and below the injured body part.

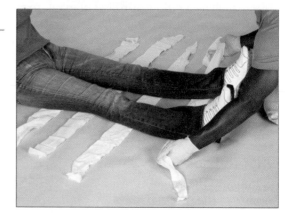

5 ALIGN BODY PARTS

Place the uninjured body part next to the injured body part.

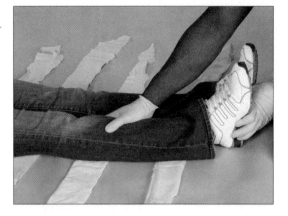

6 TIE BANDAGES SECURELY

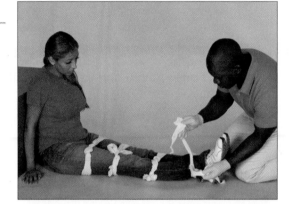

7 RECHECK CIRCULATION

Recheck for feeling, warmth and color.

> **TIP:** *If you are not able to check warmth and color because a sock or shoe is in place, check for feeling.*

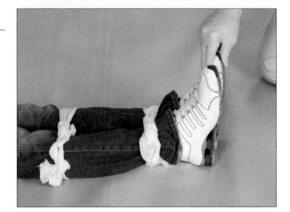

APPLYING A SOFT SPLINT

AFTER CHECKING THE SCENE AND THE INJURED PERSON:

1 GET CONSENT

2 SUPPORT INJURED PART

Support both above and below the site of the injury.

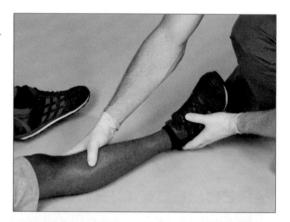

3 CHECK CIRCULATION

Check for feeling, warmth and color beyond the injury.

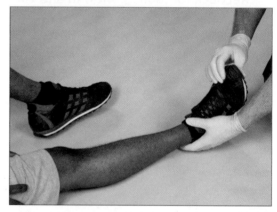

4 POSITION BANDAGES

Place several folded triangular bandages above and below the injured body part.

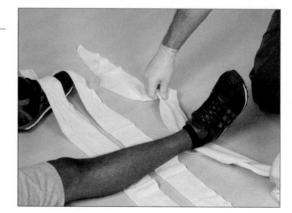

5 WRAP WITH SOFT OBJECT

Gently wrap a soft object (e.g., a folded blanket or pillow) around the injured body part.

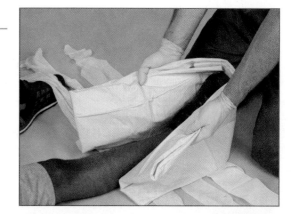

6 TIE BANDAGES SECURELY

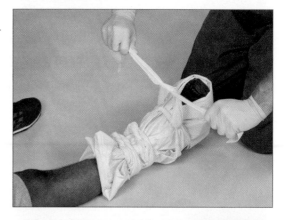

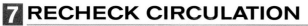

7 RECHECK CIRCULATION

Recheck for feeling, warmth and color.

> **TIP:** *If you are not able to check warmth and color because a sock or shoe is in place, check for feeling.*

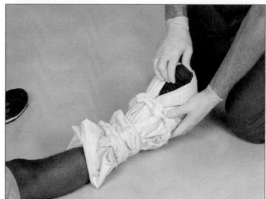

APPLYING A RIGID SPLINT

AFTER CHECKING THE SCENE AND THE INJURED PERSON:

1 GET CONSENT

2 SUPPORT INJURED PART

Support both above and below the site of the injury.

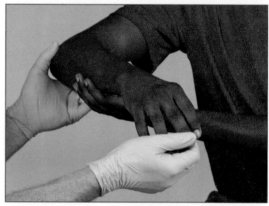

3 CHECK CIRCULATION

Check for feeling, warmth and color beyond the injury.

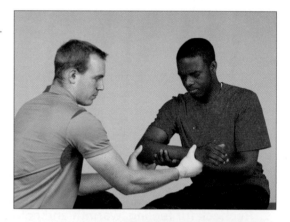

4 PLACE SPLINT

Place an appropriately sized rigid splint (e.g., padded board) under the injured body part.

TIP: *Place padding such as roller gauze under the palm of the hand to keep it in a natural position.*

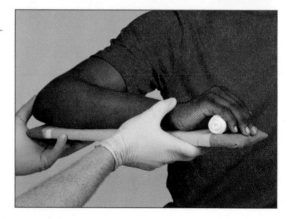

5 SECURE BANDAGES

Tie several folded triangular bandages above and below the injured body part.

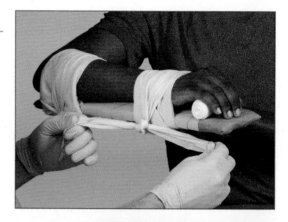

6 RECHECK CIRCULATION

Recheck for feeling, warmth and color.

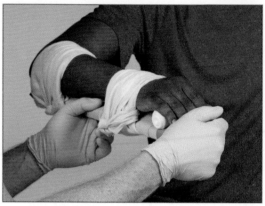

> **TIP:** *If a rigid splint is used on an injured forearm, immobilize the wrist and elbow. Bind the arm to the chest using folded triangular bandages or apply a sling. If splinting an injured joint, immobilize the bones on either side of the joint.*

APPLYING A SLING AND BINDER

AFTER CHECKING THE SCENE AND THE INJURED PERSON:

1 GET CONSENT

2 SUPPORT INJURED PART

Support both above and below the site of the injury.

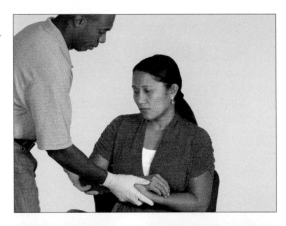

3 CHECK CIRCULATION

Check for feeling, warmth and color beyond the injury.

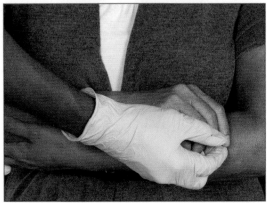

4 POSITION SLING

Place a triangular bandage under the injured arm and over the uninjured shoulder to form a sling.

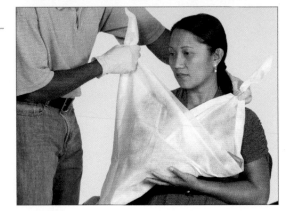

5 SECURE SLING

Tie the ends of the sling at the side of the neck.

> **TIP:** *Pad the knots at the neck and side of the binder for comfort.*

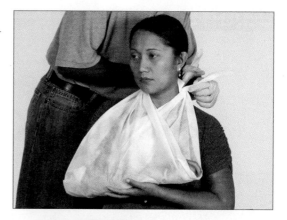

6 BIND WITH BANDAGE

Bind the injured body part to the chest with a folded triangular bandage.

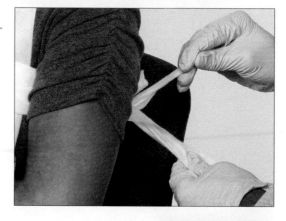

7 RECHECK CIRCULATION

Recheck for feeling, warmth and color.

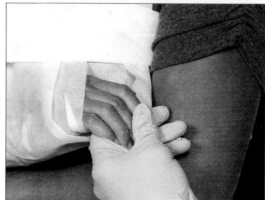

CHAPTER 9

Special Situations and Circumstances

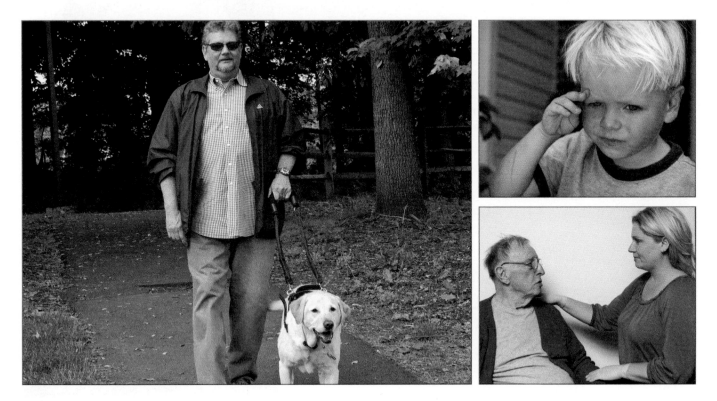

In an emergency, it is helpful to be aware of any unique needs and considerations of the person involved. For example, children, older adults, persons with disabilities and persons who speak a different language than your own have special needs and considerations that affect the care you give. In some emergencies, special circumstances, such as an emergency childbirth or a hostile situation, create additional challenges. In any case, there are steps you can take to be better prepared to respond appropriately.

In this chapter, you will explore ways to recognize and respond to special situations and circumstances. This will help you to better understand the nature of the emergency and give appropriate, effective care.

CHILDREN AND INFANTS

Children and infants have unique needs that require special care. For example, checking the condition of a conscious child or infant can be difficult, especially if the child does not know you. At certain ages, children and infants do not readily accept strangers. Very young children and infants cannot tell you what is wrong.

Communication

We tend to react more strongly and emotionally to a child who is in pain or terrified. In such a situation, try hard to remain calm and avoid showing panic or fear through your actions, speech or facial expressions. Doing so will help both the child and concerned adults.

To help an injured or ill child, try to imagine how the child might feel. A child is afraid of the unknown. This includes being ill or hurt, touched by strangers and being separated from his or her parents. Try not to separate the child or infant from loved ones, if possible. Often a parent will be holding a crying child or an infant, in which case, you perform your assessment while the adult continues to hold him or her.

How you interact with an injured or ill child or infant is very important. You need to reduce the child's anxiety and panic and gain the child's trust and cooperation, if possible. Approach the child slowly. Your sudden appearance may upset the child or infant. Get as close to eye level of the child or infant as you can and keep your voice calm (Fig. 9-1). Smile at the child. Ask the child's name and use it when you talk with him or her. Talk slowly and distinctly, and use words the child will easily understand. Ask questions that the child will be able to answer easily. Explain to the child and the parent what you are going to do. Reassure the child that you are there to help and will not leave.

To be able to effectively check children and infants, it is helpful to be aware of certain characteristics of children in specific age groups. It also is important to communicate effectively with parents. In addition, your care will be more effective if you know how to address the specific communication issues of a child with special needs.

Characteristics of Children and Infants

Children up to 1 year of age are commonly referred to as *infants*. Infants younger than 6 months are relatively easy to approach and are unlikely to be fearful of strangers. However, older infants often show "stranger anxiety." They may turn away from you, cry and cling to their parent. If the parent is calm and cooperative, ask for his or her assistance. Try to check the infant while he or she is held by or seated in the parent's lap.

One- and 2-year-old children commonly are referred to as *toddlers*. Toddlers may not cooperate with your attempts to check them. They usually are concerned about being separated from a loved one. If you reassure the toddler that he or she will not be separated from the parent, the toddler may be comforted. If possible, give the toddler a few minutes to get used to you before attempting to check him or her, and check the toddler in the parent's lap. A toddler also may respond to praise or be comforted by holding a special toy or blanket.

Three- to 5-year-old children commonly are referred to as *preschoolers*. Children in this age group usually are easy to check if you make use of their natural curiosity. Allow them to inspect items such as bandages. Opportunities to explore can reduce children's fears and distract them while you are checking them and giving care. Reassure the child that you are going to help and will not leave him or her. Sometimes you can show what you are going to do on a stuffed animal or doll (Fig. 9-2). If the child is injured, he or she may be upset by seeing

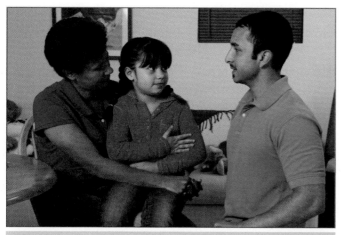

FIGURE 9-1 *To communicate with a child, get as close to eye level as you can.*

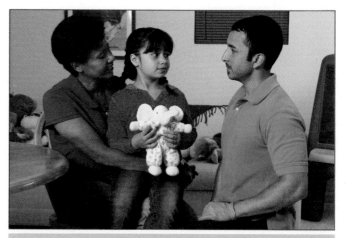

FIGURE 9-2 *Demonstrating first aid steps on a stuffed animal or doll helps a child to understand how you will care for him or her.*

the cut or injury, so cover it with a dressing as soon as possible.

School-age children are between 6 and 12 years of age. They often are more comfortable speaking with adults and can be a good source of information concerning what happened. Usually you can talk readily with school-age children. However, do not expect a child to always behave in a way that is consistent with his or her chronological age. Be especially careful not to "talk down" to school-age children. Let them know if you are going to do anything that may be painful. Children in this age group are becoming conscious of their bodies and may not like exposure. Respect their modesty.

Children between 13 and 18 years of age are considered *adolescents*. Typically they behave more like adults than children. Direct your questions to the adolescent rather than to a parent but allow input from a parent. Adolescents are modest and often react better to a responder of the same gender.

Interacting with Parents, Guardians and Caregivers

If the family is excited or agitated, the child is likely to be so. When you can calm the family, the child often will calm down as well. Remember to get consent to give care from any adult responsible for the child when possible. Concerned adults need your support too, so behave as calmly as possible.

Communicating with Children Who Have Special Health Care Needs

When communicating with children and parents, remember to observe the whole situation and ask questions to determine if the child has special physical or developmental needs.

If the child has special needs, ask the parent or caregiver if there is a list summarizing vital emergency information such as any unique or specific care procedures associated with the child's condition or allergies and other medical problems or issues.

Generally, the parents and caregivers can give you the best information since they are the most familiar with any medical equipment needed by the child.

When you attempt to communicate with children who have a developmental disability, the child's age and developmental level may not be obvious. Do not assume the child has a mental disability because he or she is unable to express thoughts or words. Ask the parents what the child is capable of understanding. Speak directly to the child. Do not speak to the parents as if the child is not in the room.

Observing Children and Infants

You can obtain a lot of information by observing children or infants before actually touching them. Look for signals that indicate changes in the level of consciousness, trouble breathing, and apparent injuries and conditions. Realize that the situation may change as soon as you touch the child or infant because he or she may become anxious or upset.

Unlike some injured or ill adults, a child or an infant is unlikely to try to cover up or deny how he or she feels. A child or an infant in pain, for example, generally will let you know that he or she hurts and will point out the source of the pain.

Ask a young child to point to any place that hurts. An older child can tell you the location of painful areas. If you need to hold an infant, always support the head when you pick up the infant. If a child becomes extremely upset, conduct your check from toe to head instead of head to toe. For more information on checking a child or an infant see Chapter 1.

Common Childhood Injuries and Illnesses

Certain problems are unique to children, such as specific kinds of injury and illness. The following sections highlight some of these concerns.

Abdominal Pain

Abdominal pain in children can be the signal of a large range of conditions. Fortunately, most are not serious and usually go away on their own.

What to Look For

Abdominal pain accompanied by any of the following signals could indicate that the child is suffering from a serious condition or illness:

- A sudden onset of severe abdominal pain or pain that becomes worse with time
- Excessive vomiting or diarrhea
- Blood in the vomit or stool
- Bloated or swollen abdomen
- A change in the child's level of consciousness, such as drowsiness or confusion
- Signals of shock

When to Call 9-1-1

Call 9-1-1 or the local emergency number if you think the child has a life-threatening condition.

What to Do Until Help Arrives

- Help the child rest in a comfortable position.
- Keep the child from becoming chilled or overheated.
- Comfort and reassure the child.
- Give care based on any conditions found.

Child Abuse

At some point, you may encounter a situation involving an injured child in which you have reason to suspect child abuse. *Child abuse* is the physical, psychological or sexual assault of a child resulting in injury and emotional trauma. Child abuse involves an injury or a pattern of injuries that do not result from an accident. *Child neglect* is a type of child abuse in which the parent or guardian fails to provide the necessary age-appropriate care to a child.

What to Look For

The *signals of child abuse* include:

- An injury whose cause does not fit the explanation of the parent, guardian or caregiver.
- Obvious or suspected fractures in a child younger than 2 years.
- Any unexplained fractures.
- Injuries in various stages of healing, especially bruises and burns.
- Bruises and burns in unusual shapes, such as bruises shaped like belt buckles or handprints or burns the size of a cigarette tip.
- Unexplained lacerations or abrasions, especially to the mouth, lips and eyes.
- Injuries to the genitalia.
- Pain when the child sits down.
- A larger number of injuries than is common for a child of the same age.

The *signals of child neglect* include:

- Lack of adult supervision.
- A child who looks malnourished.
- An unsafe living environment.
- Untreated chronic illness (e.g., a child with asthma who has no medications).

Giving Care

When caring for a child who may have been abused or neglected, your first priority is to care for the child's injuries or illnesses. An abused child may be frightened, hysterical or withdrawn. He or she may be unwilling to talk about the incident in an attempt to protect the abuser. If you suspect abuse, explain your concerns to responding police officers or emergency medical services (EMS) personnel if possible.

If you think you have reasonable cause to believe that abuse has occurred, report your suspicions to a community or state agency, such as the Department of Social Services, the Department of Child and Family Services or Child Protective Services.

You may be afraid to report suspected child abuse because you do not wish to get involved or are concerned about being sued. However, in most states, when you make a report in good faith, you are immune from any civil or criminal liability or penalty, even if you made a mistake. In this instance, *good faith* means that you honestly believe that abuse has occurred or the potential for abuse exists and a prudent and reasonable person in the same position would also honestly believe that abuse has occurred or the potential for abuse exists. You do not need to identify yourself when you report child abuse, although your report will have more credibility if you do. In some areas, certain professions are *legally obligated* to report suspicions of child abuse such as daycare workers or school employees. For more information on reporting child abuse at your workplace, contact your supervisor.

Colic

Colic is a condition in which an otherwise healthy infant cries more than 3 hours a day, for more than 3 days a week, between the ages of 3 weeks and 3 months. The crying usually starts suddenly at about the same time each day. Colic generally starts to improve at about 6 weeks. It often disappears by the time a baby is 12 weeks old.

Causes of colic may include intestinal gas, food sensitivity or allergy, or an immature nervous system. A baby with colic may have a red face and tense, hard belly because the stomach muscles tighten during crying. A baby with colic also may clench his or her legs, feet and fists when crying.

Giving Care

Movement, including walking and driving in a car, may help. White noise, such as the sound of a vacuum in the next room or the clothes dryer, also may be helpful. You also can hold the baby using certain techniques to help relieve gas pain. Consult your health care provider to rule out more serious medical conditions.

Conjunctivitis

Conjunctivitis is commonly known as "pink eye." It is a common childhood eye infection that is contagious. Signals, found in one or both eyes, include redness, swelling, itchiness, a gritty feeling, tearing and a discharge that forms a crust during the night. Seek care from a health care provider as soon as possible for diagnosis. Medication is necessary when the cause of the infection is bacterial.

Diarrhea and Vomiting

Diarrhea, or loose stools, often accompanies an infection in children. Vomiting can be frightening for a young child, but it is rarely a serious problem. However, diarrhea and vomiting both can lead to dehydration. This is more likely to occur in young children.

When to Seek Professional Medical Care

A health care provider should be contacted if:

- Diarrhea or vomiting persists for more than a few days.
- The child is not replacing lost liquids or cannot retain liquids.
- The child has not had a wet diaper in 3 or more hours or, if older, has not had any urine output for more than 6 hours.
- The child has a high fever.
- The child has bloody or black stools.
- The child is unusually sleepy, drowsy, unresponsive or irritable.
- The child cries without tears or has a dry mouth.
- The child has a sunken appearance to the abdomen, eyes or cheeks, or, in a very young infant, has a sunken soft spot at the top of the head.
- The child has skin that remains "tented" if pinched and released.

Giving Care

Remember the following when caring for children and infants with *diarrhea*:

- If the infant will not tolerate his or her normal feedings or if a child is drinking less fluid than normal, add a commercially available oral rehydration solution specially designed for children and infants.
- Do not give over-the-counter anti-diarrhea medications to children younger than 2 years. Use these with the guidance of the health care provider in older children.
- Maintain the child's normal diet. Try to limit sugar and artificial sweeteners. In addition, encourage the child to eat items like bananas, rice, applesauce and toast.

Remember the following when caring for children and infants who are *vomiting*:

- For a very young child or infant, lay the child on his or her side so that the child does not swallow or inhale the vomit.
- Halt solid foods for 24 hours during an illness involving vomiting and replace with clear fluids, such as water, popsicles, gelatin or an oral rehydration solution specially designed for children and infants.
- Introduce liquids slowly. For instance, wait 2 to 3 hours after a vomiting episode to offer the child some cool water. Offer 1 to 2 ounces every half hour, four times. Then alternate 2 ounces of rehydration solution with 2 ounces of water every 2 hours.
- After 12 to 24 hours with no vomiting, gradually reintroduce the child's normal diet.

Ear Infections

Ear infections are common in young children. Nearly 90 percent of young children have an ear infection at some time before they reach school age.

What to Look For

Common signals of an ear infection include:

- Pain. Older children can tell you that their ears hurt, but younger children may only cry or be irritable or tug on the affected ear.
- Loss of appetite.
- Trouble sleeping.
- Fever.
- Ear drainage.
- Trouble hearing.

When to Seek Professional Medical Care

A health care provider should be contacted if:

- The child's signals last longer than a day.
- You see a discharge of blood or pus from the ear. This could indicate a ruptured eardrum.
- The child's signals do not improve or get worse after he or she has been diagnosed by a health care provider.

Giving Care

Pain symptoms may be treated with ibuprofen or acetaminophen. In children younger than 2 years, watch for sleeplessness and irritability during or after an upper respiratory infection, such as a cold. Always consult the child's health care provider before giving any over-the-counter pain relievers.

Fever

Fever is an elevated body temperature of 100.4° F or greater. Fever indicates a problem, and in a child or an infant, it often means there is a specific problem. Usually these problems are not life threatening, but some can be. A high fever in a child or an infant often indicates some form of infection. In a young child, even a minor infection can result in a high fever, usually defined as a temperature 103° F and above.

Fevers that last a long time or are very high can result in seizures. A *febrile seizure* is a convulsion brought on by a fever in infants or small children. It is the most common type of seizure in children. Most febrile seizures last less than 5 minutes and are not life threatening. However, there are conditions where the child may require additional care (see When to Call 9-1-1 for more information on febrile seizures). Immediately after a febrile seizure, it is important to cool the body if a fever is present (see Chapter 5 for more information on signals of and care for seizures).

What to Look For

Older children with fever will often:

- Feel hot to the touch.
- Complain of being cold or chilled.
- Complain of body aches.
- Have a headache.
- Have trouble sleeping or sleep more than usual.
- Appear drowsy.
- Have no appetite.

Infants with fever will often:

- Be upset or fussy, with frequent crying.
- Be unusually quiet.
- Feel warm or hot.
- Breathe rapidly and have a rapid heart rate.
- Stop eating or sleeping normally.

Taking a Temperature

If children or infants have any of the signals listed above, you will need to take their temperature to determine if they have a fever. A rectal temperature gives the most reliable reading for children younger than 5 years. (*NOTE*: Before taking a rectal temperature, child care providers should make sure that doing so is not prohibited by state regulations.)

For children age 5 and older, an oral temperature (in the mouth and under the tongue) is the recommended method. You also may take an oral temperature for children age 3 and older.

A child's or an infant's temperature also can be taken in the ear (known as the *tympanic method*) or under the armpit (known as the *axillary method*).

Multiple types of thermometers are available. Do not use glass thermometers, and, whenever possible, use an electronic (digital) thermometer. Also, use a thermometer that is specifically designed for the type of temperature being taken. For example, do not use an oral thermometer to take a rectal temperature. Read the manufacturer's directions carefully so you know how to use the thermometer appropriately.

Always stay with a child while taking a temperature to make sure that the child does not move so the thermometer does not break or cause injury.

When to Call 9-1-1

Call 9-1-1 or the local emergency number if the child or infant has signals of life-threatening conditions, such as unconsciousness or trouble breathing. Also, call if this is the first time that a child has had a febrile seizure, the seizure lasts longer than 5 minutes or is repeated, or the seizure is followed by a quick rise in the temperature of the child or infant. Child care providers should follow state or local regulations regarding emergency care and contact procedures whenever a child in their care becomes injured or ill.

When to Seek Professional Medical Care

A health care provider should be contacted for:

- Any infant younger than 3 months with a fever (100.4° F or greater).
- Any child younger than 2 years with a high fever (103° F or greater).
- Any child or infant who has a febrile seizure.

Giving Care

If the child or infant has a fever, make him or her as comfortable as possible. Encourage the child to rest. Make sure that the child or infant is not overdressed or covered with too many blankets. A single layer of clothing and a light blanket usually is all that is necessary. Make sure that the child or infant drinks clear fluids (e.g., water, juice or chicken broth) or continues nursing or bottle-feeding to prevent dehydration.

Acetaminophen or ibuprofen may be given for a fever. *Do not give the child aspirin for fever or other signals of flu-like or other viral illness.* For a child, taking aspirin can result in an extremely serious medical condition called *Reye's syndrome*. Reye's syndrome is an illness that affects the brain and other internal organs. Always consult the child's health care provider before giving any over-the-counter pain relievers.

If the child has a *high fever*, it is important to gently cool the child. Never rush cooling down a child. If the fever is caused a febrile seizure, rapid cooling could bring on other complications. Instead, remove any excessive clothing or blankets and sponge the child with lukewarm water. Do *not* use an ice water bath or rubbing alcohol to cool down the body. Both of these approaches are dangerous. Continue caring for the child or infant with a high fever as described above.

Foreign Objects in the Nose

If a child has an object in the nose, *do not* try to remove the object. Special lighting and instruments are necessary. It is important to go to a health care provider for removal of the object. Also, try to calm the child and parents as best as possible.

Injury

Injury is the number one cause of death for children in the United States. Many of these deaths are the result of motor-vehicle crashes. The greatest dangers to a child involved in a motor-vehicle crash are airway obstruction and bleeding. Severe bleeding must be controlled as quickly as possible. A relatively small amount of blood lost by an adult is a large amount for a child or an infant to lose.

Because a child's head is large and heavy in proportion to the rest of the body, the head is the area most often injured. A child injured as the result of force or a blow also may have damage to the organs in the abdominal and chest cavities. Such damage can cause severe internal bleeding. A child secured only by a lap belt may have serious abdominal or spinal injuries in a motor-vehicle crash. Try to find out what happened because a severely injured child may not immediately show signals of injury.

To avoid needless deaths of children caused by motor vehicle crashes, laws have been enacted requiring that children ride in the backseat of the car in approved safety seats or wearing safety belts (see the Appendix: Injury Prevention and Emergency Preparedness for detailed information on vehicle safety). As a result of these laws, more children's lives have been saved. You may have to check and care for an injured child while he or she is in a safety seat. A safety seat does not normally pose problems while you are checking a child. Leave the child in the seat if the seat has not been damaged. If the child is to be transported to a medical facility for examination, he or she often can be safely secured and transported in the safety seat.

Meningitis

Meningitis is a disease that occurs when the tissues that cover the brain and spinal cord become inflamed. It is caused by viruses or bacteria. The bacterial form of the disease is less common but more serious.

What to Look For

Signals of meningitis include the following:

- Fever
- Irritability
- Loss of appetite
- Sleepiness
- In addition, older children may complain of a stiff neck, back pain or a headache.

When to Seek Professional Medical Care

A health care provider should be contacted if a child has been in contact with a person who has been diagnosed with bacterial meningitis. The health care provider may prescribe preventative antibiotics.

If the child shows any signals of meningitis, go immediately to a health care provider. It is important to find out whether the illness is caused by bacteria or a virus. Bacterial meningitis requires prompt treatment with antibiotics.

There is no medication to treat viral meningitis. Give supportive care for the fever and pain with acetaminophen or ibuprofen.

Poisoning

Poisoning is one of the top 10 causes of unintentional death in the United States for adolescents, children and infants.

Children younger than 6 years account for half of all exposures to poisonous substances in the United States. Children in this age group often are poisoned by ingesting household products or medications (typically those intended for adults). Although children in this age group are exposed more often than any other, only 3 percent of these cases result in death.

There has been a decrease in child poisonings in recent years due in part to child-resistant packaging for medications. This packaging makes it harder for children to get into these substances. The decrease also is a result of preventive actions taken by parents and others who care for children. For more information on poisoning, refer to Chapter 5.

Rashes

Young children and infants have sensitive skin. Their skin develops rashes easily. Two common rashes in young children and infants are heat rash and diaper rash.

Heat Rash

Heat rash is a red or pink rash that forms on any skin covered by clothing. It is most common in infants and looks like red dots or small pimples.

If the child or infant develops heat rash, give care by:

- Removing or loosening clothing to cool down the child or infant.
- Moving the child or infant to a cool location.
- Cooling the area with wet washcloths or a cool bath and letting the skin air-dry.

If the area remains irritated, use calamine lotion or a hydrocortisone cream if the child is not sensitive or allergic to these products. Avoid ointments or other lotions. They could further irritate the skin.

Diaper Rash

Diaper rash is another common rash in young children and infants. When skin is wet for too long, it begins to break down. When wet skin is rubbed, it becomes more

SIDS

Infants who sleep on their stomach at night or naptime seem to have an increased risk for SIDS. Therefore, to help reduce the risk of SIDS:

- *Always place an infant on his or her back at night or naptime, using a firm mattress in a safety-approved crib or bassinet.*

- *Make sure that there is no soft bedding, such as pillows, blankets and bumpers, or soft toys, such as stuffed animals, in the crib. These items could cause suffocation.*

- *Check the sleeping infant frequently.*

---

damaged. Moisture from a dirty diaper can harm the skin of a toddler or infant, making it more irritated. This causes diaper rash to develop.

Seek care from a health care provider if diaper rash:

- Develops blisters or pus-filled sores.
- Does not go away within 2 to 3 days.
- Gets worse.

Give care for diaper rash in toddlers and infants by applying a thick layer of over-the-counter zinc oxide or petroleum jelly to the affected area. This creates a barrier between the infant's delicate skin and the urine or feces.

To prevent diaper rash and help it to heal:

- Keep the area as dry as possible by changing wet or soiled diapers immediately.
- Clean the area with water and a soft washcloth. Avoid wipes that can dry the child's skin.
- Pat the skin dry or let it air dry.
- Keep the diaper loose so wet and soiled parts do not rub against the skin.

Sudden Infant Death Syndrome

Sudden infant death syndrome (SIDS) is the sudden, unexpected and unexplained death of a seemingly healthy infant. In the United States, approximately 2300 infants die every year of SIDS. SIDS is the third leading cause of death for infants between 1 month and 1 year of age. It occurs most often in infants between 4 weeks and 7 months of age. SIDS usually occurs while the infant is sleeping.

The condition does not seem to be linked to a disease. In addition, the cause(s) of SIDS are not yet understood. It is not thought to be hereditary, but it does tend to recur in families. Because of these factors, there is no way of knowing if a child is at risk for SIDS. Sometimes it is mistaken for child abuse because of the unexplained

death in an apparently healthy child. In addition, SIDS sometimes causes bruise-like blotches to appear on the infant's body. However, SIDS is not related to child abuse.

When to Call 9-1-1

By the time the infant's condition has been discovered, he or she may be in cardiac arrest. If you encounter an infant in this condition, make sure that someone has called 9-1-1 or the local emergency number or call yourself.

What to Do Until Help Arrives

If there is no breathing, perform CPR until EMS personnel take over, an automated external defibrillator (AED) becomes available or you see an obvious sign of life, such as breathing.

After a SIDS Incident

An incident involving a severely ill child or infant or one who has died can be emotionally upsetting. After such an episode, find someone whom you trust to talk about the experience and express your feelings. If you continue to be distressed, seek professional counseling. The feelings caused by such incidents need to be dealt with and understood or they can result in serious stress reactions.

EMERGENCY CHILDBIRTH

Words such as exhausting, stressful, exciting, fulfilling, painful and scary sometimes are used to describe a planned childbirth. A planned childbirth is one that occurs in the hospital or at home under the supervision of a health care provider. If you find yourself assisting with the delivery of a newborn, however, it probably will not be happening in a planned situation. Therefore, your feelings, as well as those of the expectant mother, may be intensified by fear of the unexpected or the possibility that something might go wrong.

Take comfort in knowing that things rarely go wrong. Childbirth is a natural process. Thousands of children all over the world are born without complications each day, in areas where no medical care is available.

When to Call 9-1-1

If a woman is giving birth, call 9-1-1 or the local emergency number immediately. Give the EMS call taker the following important information:

- The woman's name, age and expected due date
- How long she has been having labor pains
- Whether this is her first child

What to Do Until Help Arrives

By following a few simple steps, you can effectively assist in the birth process while you wait for EMS personnel to arrive. If a woman is giving birth:

- Talk with the woman to help her remain calm.
- Place layers of clean sheets, towels or blankets under her and over her abdomen.
- Control the scene so that the woman will have privacy.
- Position the woman on her back with her knees bent, feet flat and legs spread wide apart.
- Avoid contact with body fluids; wear disposable gloves and protective eyewear if possible.
- Remember, the woman delivers the baby, so be patient and let it happen naturally.
- The baby will be slippery; use a clean towel to receive and hold the baby; avoid dropping the baby.
- Keep the baby warm; have a clean, warm towel or blanket handy to wrap the newborn.

CAUTIONS:

- Do not let the woman get up or leave to find a bathroom (most women want to use the restroom).
- Do not hold the woman's knees together; this will not slow the birth process and may complicate the birth or harm the baby.
- Do not place your fingers in the vagina for any reason.
- Do not pull on the baby.

OLDER ADULTS

Older adults, or the elderly, generally are considered to be those older than 65 years. They are quickly becoming the fastest growing age group in the United States. Since 1900, life expectancy in the United States has increased by over 60 percent. In 1900, for example, the average life expectancy was 46 years for men and 48 years for women. Today, it is 75 years for men and 80 years for women. The main explanations for the increase in life expectancy are medical advancements and improvements in health care.

Normal aging brings about changes. People age at different rates, and each person's organs and body parts age at different rates as well. For example, a person with wrinkled, fragile skin may have strong bones or excellent respiratory function.

Overall, however, body function generally declines as we age. Some changes begin as early as age 30 years. The lungs become less efficient, so older people are at higher risk of developing pneumonia and other lung diseases. The amount of blood pumped by the heart with each beat decreases, and the heart rate slows. The blood vessels harden, causing increased work for the heart. Hearing and vision usually decline, often causing some degree of sight and hearing loss. Reflexes become slower, and arthritis may affect joints, causing movement to become painful.

Checking an Older Adult

The physical and mental changes associated with aging may require you to adapt your way of communicating and to be aware of certain potential age-related conditions, such as hearing loss.

To check an injured or ill older adult, attempt to learn the person's name and use it when you speak to him or her. Consider using "Mrs.," "Mr." or "Ms." as a sign of respect. Make sure that you are at the person's eye level so that he or she can see and hear you more clearly (Fig. 9-3).

If the person seems confused at first, the confusion may be the result of impaired vision or hearing. If he or she usually wears eyeglasses and cannot find them, try to locate them. Speak slowly and clearly, and look at the person's face while you talk. Notice if he or she has a hearing aid. Someone who needs glasses to see or a hearing aid to hear is likely to be very anxious without them. If the person is truly confused, try to find out if the confusion is the result of the injury or an

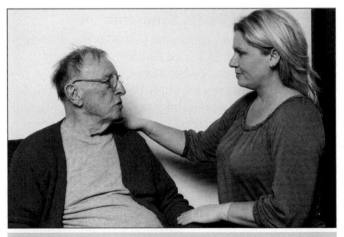

FIGURE 9-3 *Speak to an elderly person at eye level so that he or she can see and hear you more clearly.*

existing condition. Be sure to get as much information as possible from family members or bystanders. The person may be afraid of falling, so if he or she is standing, offer an arm or hand. Remember that an older person may need to move slowly.

Try to find out what medications the person is taking so that you can tell EMS personnel. Look for a medical identification (ID) tag, bracelet or necklace that lists the person's name, address and medical information. Be aware that an elderly person may not recognize the signals of a serious condition. An elderly person also may minimize any signals for fear of losing his or her independence or being placed in a nursing home.

Common Injuries and Illnesses in Older Adults

Certain problems are more prevalent in older adults, such as specific kinds of injury and illness. The following sections discuss some of these concerns.

Confusion

Older adults are at increased risk of altered thinking patterns and confusion. Some of this change is the result of aging. Certain diseases, such as Alzheimer's disease, affect the brain, resulting in impaired memory and thinking and altered behavior. Confusion that comes on suddenly, however, may be the result of medication, even a medication the person has been taking regularly. An injured or ill person who has problems seeing or hearing also may become confused when injured or ill. This problem increases when the person is in an unfamiliar environment. A head injury also can result in confusion.

Confusion can be a signal of a medical emergency. An elderly person with pneumonia, for example, may not run a fever, have chest pain or be coughing, but because not enough oxygen is reaching the brain, the person may be confused. An older person can have a serious infection without fever, pain or nausea. An elderly person having a heart attack may not have chest pain, pale or ashen skin or other classic signals but may be restless, short of breath and confused.

Depression is common in older adults. A depressed older adult may seem to be confused initially. A person suffering from depression also may show signals that have no apparent cause, such as sudden shortness of breath or chest pain. Whatever the reason for any the confusion, be respectful and do not talk down to or treat him or her like a child.

Falls

Older adults are at increased risk of falls. In fact, falls are the leading cause of death from injury for older adults.

Falls in older adults are due to slower reflexes, failing eyesight and hearing, arthritis and problems such as unsteady balance and movement. Falls frequently result in fractures because the bones become weaker and more brittle with age.

Head Injuries

An older adult is at greater risk of serious head injury. As we age, the size of the brain decreases. This decrease results in more space between the surface of the brain and the inside of the skull. This space allows more movement of the brain within the skull, which can increase the likelihood of serious head injury. Occasionally, an older adult may not develop the signals of a head injury until days after a fall. Therefore, unless you know the cause of a behavior change, you should always suspect a head injury as a possible cause of unusual behavior in an elderly person. This is especially true if you know that the person had a fall or a blow to the head.

Problems with Heat and Cold

An elderly person is more susceptible to extremes in temperature. The person may be unable to feel temperature extremes because his or her body may no longer regulate temperature effectively. Body temperature may change rapidly to a dangerously high or low level.

The body of an elderly person retains heat because of a decreased ability to sweat and the reduced ability of the circulatory system to adjust to heat. This can lead to heat exhaustion or heat stroke.

An elderly person may become chilled and suffer hypothermia simply by sitting in a draft or in front of a fan or air conditioner. Hypothermia can occur at any time of the year. People can go on for several days suffering from mild hypothermia without realizing it. The older person with mild hypothermia will want to lie down frequently; however, this will lower the body temperature even further.

Giving Care for a Heat-Related Illness

See Chapter 6 for information about caring for heat-related illnesses.

Giving Care for a Cold-Related Emergency

See Chapter 6 for information about caring for cold-related emergencies.

PEOPLE WITH DISABILITIES

According to the American with Disabilities Act (ADA), a person with a disability is someone who has a physical or mental impairment that substantially limits one or more major life activities such as walking, talking, seeing, hearing or learning. This includes, for example, a blind person who cannot read information posted on a bulletin board or a deaf person who may need a sign language interpreter.

The Centers for Disease Control and Prevention (CDC) estimates that over 33 million people in the United States have disabilities. When giving care to people with disabilities, communication can be a challenge. It may be difficult to find out what has happened and what might be wrong in an emergency situation.

Physical Disability

A person is considered to have a physical disability if his or her ability to move (also called *motor function*) is impaired. A person also is considered to have a physically disability if his or her sensory function is impaired. Sensory function includes all of the senses: sight, hearing, taste, smell and touch. A person with a physical disability may have impairments in motor function, sensory function or both.

General hints for approaching an injured or ill person whom you suspect may have a physical disability include:

- Speak to the person before touching him or her.
- Ask, "How can I help?" or "Do you need help?"
- Ask for assistance and information from the person who has the disability—he or she has been living with the disability and best understands it. If you are not able to communicate with the person, ask family members, friends or companions who are available to help.
- Do not remove any braces, canes, other physical support, eyeglasses or hearing aids. Removal of these items may take away necessary physical support for the person's body.
- Look for a medical ID tag, bracelet or necklace at the person's wrist or neck.

- A person with a disability may have a service animal, such as a guide or signal dog. Be aware that this animal may be protective of the person in an emergency situation. Allow the animal to stay with the person if possible, which will help to reassure both of them.

Deaf and Hard of Hearing

Hearing loss is defined as a partial or total loss of hearing. Some people are born with a hearing loss. Hearing loss also can result from an injury or illness affecting the ear, the nerves leading from the brain to the ear or the brain itself. You may not immediately realize that the injured or ill person has a hearing loss. Often the person will tell you, either in speech or by pointing to the ear and shaking the head no. Some people carry a card stating that they have a hearing loss. You may see a hearing aid in a person's ear.

The biggest obstacle you must overcome in caring for a person with a hearing loss is communication. You will need to figure out how to get that person's consent to give care, and you will need to assess the problem.

Sometimes the injured or ill person will be able to read lips. To assist him or her, position yourself where the person can clearly see your face. Look straight at the person while you speak, and speak slowly. Do not exaggerate the way you form words. Do not turn your face away while you speak. Many people with a hearing impairment, however, do not read lips. In these cases, using gestures and writing messages on paper may be the most effective way to communicate.

If you and the person know sign language, use it. Some people who are deaf or hard of hearing have a machine called a telecommunications device for the deaf (TDD). You can use this device to type messages and questions, and the person can type replies back to you (Fig. 9-4, A–B). Many people who have a hearing

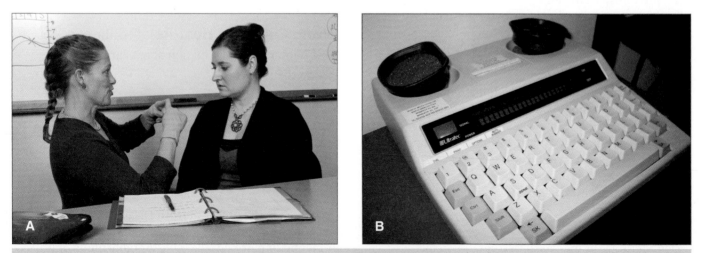

FIGURE 9-4, A–B *Communicate with a person who has a hearing loss in the best way possible.* **A,** *Use sign language, lip reading or writing to communicate.* **B,** *You may also use a telecommunications device for the deaf.*

impairment can speak, some distinctly, some not so clearly. If you have trouble understanding, ask the person to repeat what he or she said. Do not pretend to understand.

Blind or Visually Impaired

Vision loss is a partial or total loss of sight. Vision loss can have many causes. Some people are born with vision loss. Others lose vision as a result of disease or injury. Vision loss is not necessarily a problem with the eyes. It can result from problems with the vision centers in the brain.

It is no more difficult to communicate verbally with a person who has a partial or total loss of sight than with someone who can see. You do not need to speak loudly or in overly simple terms. The person may not be able to tell you certain things about how an injury occurred but usually can give an accurate account based on his or her interpretation of sound and touch.

When caring for a person with vision loss, help to reassure him or her by explaining what is going on and what you are doing. If you must move a visually impaired person who can walk, stand beside the person and have him or her hold onto your arm. Walk at a normal pace, alert the person to obstacles in the way, such as stairs, and let the person know whether to step up or down. If the person has a service animal, try to keep them together. Ask the person to tell you how to handle the dog or ask him or her to do it.

Motor Impairment

A person with motor impairment is unable to move normally. He or she may be missing a body part or have a problem with the bones or muscles or the nerves that control movement. Causes of motor impairment could include stroke, muscular dystrophy, multiple sclerosis, paralysis, cerebral palsy or loss of a limb.

Determining which problems are pre-existing and which are the result of immediate injury or illness can be difficult. Care for all problems you detect as if they are new.

Mental Impairment

Mental, or cognitive, function includes the brain's capacity to reason and process information. A person with a mental impairment has problems performing these operations. Some types of mental impairment are genetic. Others result from injuries or infections that occur during pregnancy, shortly after birth or later in life. Some causes never are determined.

In some situations, you will not be able to determine if a person has a mental impairment; in others, it will be obvious. If you suspect that a person has a mental impairment, approach him or her as you would any other person in his or her age group. If the person appears not to understand you, rephrase what you were saying in simpler terms. Listen carefully to what the person says. An injury or a sudden illness can be disruptive to some individuals who have a cognitive impairment, causing them a great deal of anxiety and fear. Take time to explain who you are and what you are going to do. Offer reassurance. Try to gain the person's trust. If a parent, guardian or caregiver is present, ask that person to help you give care to the person.

People with certain types of mental illness might misinterpret your actions as being hostile. If the scene becomes unsafe, you may need to remove yourself from the immediate area. Call 9-1-1 or the local emergency number and explain your concerns about a potential psychiatric emergency. If possible, keep track of the person's location and what he or she is doing. Report this information to the emergency responders.

LANGUAGE BARRIERS

Getting consent to give care to a person with whom you have a language barrier can be a problem. Find out if any bystanders speak the person's language and can help to translate. Do your best to communicate nonverbally. Use gestures and facial expressions. If the person is in pain, he or she probably will be anxious to show you where the pain is located. Watch his or her gestures and facial expressions carefully. When you speak to the person, speak slowly and in a normal tone. The person probably will have no trouble hearing you.

When you call 9-1-1 or the local emergency number, explain that you are having difficulty communicating with the person and tell the call taker which language you believe the person speaks. The EMS system may have someone available who can help with communication. If the person has a life-threatening condition, such as severe bleeding, consent is implied.

CRIME SCENES AND HOSTILE SITUATIONS

In certain situations, such as a giving care to a person in a crime scene or an injured person who is hostile, you will need to use extreme caution. Although your first reaction may be to go to the aid of a person, in these situations you should call 9-1-1 or the local emergency number and stay at a safe distance.

Do not enter the scene of a suicide. If you happen to be on the scene when an unarmed person threatens suicide, call 9-1-1 or the local emergency number. Do not argue with the person. Remain at a safe distance.

Leave or avoid entering any area considered to be a crime scene, such as one where there is a weapon, or the scene of a physical or sexual assault. Call 9-1-1 or the local emergency number and stay at a safe distance.

You may encounter a situation where there is a hostile or angry person. A person's rage or hostility may be caused by the injury, pain or fear. Some individuals, afraid of losing control, may act resentful and suspicious. Hostile behavior also may result from the use of alcohol or other drugs, a lack of oxygen or a medical condition. If a person refuses your care or threatens you, remove yourself from the situation and stay at a safe distance. Never argue with or restrain an injured or ill person. Call 9-1-1 or the local emergency number if someone has not already done so. Never put your own safety at risk.

Uninjured family members also may display anger. This anger may stem from panic, anxiety or guilt. Try to remain calm and explain what you plan to do in giving emergency care. If possible, find a way that family members can help, such as by comforting the person.

PUTTING IT ALL TOGETHER

It is important to be aware of the special needs and considerations of children and infants, older adults, people with disabilities and people who speak a different language than your own. In rare circumstances, you could find yourself in a position to give help in an emergency childbirth or help an older person who has become suddenly ill. Knowing what to do in these types of situations will help you to act calmly and give the right care. Interacting and communicating with all types of people in many different situations will enable you to respond quickly and effectively in an emergency.

CHAPTER 10

Asthma

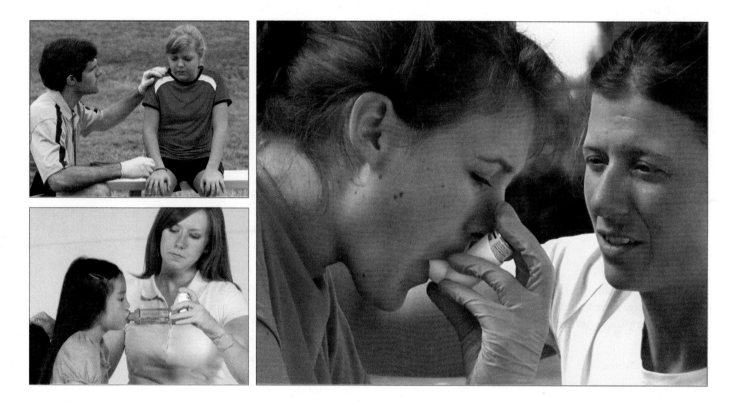

Note: *The instructions for administering asthma medication found in this chapter should not be substituted for those given by a medical professional to an individual person. Nor should these instructions be substituted for directions given by a medical professional in consultation with a site where asthma medication will be administered. Consult a health care professional for specific advice on the use of asthma inhalers and nebulizers.*

Asthma is a life-long lung disease. It affects millions of adults and children in the United States. Cases of severe asthma and deaths from asthma are increasing. As a first aid responder, there is a good chance that you could be asked to help a person with a breathing emergency caused by asthma.

In this chapter, you will read about how to identify the signals of an asthma attack. This chapter also covers how to give care to a person having an asthma attack, which includes helping the person to use an inhaler to administer quick-relief medications.

ASTHMA

Asthma is an illness in which certain substances or conditions, called "triggers," cause inflammation and constriction of the *airways* (small tubes in the lungs through which we breathe), making breathing difficult. Triggers of an asthma attack include exercise, cold air, allergens or irritants, such as perfume.

In 2008, the Centers for Disease Control and Prevention (CDC) estimated that over 23 million Americans were affected by asthma. Asthma is more common in children and young adults. However, its frequency and severity is increasing in all age groups in the United States. Asthma is the third-ranking cause of hospitalization among those younger than 15 years.

People diagnosed with asthma can reduce the risk of an attack by controlling environmental variables when possible. This helps to limit exposure to the triggers that can start an asthma attack.

When an attack does occur, they can use medications and other forms of treatment. Asthma medications stop the muscle spasm and open the airway, which makes breathing easier.

Asthma Triggers

A trigger is anything that sets off or starts an asthma attack. A trigger for one person is not necessarily a trigger for another. Asthma triggers include the following:

- Dust and smoke
- Air pollution
- Respiratory infections
- Fear or anxiety
- Perfume
- Exercise
- Plants and molds
- Medications, such as aspirin
- Animal dander
- Temperature extremes
- Changes in weather

These are only a few of the things that can trigger asthma in people.

Preventing Asthma Attacks

Prevention is key. A person can follow these preventative measures to reduce his or her risk of an attack:

- Limit triggers in the home.
- Control emotions.
- Prevent infections.
- Reduce environmental triggers.
- Exercise carefully.

Limiting Triggers in the Home

You can reduce the chances of triggering an asthma attack at home by:

- Keeping plants outside.
- Washing bedclothes and pajamas weekly in hot water.
- Using hypoallergenic covers on mattresses and pillows.
- Eliminating or reducing the number of carpets and rugs.
- Regularly steam cleaning all carpets, rugs and upholstery.
- Keeping the home clean and free of dust and pests—wet dusting can be more effective than dry dusting.
- Not allowing, or being around, smoke.
- Regularly changing the air filter in the central air conditioning or heating unit.
- Eliminating or minimizing the number of stuffed toys.
- Using hypoallergenic health and beauty products.
- Washing pets weekly.
- Keeping pets outside of the house.

Controlling Emotions

Certain strong emotions can trigger an asthma attack. When you feel a strong emotion, such as anger or fear, the following suggestions can reduce the chances that the emotions will trigger an asthma attack:

- Take a long deep breath in through the nose and slowly let it out through the mouth.
- Count to 10.
- Talk with a family member, trusted friend or health care provider.
- Do a relaxing activity.

Preventing Infections

Colds and other respiratory infections can make an asthma condition worse. One of the most common ways to catch colds is by rubbing the nose or eyes with hands contaminated with a cold virus. Contamination often occurs by touching surfaces (such as doorknobs) or objects that other people have touched.

Some ways to reduce the chances of getting a cold or other respiratory infection include:

- Washing hands regularly, especially after using the restroom or shaking hands with other people and before eating.

- Cleaning environmental surfaces, such as telephones and counters, with a virus-killing disinfectant. The viruses that cause colds can survive up to 3 hours on objects such as telephones, counters and stair railings. Disinfecting them regularly can help to prevent the spread of colds and viruses.
- Getting vaccinated for illnesses when a vaccine is available, such as for influenza and whooping cough (pertussis).

Your health care provider might have other suggestions based on your medical history.

Reducing Environmental Triggers

Sudden changes in the weather, heavy mold or pollen content in the air and pollution can trigger an asthma attack. To avoid attacks brought on by triggers in the environment:

- Wear the right clothing for the weather conditions.
- Stay indoors on days when there is a high risk of respiratory trouble.
- Take preventative medications, as prescribed by your health care provider.
- Stay away from places with high amounts of dirt, smoke and other irritants.
- Know how the weather affects your condition.
- Talk to your health care provider about other prevention strategies.

Exercising Carefully

Exercise-induced asthma happens during or shortly after exercise. Having this type of asthma does not mean one cannot or should not exercise or play sports. It is, however, important to know what to do to prevent an asthma attack. Things to keep in mind when you have exercise-induced asthma include the following:

- Take prescribed medications 30 to 60 minutes before exercising.
- Slowly warm up before exercising. Cool down gently after exercising.
- Make sure that you drink plenty of fluids during exercise.
- Seek and follow the advice of your health care provider.
- If participating in organized sports, notify the coach of your condition.

Using Medications to Control Asthma

People who have been diagnosed with asthma will have a personalized medication plan. They should take all medications exactly as prescribed by their health care provider.

Asthma medications are available in two forms: long-term control and quick relief.

Long-Term Control Medications

Long-term control medications prevent or reverse *inflammation* (swelling) in the airway. They also help to decrease sensitivity, which helps to keep the airways from reacting to asthma triggers.

The long-term control medicines work slowly. They help to control asthma over many hours. They should be taken every day whether or not signals of asthma are present.

Quick-Relief Medications

Quick-relief or *rescue medications* are used to stop an asthma attack. These medications work quickly to relieve the sudden swelling. They lessen wheezing, coughing and chest tightness. This allows the person to breathe easier. They also are called *short-acting bronchodilators*.

Methods of Delivery

The most common way to take long-term control and quick-relief asthma medications is by inhaling them. Inhalation allows the medication to reach the airways faster and work quickly. There also are fewer side effects.

Medications are inhaled using a metered dose inhaler (MDI), a dry powder inhaler (DPI) or a small-volume nebulizer (Fig. 10-1). Both long-term and quick-relief medications also are available in pill and liquid form. In addition, long-term medications are available in the form of an injection given just under the skin.

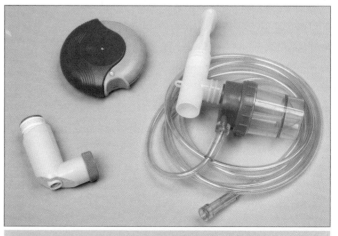

FIGURE 10-1 *Long-term and quick-release medications are inhaled using an MDI, a DPI or a small-volume nebulizer.*

MDI

An MDI sends a measured dose of medicine in mist form directly into the person's mouth. The person gently presses down the top of the inhaler. This causes a small amount of pressurized gas to push the medicine out quickly. Sometimes a "spacer" is used to control the amount of medication that is inhaled. The medicine goes into the spacer and then the person inhales the medication through the mouthpiece on the spacer.

DPI

A DPI is similar to an MDI. It is a hand-held device that delivers a dry powder form of the medication. Some dry powders are tasteless. Others are mixed with lactose to give them a sweet taste. The DPI is administered by breathing in quickly to activate the inhaler. The person does not have to press down the top of the inhaler. DPIs may be difficult for some people to use because of the need to take in a quick, strong breath.

Small-Volume Nebulizers

Small-volume nebulizers deliver medication in the form of a mist. The mist is delivered over several minutes. This is especially helpful when the person is unable to take deep breaths. Nebulizers are commonly used for children younger than 5 years and the elderly. They also are used for people who have trouble using inhalers and for those with severe asthma.

What to Look For

You often can tell when a person is having an asthma attack by the hoarse whistling sound made while exhaling. This sound, known as *wheezing*, occurs because air becomes trapped in the lungs. Coughing after exercise, crying or laughing are other signals that an asthma attack could begin.

Signals of an asthma attack include:

- Trouble breathing or shortness of breath.
- Rapid, shallow breathing.
- Sweating.
- Tightness in the chest.
- Inability to talk without stopping for a breath.
- Feelings of fear or confusion.

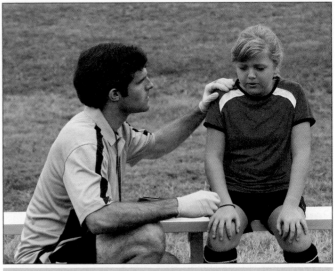

FIGURE 10-2 *To assist a person having an asthma attack, remain calm and help the person to sit comfortably.*

When to Call 9-1-1

Call 9-1-1 or the local emergency number if the person's breathing trouble does not improve in a few minutes after using the quick-relief medication.

What to Do Until Help Arrives

Remain calm. This will help the person to remain calm and ease breathing troubles. Help the person to sit comfortably (Fig. 10-2). Loosen any tight clothing around the neck and abdomen. Assist the person with his or her prescribed quick-relief medication if requested and if permitted by state or local regulations.

PUTTING IT ALL TOGETHER

Asthma is a life-long lung disease that affects millions of adults and children in the United States. Asthma can be controlled. Knowing the triggers for asthma and how to limit those triggers, and taking prescribed medications as directed can help to prevent an asthma attack.

It is important to be prepared to help people with breathing emergencies caused by asthma. The first step is to know the signals of an asthma attack. When you recognize the signals, act quickly and give appropriate care. Your care could help to save the life of a person with asthma.

ASSISTING WITH AN ASTHMA INHALER

> **TIP:** *Always obtain consent and wash your hands immediately after giving care. Read and follow all instructions printed on the inhaler prior to administering the medication to the person.*

IF THE PERSON HAS MEDICATION FOR ASTHMA, HELP HIM OR HER TAKE IT IF ASKED:

1 HELP PERSON SIT UP

Help the person sit up and rest in a position comfortable for breathing.

2 CHECK PRESCRIPTION

- Ensure that the prescription is in the person's name and is prescribed for "quick relief" or "acute" attacks.
- Ensure that the expiration date has not passed.

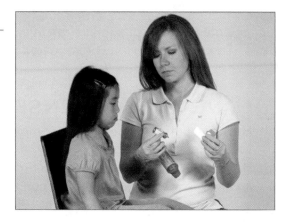

3 SHAKE INHALER

4 REMOVE MOUTHPIECE COVER

If an extension tube (spacer) is available, attach and use it.

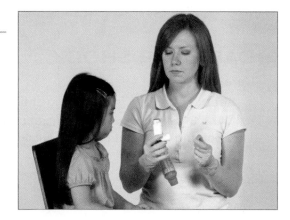

5 INSTRUCT PERSON TO BREATHE OUT

Tell the person to breathe out as much as possible through the mouth.

> **TIP:** *The person may use different techniques, such as holding the inhaler two-finger lengths away from the mouth.*

Continued on next page

6 ADMINISTER MEDICATION

Have the person place his or her lips tightly around the mouthpiece and take a long, slow breath.

- As the person breathes in slowly, administer the medication by quickly pressing down on the inhaler canister, or the person may self-administer the medication.
- The person should continue a full, deep breath.
- Tell the person to try to hold his or her breath for a count of **10**.
- When using an extension tube (spacer) have the person take **5** to **6** deep breaths through the tube without holding his or her breath.

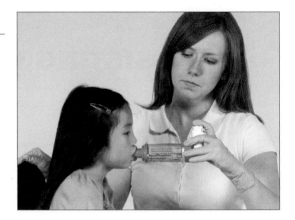

7 RECORD TIME OF ADMINISTRATION

- Note the time of administration and any change in the person's condition.
- The medication may be repeated once after **1** to **2** minutes.

8 HAVE PERSON RINSE MOUTH

Have the person rinse his or her mouth out with water to reduce side effects.

- Stay with the person and monitor his or her condition and give **CARE** for any other conditions.

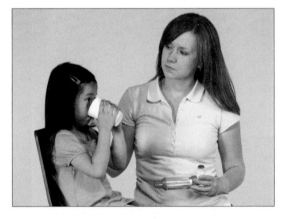

9 CARE FOR SHOCK

Care for shock.

- Keep the person from getting chilled or overheated.
- **CALL** 9-1-1 or the local emergency number if trouble breathing does not improve quickly.

> **TIP:** *These medications might take **5** to **15** minutes to reach full effectiveness. Follow label instructions regarding additional doses of the medication.*

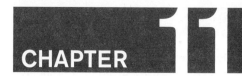
Anaphylaxis and Epinephrine Auto-Injectors

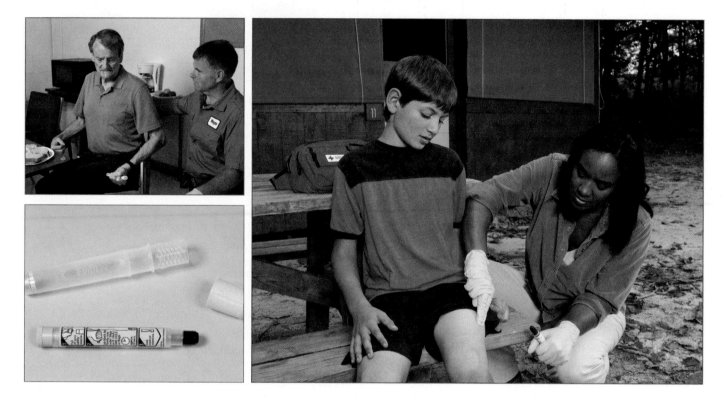

Note: *The instructions in this chapter are not a substitute for the directions given by a medical professional to an individual person. Nor should these instructions be substituted for directions given by a medical professional in consultation with a site where epinephrine auto-injectors will be used. Consult a health care professional for specific advice on the use of epinephrine auto-injectors.*

A severe allergic reaction can bring on a condition called *anaphylaxis,* also known as *anaphylactic shock.* Anaphylaxis can quickly cause trouble breathing. It is a life-threatening emergency that must be recognized and cared for immediately.

In this chapter you will learn to identify the signals of anaphylaxis. You also will learn what care to give to a person in anaphylactic shock. Part of giving care may mean helping the person use an epinephrine auto-injector.

ANAPHYLAXIS

Every year in the United States, between 400 and 800 deaths are caused by anaphylaxis. Respond quickly if a person is exposed to an *antigen*—a foreign substance that brings on an allergic reaction. Fortunately, some deaths can be prevented if anaphylaxis is recognized immediately and cared for quickly.

Allergic Reactions

Allergic reactions are caused by the activity of the *immune system*. The body recognizes and protects itself from antigens by producing *antibodies*. These antibodies fight antigens. Antibodies are found in the liver, bone marrow, spleen and lymph glands. When the immune system recognizes an antigen, it releases chemicals to fight these foreign substances and eliminate them from the body.

Antigens that cause an allergic reaction—are called *allergens*. Allergic reactions range from mild to very severe. A common mild reaction is skin irritation from contact with poison ivy. A severe, life-threatening reaction is swelling of the airway, trouble breathing and an obstructed airway.

Some common allergens include bee or insect venom, certain antibiotics, pollen, animal dander and sulfa drugs.

Over 12 million people in the United States have food allergies. Every year there are over 30,000 cases of food-related anaphylaxis. Certain types of food commonly cause an allergic reaction in individuals with sensitivities to those foods. Peanuts and tree nuts cause the most cases of fatal and near-fatal allergic reactions to food. Other common food allergens include cow's milk, eggs, seafood (especially shellfish), soy and wheat.

What to Look For

Anaphylaxis usually occurs suddenly, within seconds or minutes after contact with the substance. The skin or area of the body that comes in contact with the substance usually swells and turns red (Fig. 11-1). Other signals include the following:

- Difficulty breathing, wheezing or shortness of breath
- Tight feeling in the chest and throat
- Swelling of the face, throat or tongue
- Weakness, dizziness or confusion
- Rash or hives
- Low blood pressure
- Shock

Trouble breathing can progress to a blocked airway due to swelling of the lips, tongue, throat and larynx (voice box). Low blood pressure and shock may accompany

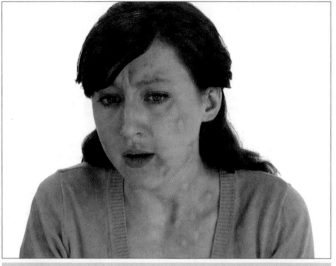

FIGURE 11-1 *In anaphylaxis, air passages can swell, restricting breathing.*

these reactions. Death from anaphylaxis may happen because the person's breathing is severely restricted.

When to Call 9-1-1

Call 9-1-1 or the local emergency number if the person:

- Has trouble breathing.
- Complains of the throat tightening.
- Explains that he or she is subject to severe allergic reactions.
- Is or becomes unconscious.

What to Do Until Help Arrives

If you suspect anaphylaxis, and have called 9-1-1 or the local emergency number, follow these guidelines for giving care:

- Monitor the person's breathing and for changes in his or her condition.
- Give care for life-threatening emergencies.
- Check a conscious person to determine:
  - The substance (antigen) involved.
  - The route of exposure to the antigen.
  - The effects of the exposure.

If the person is conscious and is able to talk, ask:

  - What is your name?
  - What happened?
  - How do you feel?
  - Do you feel any tingling in your hands, feet or lips?
  - Do you feel pain anywhere?
  - Do you have any allergies? Do you have prescribed medications to take in case of an allergic reaction?
  - Do you know what triggered the reaction?

- How much and how long were you exposed?
- Do you have any medical conditions or are you taking any medications?

Quickly check the person from head to toe. Visually inspect the body:

- Observe for signals of anaphylaxis including respiratory distress.
- Look for a medical identification (ID) tag, bracelet or necklace.

Check the person's head.

- Look for swelling of the face, neck or tongue.
- Notice if the person is drowsy, not alert, confused or exhibiting slurred speech.

Check skin appearance. Look at person's face and lips. Ask yourself, is the skin:

- Cold or hot?
- Unusually wet or dry?
- Pale, ashen, bluish or flushed?

Check the person's breathing.

- Ask if he or she is experiencing pain during breathing.
- Notice rate, depth of breaths, wheezes or gasping sounds.

Care for respiratory distress.

- Help the person to rest in the most comfortable position for breathing, usually sitting.
- Calm and reassure the person.

- Assist the person with using a prescribed epinephrine auto-injector, if available and if permitted by state regulations.
- Document any changes in the person's condition over time.

Assisting with an Epinephrine Auto-Injector

People who know they are extremely allergic to certain substances usually try to avoid them. However, sometimes this is impossible. These people may carry an anaphylaxis kit in case of a severe allergic reaction.

These kits are available by prescription only. They contain a dose (or two) of the drug *epinephrine*. This drug works in the body to counteract the anaphylactic reaction. Two injectable epinephrine systems are available: the *Epi-Pen®*, which includes one dose; and *Twinject®*, which includes two doses (Fig. 11-2, A–B). The instructions provided by the manufacturer and health care provider always

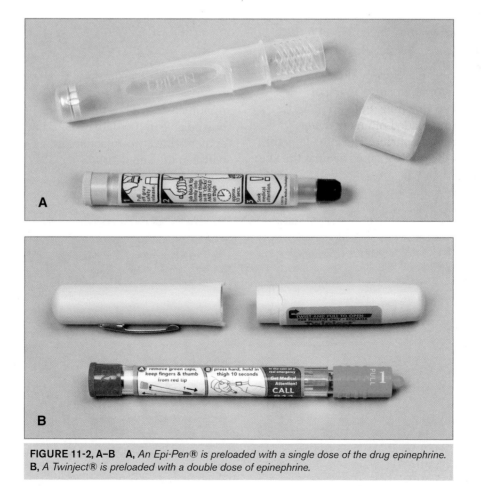

FIGURE 11-2, A–B **A,** *An Epi-Pen® is preloaded with a single dose of the drug epinephrine.* **B,** *A Twinject® is preloaded with a double dose of epinephrine.*

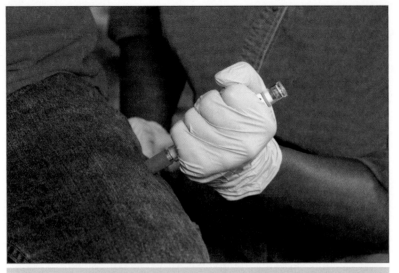

FIGURE 11-3 *Forcefully pushing the auto-injector against the skin activates the device. It should be used on a muscular area, usually the person's mid-outer thigh.*

should be followed when assisting someone with their prescribed epinephrine auto-injector. A second dose should not be given unless recommended by advanced medical personnel or in extremely unusual circumstances, where advanced medical care is not available or is significantly delayed and signals of anaphylaxis persist after a few minutes.

Note: *Only the person having the reaction should self-administer the second dose included with the Twinject® injector.*

An auto-injector contains a preloaded dose of 0.3 mg of epinephrine for adults or 0.15 mg of epinephrine for children weighing 33 to 66 pounds. The injector has a spring-loaded plunger. When activated, it injects the epinephrine. The auto-injector is activated when it is forcefully pushed against the skin.

It should be used on a muscular area, usually the person's mid-outer thigh (Fig. 11-3). The injector needs to stay in place for 10 seconds. This allows the medication to fully empty. When the auto-injector is removed, handle it carefully and do not touch the needle if it is exposed.

If a person is conscious and able to use the auto-injector, help him or her in any way asked. If you know that a person has a prescribed auto-injector and is unable to administer it him- or herself, then you may help the person use it where allowed by state or local laws or regulations. Remember, for a person experiencing anaphylaxis, time is of the essence.

Helping the Person Self-Administer an Antihistamine

Some anaphylaxis kits also contain an *antihistamine* in pill form. An antihistamine is a type of medication. It lessens the effects of compounds released by the body during an allergic reaction.

The person should read and follow all medication labels. It also is important for the person to follow any instructions given by the health care provider. Check state and local regulations about assisting someone with the use of prescription and over-the-counter medications.

PUTTING IT ALL TOGETHER

Anaphylaxis is a life-threatening emergency. Knowing how to give immediate care and help someone use an epinephrine auto-injector could mean the difference between life and death.

ASSISTING WITH AN EPINEPHRINE AUTO-INJECTOR

Determine whether the person has already taken epinephrine or antihistamine. If so, administer a second dose only when EMS personnel are not present or delayed and if signals of anaphylaxis persist after a few minutes. Check the label to confirm that the prescription of the auto-injector is for this person.

Check the expiration date of the auto-injector. If it has expired, DO NOT USE IT. If the medication is visible, confirm that the liquid is clear and not cloudy. If it is cloudy, DO NOT USE IT.

NOTE: *If possible, help the person self-administer the auto-injector.*

TO CARE FOR A CONSCIOUS PERSON WHO IS UNABLE TO SELF-ADMINISTER THE AUTO-INJECTOR, AND LOCAL OR STATE REGULATIONS ALLOW:

1 LOCATE INJECTION SITE

Locate the outside middle of one thigh to use as the injection site.

NOTE: *If injecting through clothing, press on the area with a hand to determine that there are no obstructions at the injection site, such as keys, coins, the side seam of trousers, etc.*

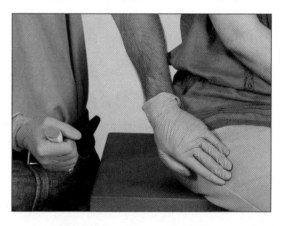

2 REMOVE SAFETY CAP

Grasp the auto-injector firmly in your fist, and pull off the safety cap with your other hand.

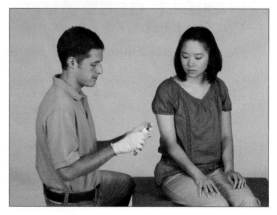

3 POSITION AUTO-INJECTOR

Hold the tip (needle end) near the patient's outer thigh so that the auto-injector is at a 90-degree angle to the thigh.

Continued on next page

4 ADMINISTER INJECTION

Quickly and firmly push the tip straight into the outer thigh. You will hear a click.

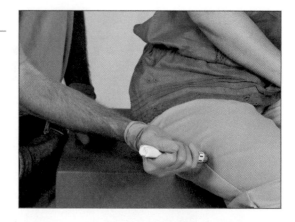

5 HOLD IN PLACE

Hold the auto-injector firmly in place for **10** seconds, then remove it from the thigh and massage the injection site with a gloved hand for several seconds.

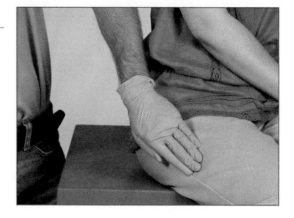

6 RECHECK BREATHING

Recheck the person's breathing and observe his or her response to the medication.

7 HANDLE USED AUTO-INJECTOR CAREFULLY

Handle the used auto-injector carefully, placing it in a safe container. Give it to EMS personnel when they arrive.

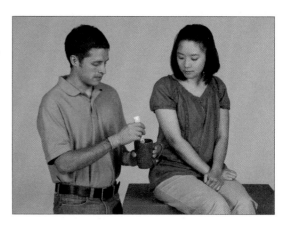

Injury Prevention and Emergency Preparedness

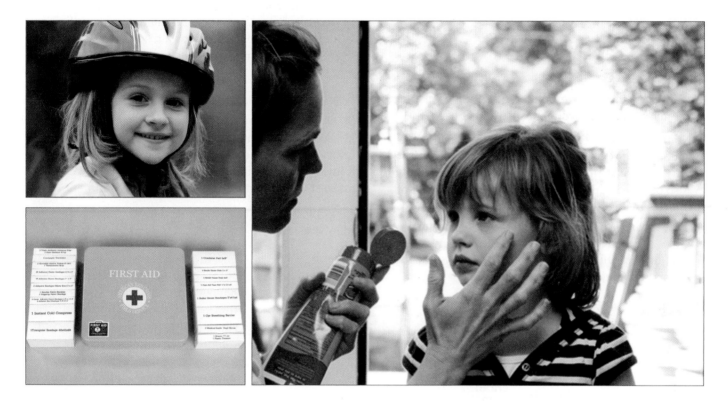

Unintentional injuries cause disability and death for thousands of people in the United States each year. These injuries incur billions of dollars in lost wages, medical expenses, insurance, property damage and other indirect costs.

Injuries are not always inevitable. Being prepared and following established safety precautions can reduce risk, prevent injuries and save lives.

INJURIES

Every year in the United States millions of people suffer an unintentional injury. In 2007, nearly 124,000 Americans died from these injuries. That year, unintentional injury was the leading cause of death for people 1 to 44 years of age; of these, motor-vehicle crashes were the number one cause of death from unintentional injury, followed by poisoning and falls (Fig. A-1). In 2007, American also sustained approximately 34.3 million nonfatal injuries that required medical attention.

Injury Risk Factors

Several factors affect a person's risk of being injured. These factors include age, gender, geographic location, economic status and alcohol misuse and abuse.

■ Nonfatal injury rates remain highest among people younger than 39 years; however, deaths from injury are more common in people 40 years of age and older. Also of note is this age group has the highest rate of injuries that result in death.

■ Gender also is a significant factor in risk of injury. Males are at greater risk than females for any type of injury. In general, men are about twice as likely to suffer a fatal injury as women.

■ Environmental and economic factors influence injury rates. Living on a farm or in the city, having a home made of wood or brick, using a specific type of heat in your home and your local climate all affect your degree of risk. For instance, death rates from injury are higher in rural areas as opposed to metropolitan areas. The death rate from injuries is twice as high in low-income areas as in high-income areas.

■ Alcohol misuse and abuse is a significant factor in many injuries and fatalities, in both teenagers and adults. In 2008, 32 percent of all motor-vehicle deaths were alcohol related. It is estimated that a significant number of victims who die as a result of falls, drowning and fires were under the influence of alcohol.

Reducing Your Risk of Injury

Statistics show that people of certain ages and gender are injured more often than others. However, the chances of injury have more to do with a person's behavior. Many injuries are preventable and result from the way people interact with potential dangers in the environment.

Risks of an injury can be reduced by taking the following steps:

■ Know the risk.

■ Take measures that make a difference. Change behaviors that increase your risk of injury and your risk injuring others.

■ Think safety. Be alert for and avoid potentially harmful conditions or activities that increase your risk of injury. Take precautions, such as wearing appropriate protective devices, including helmets, padding and eyewear. Always buckle up when driving or riding in motor vehicles.

■ Learn and use first aid skills. There have been dramatic improvements in emergency medical systems nationwide over the past decade; however, you are the person who often makes the difference between life and death. Apply your first aid training when necessary.

In addition to these personal steps, laws and consumer protection regulations have been put in place to reduce or prevent injury. Examples include laws on the mandatory use of safety belts, manufacturers' requirements to build air bags into motor vehicles and restrictions on the use of cell phones while driving.

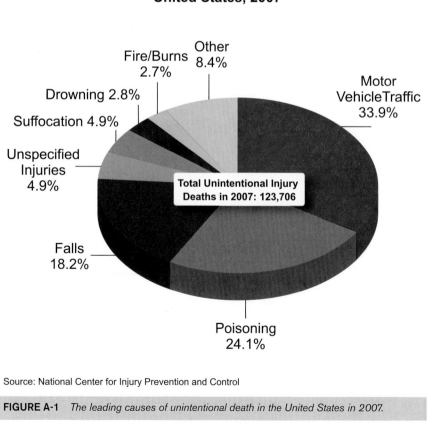

Leading Causes of Unintentional Injury Deaths United States, 2007

- Other 8.4%
- Fire/Burns 2.7%
- Drowning 2.8%
- Suffocation 4.9%
- Unspecified Injuries 4.9%
- Motor Vehicle Traffic 33.9%
- Total Unintentional Injury Deaths in 2007: 123,706
- Falls 18.2%
- Poisoning 24.1%

Source: National Center for Injury Prevention and Control

FIGURE A-1 *The leading causes of unintentional death in the United States in 2007.*

DEVELOPING A PLAN OF ACTION

Emergencies can happen quickly. There may not be time to consider what to do, only time to react. You can improve your response and the outcome of emergencies by developing a plan. Meet with your family or household members to gather information for an emergency action plan.

Think about your home:

- *Style of home (e.g., mobile, high-rise apartment, single family) and type of construction (e.g., wood, brick)*
- *Location of sleeping areas (e.g., basement, ground floor, second floor)*
- *Location of windows*
- *Number and location of smoke alarms*
- *Location of gasoline, solvent or paint storage*
- *Number and types of locks on doors*
- *Location of telephones, flashlights, fire extinguisher and first aid kit*

Think about who lives in your home:

- *Total number of people and number of people older than 65 years or younger than 6 years of age*
- *Number of people sleeping above or below the ground floor*
- *Number of people who are unable to exit without help*

Think about the types of possible emergencies that you may face:

- *Injuries (e.g., fall or cut)*
- *Illnesses (e.g., stroke or heart attack)*
- *Natural disasters (e.g., tornado or earthquake)*
- *Fire*

Write down the list of emergencies that you could face. Under each one write:

1. *How the emergency would affect your home.*
2. *How you would like the people in your home to react. Specifically, what would be the responsibilities for each member of the household in an emergency?*
3. *The steps you have already taken to prevent or minimize the effect of the emergency.*
4. *The steps you still need to take.*

Try to imagine as many situations as possible for each emergency. Gather information from sources such as insurance companies, your city or county emergency management office and your police, fire or rescue department.

When thinking about emergencies away from home:

- *Use the same process to decide what to do.*

When you reach a decision, write it down. You now have a personal emergency plan. Practice it. Keep it current.

It also is important to develop a plan of action in case of an emergency. Being prepared for an emergency before it actually occurs will help you, and those with whom you live, to react calmly in a stressful situation. See Focus on Preparedness: Developing a Plan of Action above.

Vehicle Safety

Tens of thousands of people in the United States die in motor-vehicle crashes each year. Crash injuries result in nearly 5 million emergency department visits annually. The economic burden of these motor-vehicle-related deaths and injuries is significant.

Do not drink and drive. If you are going to consume alcohol, plan ahead to find a ride, or take a cab or public transportation. If you are with a group, designate a driver who agrees not to drink on this occasion.

Do not become distracted. Doing things that take your eyes off the road, your hands off the wheel or your mind off of driving are distractions that can be dangerous or even fatal. The use of electronic devices while driving, such as talking on hand-held cell phones and text messaging, causes thousands of collisions and highway fatalities. Other distractions while driving include eating and drinking; talking to passengers; reading; using navigation systems; and operating radios and CD or MP3 players. Many states and the District of Columbia have enacted laws restricting the use of hand-held cell phones and electronic devices.

When riding in a motor vehicle, always buckle up. Although cars more often are equipped with airbags than not, wearing a safety belt is the easiest and best way to prevent injury in a motor-vehicle collision. Always wear a safety belt, including a shoulder restraint, when riding in either the front or back seat. In 49 states and the District of Columbia, wearing a safety belt is required by law. In 2007, safety belts saved more than 13,000 lives.

Although airbags have saved many lives, they pose several risks to children. The amount of force during airbag deployment can kill or severely injure children occupying the front seat. Even when in a car seat, infants could be at risk. An infant in a rear-facing car seat is close to the dashboard and therefore could easily be struck by the airbag with sufficient force to cause serious harm or even death. Always have children younger than 13 years sit in the back seat, away from airbags.

Child Safety Seats

Motor-vehicle crashes are the leading cause of injury-related deaths for children. All 50 states and the District of Columbia require the use of child safety seats and child safety belts. *Always* have infants and children ride in the back seat in safety seats that are approved for the child's weight and/or age (Fig. A-2).

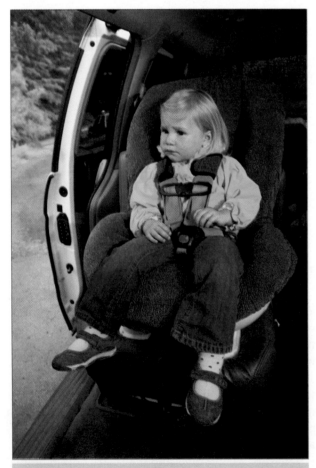

FIGURE A-2 *Infants and children always should ride in an approved safety seat.*

Choosing the proper child safety seat to fit the weight and age of your child is only the first step. Another important child-safety-seat issue is making sure that the child safety seat is installed correctly in your vehicle. The National Highway Traffic Safety Administration (NHTSA) estimates that three out of four parents do not properly use child restraints. It is essential to always read the instruction manual. Every manufacturer of child safety seats provides specific instructions about how to use and install its seat. To make sure that you installed your child safety seat correctly in your vehicle, you can have it checked by professionals. Contact NHTSA for information on finding a nearby child safety seat inspection station.

Fire Safety

Fire safety in the home and in hotels is essential. You should learn how to prevent fires but also know what to do in case a fire does occur.

Home Fire Safety Prevention and Preparation

In 2006, 3202 people died in unintentional fires in the United States. Approximately four of 10 deaths from fires occurring in the home occurred in homes without smoke alarms. To prevent fires:

- Install a smoke alarm on every floor of your home. Check the batteries once a month, and change the batteries at least twice a year.
- Keep fire extinguishers where they are most likely to be needed and keep matches out of children's reach.
- Always keep space heaters away from curtains and other flammable materials.
- Install guards around fireplaces, radiators, pipes and wood-burning stoves.

Regardless of the cause of fires, everyone needs to know how to respond in case of fire. Plan and practice a fire escape route with your family or roommates (Fig. A-3):

- Gather everyone together at a convenient time.
- Sketch a floor plan of all rooms, including doors, windows and hallways, for all floors of the home.
- Draw the escape plan with arrows showing two ways, if possible, to get out of each room. Sleeping areas are the most important, since many fires happen at night.
- Plan to use stairs only, never an elevator.
- Plan where everyone will meet after leaving the building.
- Designate who should call the fire department and from which phone.

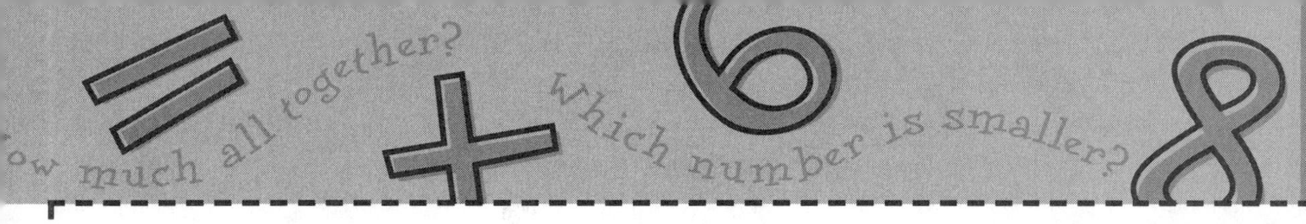

Name ______________________________

Counting

Hide-and-Seek Countdown

Jack Rabbit was playing "Hide and Seek." He was "It"! He had to count backwards from 10. Help Jack Rabbit by filling in the missing numbers.

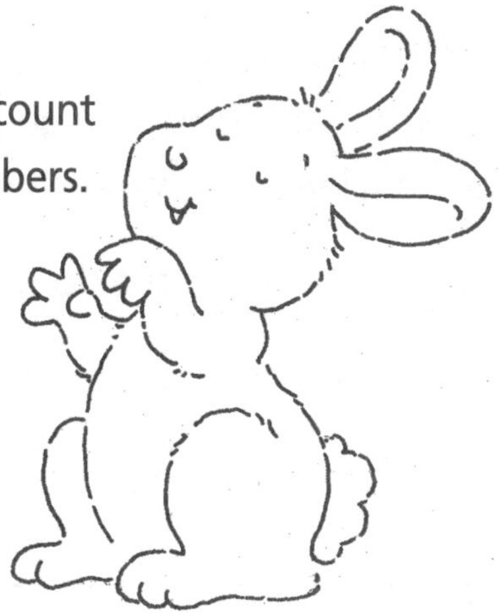

10, 9 ______, 7, 6, ______, ______, 3, ______, 1

Extra: Help Jack Rabbit count backwards from 20 to 11.

20, ______, 18, 17, ______, 15, 14, ______, ______, 11

Name ______________________________

Graphing, Comparing

Apple Colors

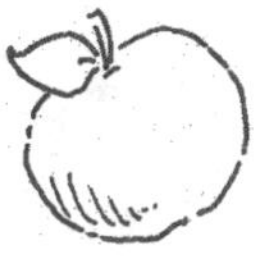

Apples can be red, yellow, or green. Ask your classmates which color apple they like best. Color in the boxes in the correct rows to show their answers.

Red																				
Yellow																				
Green																				

Which apple is the class favorite? ______________________________

Name ______________________________

Addition

Adding in Code

The number words below are missing vowels. Fill in the vowels to solve the code.

There were T H R ______ ______ plus F______ ______ R apples on my tree.
I picked them so they would not fall.

When I added them up, my total was S ______ V ______ N.
That's how many apples I had in all!

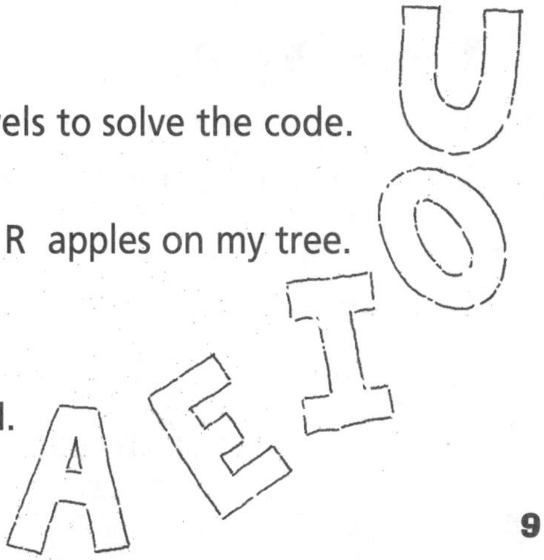

How many in each group? What patterns do you see?

Name _____

Pencil Puzzler

Katie Kangaroo started school with 6 new pencils. She lost 4.
Her friend Kenny gave her 2.

How many pencils does Katie have now? _____

Write your math equations here:

_____

_____

Name _____

One Bee in Our Classroom

Complete the poem by filling in the missing numbers.

1 bee in our classroom, and then there were 3.

Soon there were 5, straight from the hive.

Next there were _____.   That wasn't so fine.

And when the day ended, the total was _____.

Hint: Look for a pattern.

Name _____

Apple Problems

Nick needs to buy 8 apples. He needs the same number of red apples and green apples.
How many apples should he buy of each? Color in the apples to figure it out!

He needs _____ green apples and _____ red apples.

Extra: What if Nick needed 10, 12, 14, 16, or 18 apples?
Write your ideas on the back.

Name _____

Recognizing Shapes

Shapes All Around

Look around the classroom. What shapes do you see? Fill in each blank with an object.

The _____ is a rectangle.

The _____ is a square.

The _____ is a circle.

Shapes are everywhere!

Name _____

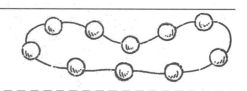

Recognizing Patterns

Red, Black, Snap, Clap

The beads on Beth's bracelet look like this: red, black, black, red, black, black, red, black, black, red.

What are the next three colors in the pattern? _____

Make the same pattern using the letters A and B. _____

Extra: Make the same pattern using snaps and claps.

Name _____

Addition

The Last Leaves

From their home in a tree, Sid Squirrel said to his little sister Sally, "The oak tree has 5 leaves left. The maple tree has 3 more leaves than the oak.   How many leaves does the maple have?"

Draw a picture on the back to find the answer.

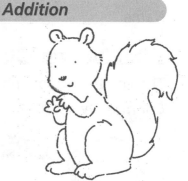

Extra: Write a math equation here: _____

Name _____

Falling Leaves

Solve this math riddle:

10 autumn leaves were hanging on a tree.
Along came the wind
and then there were 3.
How many leaves fell down on me? _____

Extra: Substitute a different number for 3.

- - -

Name _____

Classroom Zoo

These animals are in
Ms. Zooey's classroom zoo.
Cut out the animals.
Sort them into 3 groups.

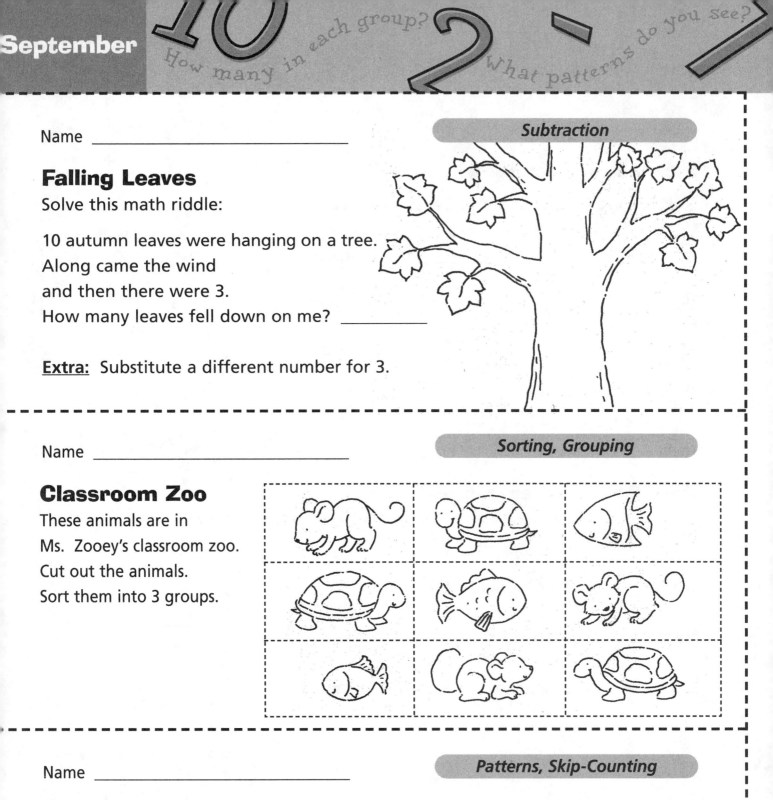

- - -

Name _____

Who Needs Glasses?

The children below had their eyes examined. How many eyes got checked? _____
Count by twos.

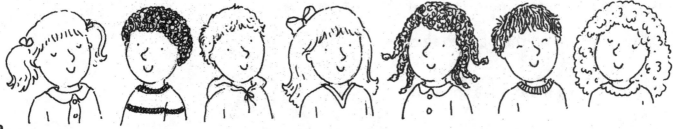

Frog School

At Frog School, Croaker Frog and his friends sit on lily pads.
Are there enough lily pads for all the frogs in Croaker's class?
Draw lines to match the frogs with the lily pads.

Extra

How many frogs need lily pads? _____.

13

Big Foot

Benny Bear needed new shoes for the first day of school.
Here is his footprint.

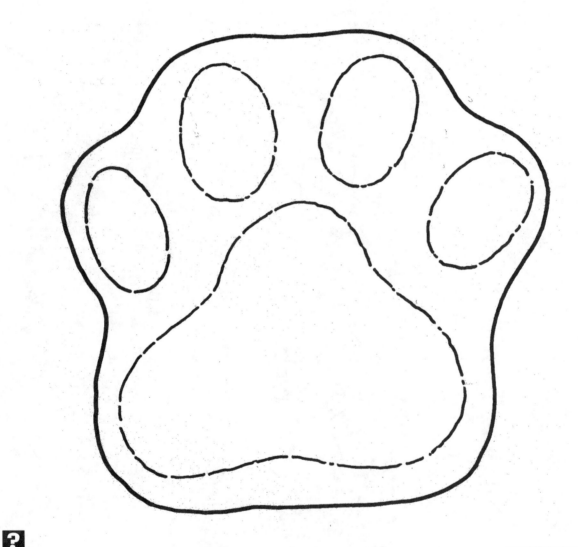

?

Estimate how many inches his foot is from top to bottom.

_____

Now measure his foot. You can use linking cubes or a ruler.

How many inches is his foot? _____

Mary Had a Little Puppy

Read the rhyme below.

Fill in the blanks with the correct words from the box.

above	followed	up	in	under

Mary had a little puppy

that _____ her to school.

The birds that flew _____ the puppy

said, "That's against the rule."

The puppy ran _____ the jungle gym.

Then he went _____ the classroom door.

He jumped _____ on the teacher's desk,

and barked and yipped and barked some more.

Extra

Color and cut out the figures below. Use them to act out the story.

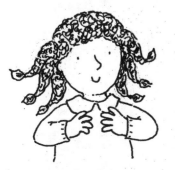

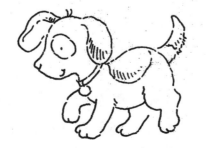

15

Name _____

Fall Leaf Patterns

Fred made a pattern using the leaves below. You can make patterns too. First, color the leaves as shown in the small boxes. Then color and cut out the bigger leaves. Use the leaves to make patterns.

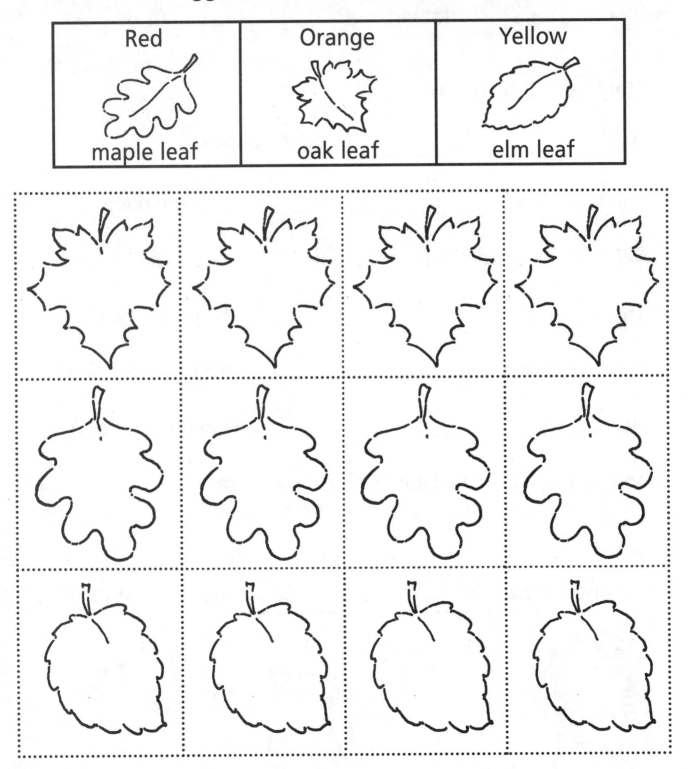

| Red | Orange | Yellow |
| maple leaf | oak leaf | elm leaf |

October

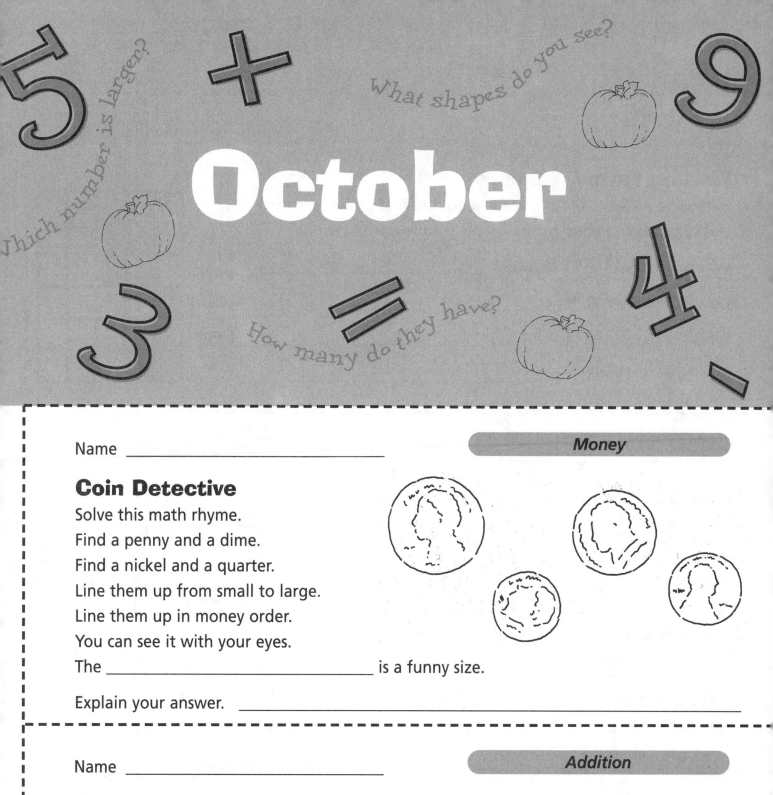

Name _____

Coin Detective

Solve this math rhyme.
Find a penny and a dime.
Find a nickel and a quarter.
Line them up from small to large.
Line them up in money order.
You can see it with your eyes.
The _____ is a funny size.

Explain your answer. _____

Name _____

Finger-Adding Game

Play this game with a partner. Say, "Ready, set, go." Then you and your partner both hold out some fingers on one hand. Try to get a sum of 5 when you add the fingers on both your hands. No talking!

How many tries does it take? _____

As a class, record the diffferent ways to make 5.

Extra: Try it with a different number, like 7 or 8!

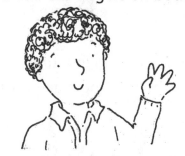

How many in each group?

What patterns do you see?

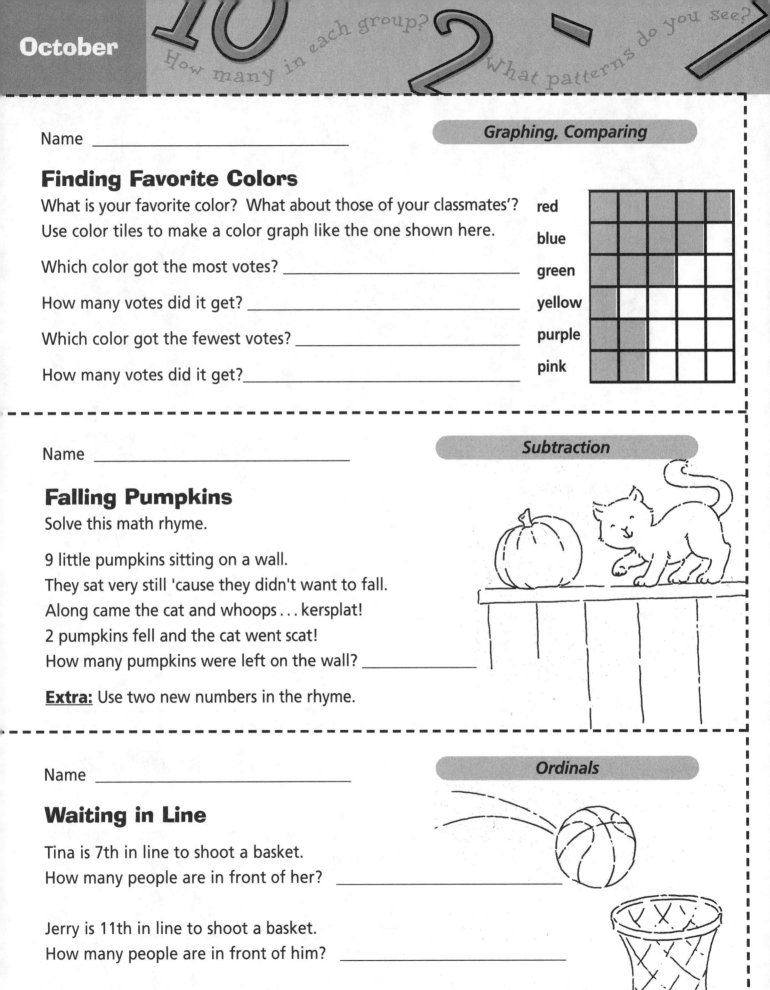

Name _____

Finding Favorite Colors

What is your favorite color? What about those of your classmates'?
Use color tiles to make a color graph like the one shown here.

Which color got the most votes? _____

How many votes did it get? _____

Which color got the fewest votes? _____

How many votes did it get?_____

red

blue

green

yellow

purple

pink

Name _____

Subtraction

Falling Pumpkins

Solve this math rhyme.

9 little pumpkins sitting on a wall.
They sat very still 'cause they didn't want to fall.
Along came the cat and whoops . . . kersplat!
2 pumpkins fell and the cat went scat!
How many pumpkins were left on the wall? _____

Extra: Use two new numbers in the rhyme.

Name _____

Ordinals

Waiting in Line

Tina is 7th in line to shoot a basket.
How many people are in front of her? _____

Jerry is 11th in line to shoot a basket.
How many people are in front of him? _____

Name _____

Subtraction

One and Only One

A silly king liked being number 1. So he made subtraction equations where all the answers were 1. He used the numbers 1, 2, 3, 4, and 5. Which equations did he make?

_____ – _____ = 1

_____ – _____ = 1

_____ – _____ = 1

_____ – _____ = 1

Name _____

Identifying Solid Shapes

Shape Hunters

Be a shape hunter. Fill in the blanks. Use the words in the box.

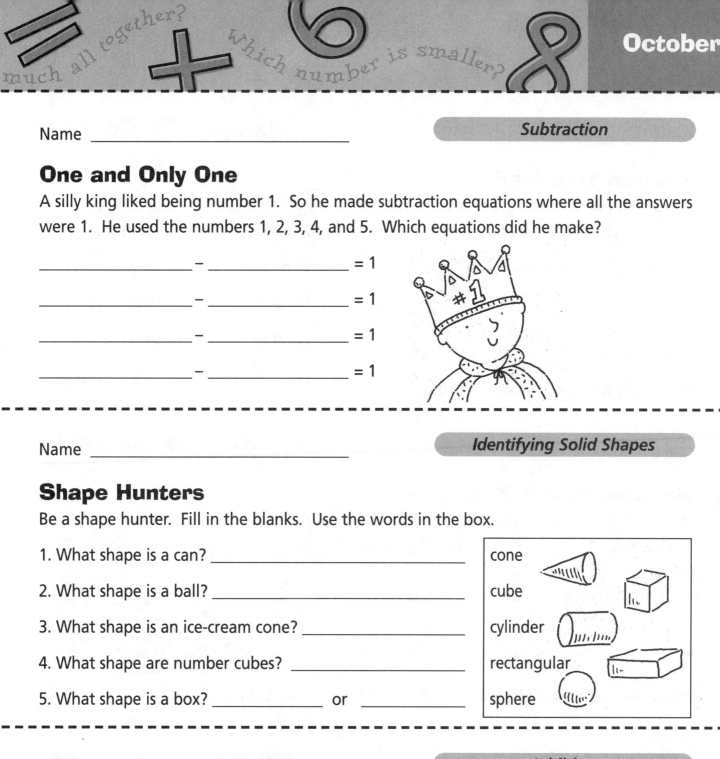

1. What shape is a can? _____

2. What shape is a ball? _____

3. What shape is an ice-cream cone? _____

4. What shape are number cubes? _____

5. What shape is a box? _____ or _____

cone

cube

cylinder

rectangular

sphere

Name _____

Addition

Poodles and Beagles

When Asheem went to the park, he counted 8 dogs. Some were poodles and some were beagles. How many poodles and how many beagles could there have been? Write as many number sentences as you can. Here is an example:

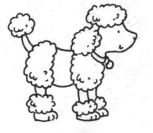

1 poodle + 7 beagles = 8 dogs in all

Use the other side or another sheet of paper to write your number sentence.

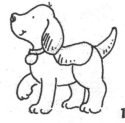

How many in each group?

What patterns do you see?

Name _____

Big Bad Wolf Math

The Big Bad Wolf is visiting the three little pigs. He is measuring their houses using his hands and feet. Circle "hand spans" or "giant steps" to show how he should measure these lengths.

1. The width of the third pig's door

   hand span   giant steps

2. The width of the third pig's house

   hand span   giant steps

3. The length from the first pig's house to the second pig's house

   hand span   giant steps

4. The width of the chimney opening

   hand span   giant steps

Name _____

National Cookie Month

October is National Cookie Month. Bethany and two friends baked 9 cookies. They divided the cookies into 3 equal piles.

How many cookies did each friend have?

_____

Extra: How many cookies would each friend have if they baked 12 cookies?

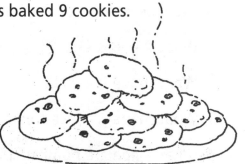

Name _____

Disappearing Counting Cubes

Play this game with a partner. Put 8 counters or cubes on a desk.

Close your eyes. Have your partner take away some of the counters.

Open your eyes. How many counters are left? _____

How many counters did your partner take? _____

Extra: Switch roles and play the game again!

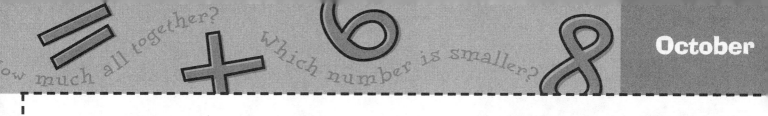
Name _____

Addition, Subtraction

Nan's Number Cubes

Nan threw two number cubes.

When she added the dots, she got 7.

One of the cubes looked like the one shown here.

What did the other cube look like?

Draw in the dots.

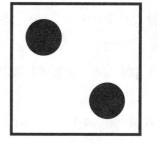

Name _____

Recognizing Shapes

Jack-O'-Lantern Designer

Make a jack-o-lantern face using 2 triangles, 2 squares
1 rectangle, and 1 circle.

Don't forget to draw teeth!

Extra: On the back make one more face.

Name _____

Adding Sums of 10

Three Halloween Kittens

Three black kittens weigh 10 pounds all together. One kitten weighs 4 pounds.

How much could each of the other two weigh?

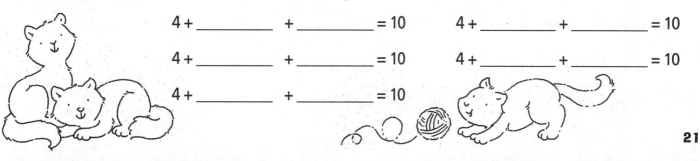

$4 + \underline{\hspace{1.5cm}} + \underline{\hspace{1.5cm}} = 10$ $4 + \underline{\hspace{1.5cm}} + \underline{\hspace{1.5cm}} = 10$

$4 + \underline{\hspace{1.5cm}} + \underline{\hspace{1.5cm}} = 10$ $4 + \underline{\hspace{1.5cm}} + \underline{\hspace{1.5cm}} = 10$

$4 + \underline{\hspace{1.5cm}} + \underline{\hspace{1.5cm}} = 10$

October
How many in each group?
What patterns do you see?

Name _____

Trick or Treat?

Ashley and Ben went trick-or-treating.

Mrs. Story gave Ashley 3 treats. Mr. Story gave her 2 more.

Mrs. Story gave Ben 2 treats. Mr. Story gave him 3 more.

Did Ashley and Ben get the same number of treats? _____

Write the equations to show how you know:

_____   _____

Name _____

Comparing Costumes

Beth went trick-or-treating with 11 friends.
8 friends were wearing scary costumes.

How many were wearing other kinds of costumes?

_____

Write the equation to show how you know:

_____

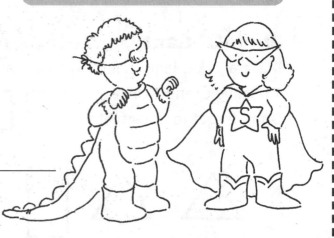

Name _____

What's Your Costume?

Make a Halloween graph of the costumes in your class. Use these categories or ones you make up: **story character, funny, scary.** Draw your graph on another sheet of paper.

Which category has the most costumes? _____

How many does it have? _____

Which category has the fewest costumes? _____

A Friendly Scarecrow

This scarecrow has 2 birds on his right arm and 2 birds on his left arm.

How many birds are there in all?_____

Write the equation to show how you know:

_____

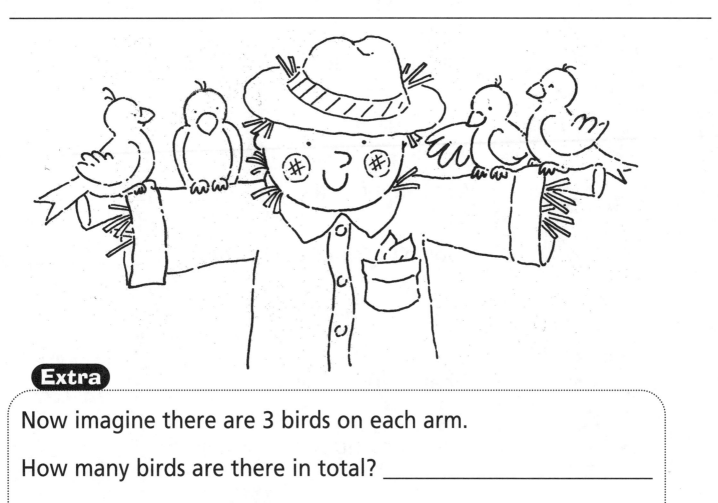

Extra

Now imagine there are 3 birds on each arm.

How many birds are there in total? _____

Imagine there are 4 birds on each arm.

How many birds are there in total? _____

What pattern do the numbers make? _____

_____

Sign Shape

Street signs come in different shapes. Use string to form the shapes below. Work with a partner. Answer the questions below about the shapes, too.

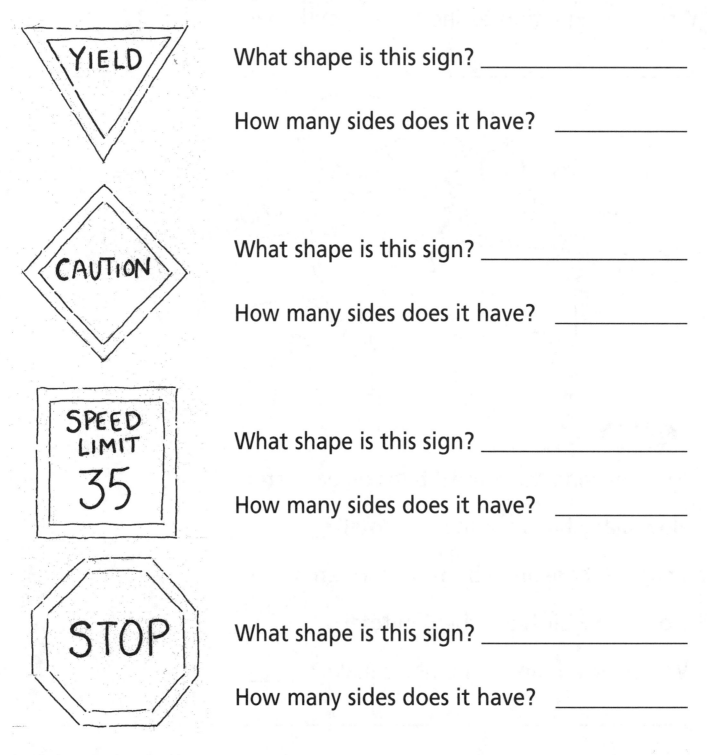

What shape is this sign? _____

How many sides does it have? _____

What shape is this sign? _____

How many sides does it have? _____

What shape is this sign? _____

How many sides does it have? _____

What shape is this sign? _____

How many sides does it have? _____

Ladybug Dots

Every year, ladybugs hibernate when the weather gets cool.
Count the dots on each ladybug wing. Then write an equation to
show the total number of dots each ladybug has. The first one has
been done for you.

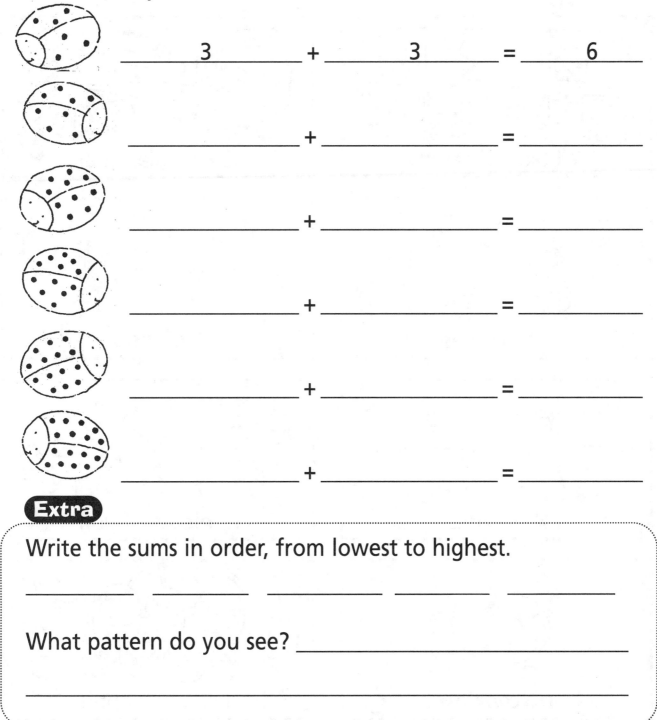

_____3_____ + _____3_____ = _____6_____

_____ + _____ = _____

_____ + _____ = _____

_____ + _____ = _____

_____ + _____ = _____

_____ + _____ = _____

Extra

Write the sums in order, from lowest to highest.

_____ _____ _____ _____ _____

What pattern do you see? _____

_____

Name _____

Sorting Treats

Look at the Halloween treats below. Cut apart the boxes.
Then sort them into 2 piles. One pile is for numbers greater
than 10. The other pile is for numbers less than 10.

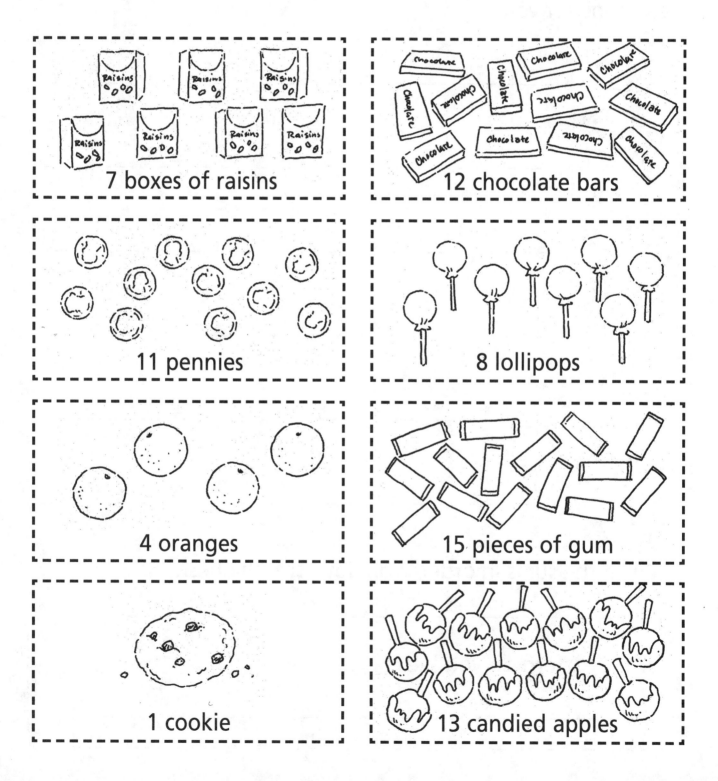

7 boxes of raisins

12 chocolate bars

11 pennies

8 lollipops

4 oranges

15 pieces of gum

1 cookie

13 candied apples

November

Which number is larger?

What shapes do you see?

How many do they have?

Name _____

Piggy Bank Puzzle

Tina heard her brother Joey counting coins.

Here's what Joey was saying: " . . . 30, 40, 50, 60 . . . "

What kind of coins was Joey counting? _____

Joey counted other coins. Tina heard, " . . . 30, 35, 40, 45 . . . "

What kind of coins was he counting now? _____

Name _____

Favorite Pet Tally

Elections are held in November. Have an election in your class. Ask your classmates to vote on which of the following animals they would like to have as a class mascot. Make tally marks next to each animal to show how your classmates voted.

dog _____   cat _____   bird _____   rabbit _____   other

Which animal was voted the mascot? _____

Name _____

Playing in the Snow

A big snow storm dropped a lot of snow! Harry and his dog played in the snow for 6 days one week. Then they played for 7 days the next week. Use "doubles +1" to find out how many days they played in all. Write your equations on the lines. First write the doubles. Then the doubles plus one.

_____

_____

Name _____

ABC Sort

Look at the letters below. How could you sort them? Come up with categories and label them. Then list the letters for each. Show your work on the back of this paper, or on another sheet.

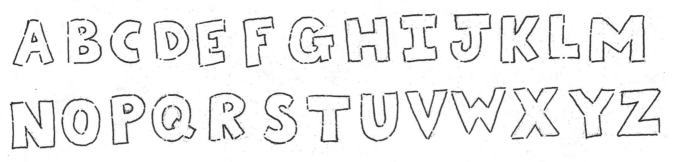

A B C D E F G H I J K L M
N O P Q R S T U V W X Y Z

Name _____

How Many Birthdays?

In November, Timmy was 7 years old. How many more birthdays will Timmy have before he is 11, like his older brother? _____

Write the equations here to show how you know:

_____

Extra: When Timmy is 11, how old will his brother be? _____

28

Name _____

Addition, Subtraction

Game and Puzzle Week

The 4th week of November is "Game and Puzzle Week." To celebrate, see how many addition and subtraction equations you can make using only the numbers 2, 7, and 9.

_____
_____
_____
_____

Name _____

Greater Than/Less Than, Addition

Birthday Riddle

Solve this math riddle.

On his birthday, David said:
"I am less than 10.
I am more than 4 + 4.
How old am I?"

_____

Name _____

Addition, Subtraction

Sledding Time

Eddie and his friends went sledding. There were 5 girls and 3 boys.
Make up an addition problem and a subtraction problem. Then solve them.

Addition: _____

_____

Subtraction: _____

_____

How many in each group?

What patterns do you see?

Name _____

Wildlife Shelter

Josie volunteers at the wildlife shelter. In one year she helped 39 squirrels, 45 birds, and 28 gophers. Fill in the blanks with these numbers to show greater than and less than.

_____ > _____   _____ < _____

_____ > _____   _____ < _____

Extra: Read your results aloud to a partner.

Name _____

Position Words, Shapes

Mystery Drawing

Follow these directions to draw a mystery animal.

1. On another sheet of paper, draw a big circle in the middle.
2. To the left of the big circle, draw a little circle that touches the big circle.
3. Inside the little circle, draw a little square.
4. At the bottom of the big circle, draw two triangles that touch the circle.
5. To the right of the big circle, draw three long, thin, rectangles that touch the circle.
6. To the left of the little circle, draw a triangle that touches the circle and looks like a beak.

What did you draw?_____

Name _____

Adding Sums of 10

Gobbler Riddle

Solve this math riddle:

10 little gobblers sitting on a wall.

How many are big?

How many are small?

Write as many equations as you can that equal 10. Use the back of this sheet.

Example: $1 + 9 = 10$

Name _____

Thanksgiving Puzzler

Every year on Thanksgiving, someone at Teresa's house makes up a puzzle.
This year, Teresa said, "Which answer has the largest number: 11 - 3, 11 - 5, or 11 - 7?"
Try to solve Teresa's puzzle! Write your answer on the lines below
and explain it.

_____

_____

_____

Name _____

Mystery Holiday

Look at a calendar. Find the 11th month.

What is it? _____

Now find the last Thursday of that month.

What is the date? _____

Which holiday do we celebrate on that day?

_____

Name _____

Mashed, Baked, or Fried?

What kinds of potatoes do you and your classmates like to eat on Thanksgiving? Draw a tally
mark next to each potato dish. If the dish is not listed, draw a tally mark next to "other."

mashed _____   baked _____

fried _____   other _____

Count up the tally marks for each potato.
Which potato dish is the class favorite? _____

Scavenger Hunt

Cut out the acorn ruler on this page.
Each acorn is 1– inch long.
Use the acorn ruler for this scavenger hunt.

1. Find an object that is 2 inches long.

_____

2. Find an object that is 4 inches long.

_____

3. Find an object that is 6 inches long.

_____

4. Find an object that is 8 inches long.

_____

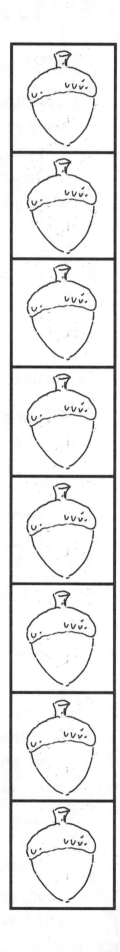

Collecting Food

Lan's class collected food to give to needy families on Thanksgiving. Cut out the cans below. Sort them into three groups. On another sheet of paper, make a bar graph to show how many cans are in each group. Name the groups.

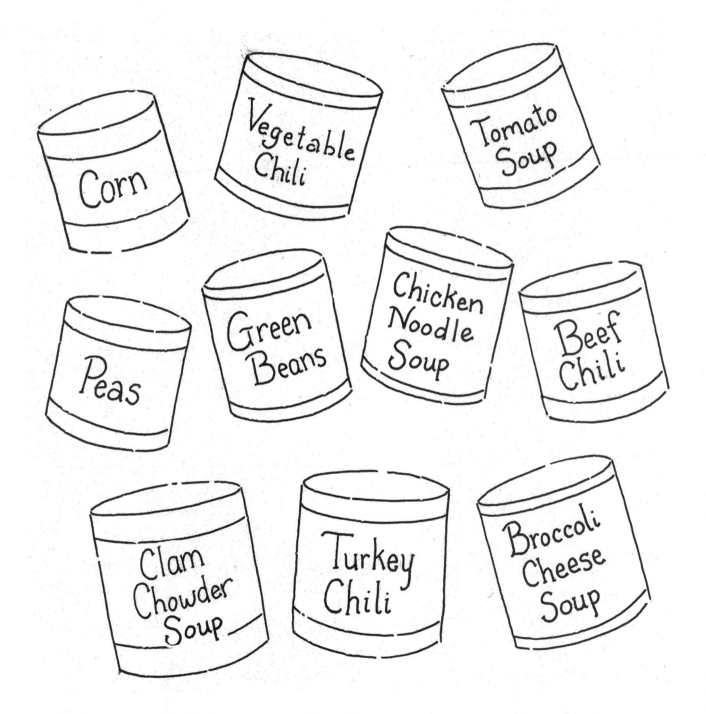

Money Matters

Alex asked his little brother Billy to trade piggy banks.

Alex's bank has these coins: Billy's has these coins:

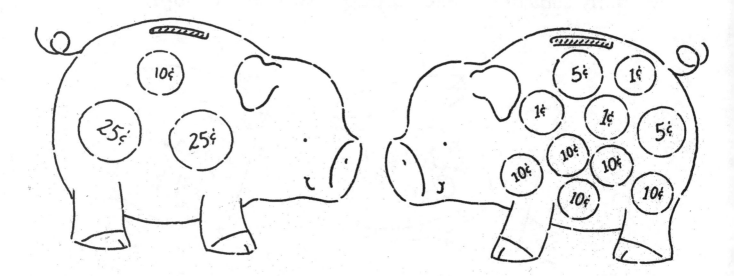

Extra

Do you think this is a fair trade? _____

Test your answer:

Add up Alex's coins: _____

Add up Billy's coins: _____

Write the totals in this Greater Than/Less Than equation:

_____ > _____

Who has more money? _____

Name _____

Penguin Family on Parade

The penguin family is part of the winter parade. They need to line up from shortest to tallest. Give them a hand! Use a ruler to measure each penguin. Label each penguin with its height. Then write the name of each penguin in size order, from smallest to tallest.

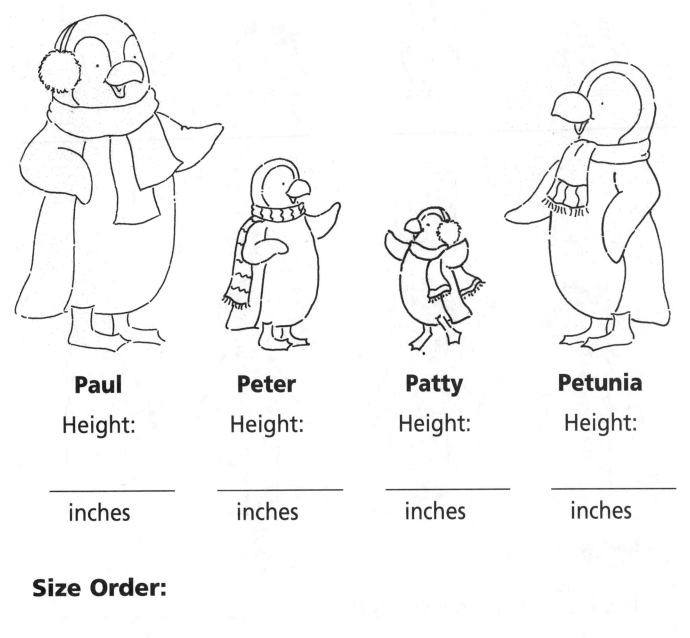

Paul

Height:

_____

inches

Peter

Height:

_____

inches

Patty

Height:

_____

inches

Petunia

Height:

_____

inches

Size Order:

_____ _____ _____ _____

(smallest)   (tallest)

Thanksgiving Play

The class put on a Thanksgiving play. Two children were playing Pilgrims. The total number of children playing Native Americans was 2 more than the number of children playing Pilgrims. Draw Pilgrim or Native American costumes on the correct number of children.

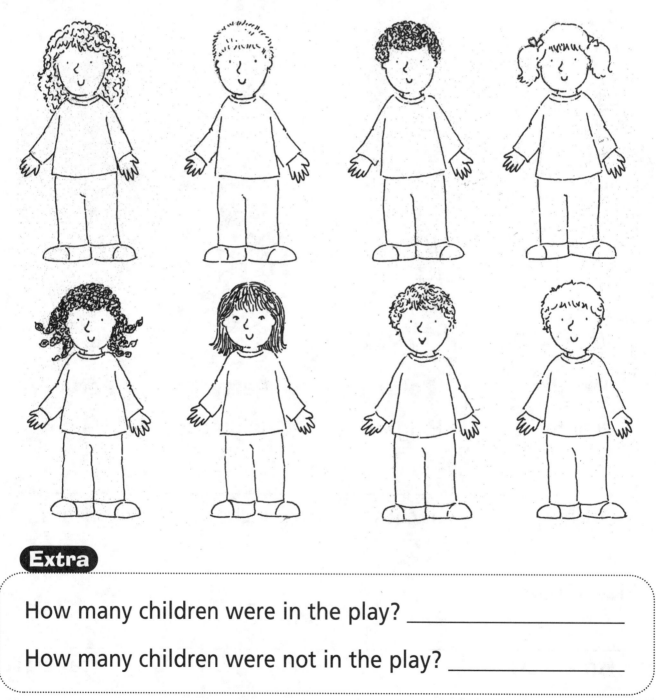

Extra

How many children were in the play? _____

How many children were not in the play? _____

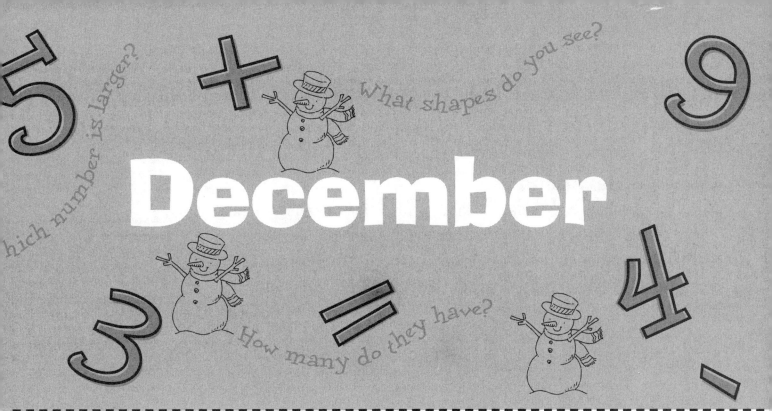

Name _____

On and Off the Bus

Solve this rhyming math riddle:

4 kids are riding on the bus.
2 kids get off, 3 more get on.
The wheels turn, the horn goes beep,
They sing a song to the driver, Ron.

How many kids sing to the driver? _____

Write your equation. _____

Name _____

Magic Tricks

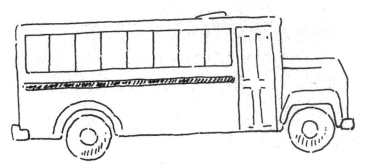

Jerry did magic tricks at his birthday party. Write equations
for the tricks below. Use 0 (zero) in each equation.

Trick 1: Jerry put 6 rabbits in a
hat and made them disappear.

Trick 2: Jerry had no birds. He stuck his
hand in his sleeve and pulled out 5 birds.

_____   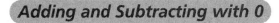_____

37

How many in each group?

2

What patterns do you see?

Name _____

Beehive Hexagons

A cell in a beehive has 6 sides. A shape with 6 sides is called a hexagon. Find a yellow hexagon among the Pattern Blocks in your classroom. Then use the other Pattern Block shapes to cover the yellow hexagon in as many ways as you can. Draw or trace the ways on another piece of paper.

Example:

How many different ways can you cover the hexagon?

_____

Name _____

Basketball Time

Help Jen get ready for her basketball game.
Fill in the blanks below with 1 minute, 5 minutes and 2 hours.

When Jen woke up, she brushed her teeth for _____. She put on all her

basketball clothes in _____. Then she headed out the door for her game.

"I'll be back in _____," she shouted to her brother.

Name _____

Barn Owl's Mistake

In the cold winter barn, Barn Owl said to the horses,
"I have found a good way to add numbers in my head. Listen to this:

If 4 + 4 = 8, then 4 + 5 = 7. If 6 + 6 = 12, then 6 + 7 = 11."

Put a star by the wrong answers. Write the correct ones here: _____ , _____

What is Barn Owl doing wrong? How can doubles help you add? Write your ideas on the back.

Name _____

Cold Fingers and Toes

Draw a picture on the back of this sheet of 4 children playing in the snow, building snow people. When they were finished, the fingers and toes of all the children were icy cold.

How many cold fingers and toes were there in all?

_____

Use skip counting or multiplication to show your answer.

_____

Name _____

Two by Two

If your class lined up in 2's, would everyone have a partner? Count everyone's name tag, or line up, to find out.

Is there an even or an odd number of kids in your class? _____

How do you know?_____

_____

Name _____

The Goldfish Gift

Greg wanted to buy a goldfish for his friend Graham. The goldfish cost 25¢. Show all the different ways Greg could pay for the goldfish using coins. Draw or write your answers below. Use the back if you need more room.

_____   _____

_____   _____

How many in each group? *What patterns do you see?*

Name _____

Exactly in the Middle

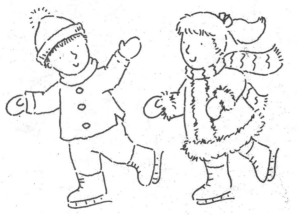

Solve this math riddle:

A group of kids went ice skating.
There were between 60 and 70 kids.
The exact number was exactly in the middle.
How many children went ice skating?

_____

Hint: You can use a number line to find out.

Name _____

Fractions, Patterns

Pie Slices

Polly was cutting peach pies.

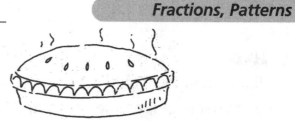

She cut one pie in 2 equal slices, or halves. How many cuts did she make? _____

She cut one pie into 4 equal slices, or fourths. How many cuts did she make? _____
Hint: draw pies on the back of this sheet to help you.

Extra: She cut one pie into 6 equal slices, or sixths. How many cuts did she make? _____

Name _____

Counting by 5's, Money

A Nickel a Month

Most people keep their money in a bank account. The money earns "interest."
This means that the bank adds money to the money in the bank account.

If the bank adds 5¢ every month for 1 year, how much extra money would there be?

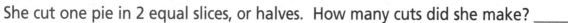

Hint: You can skip count or write the multiplication equation to find the answer.

Name _____

Thumbprints and Hand Spans

Suppose you used your thumbprint or your hand span to measure your desk.

Which measurement would be larger? _____

Use your thumbprint to measure your desk.

How many thumbprints long is your desk? _____

Now use your hand span to measure your desk.

How many hand-spans long is your desk? _____

Name _____

A Wingful of Books

Over the long holiday vacation, Owl took out a wingful of books from the library.
She read 7 the first week. How many did she have left to read?

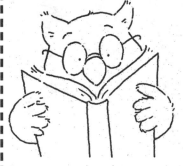

What information would you need to answer this question?

_____

Make up a number of books for Owl to take out of the library.
Write and solve your equation now.

_____

Name _____

Holiday Piggy Bank

Franny Frog was saving pennies to buy holiday gifts.
On the 1st day she saved 1 penny. On the 2nd day, she saved 2 pennies.
On the 3rd day, she saved 3 pennies.

How many pennies did she save on the 4th day? _____

How many pennies did she save on the 5th day? _____

How many pennies did she save in all? _____

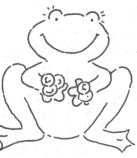

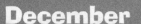

How many in each group? *What patterns do you see?*

Name _____

Family Time at Holiday Time

Holiday time is family time. Everyone's family is special.
How many people are in your family? On another sheet
of paper, make a bar graph, like the one shown here.
Color in the squares to show how many people are in
your classmates' families.

Which bar on the graph is longest? _____

What does this tell you? Write your answer on the back.

People in our Families				
2 people				
3 people				
4 people				
5 people				
6 people				
7 people				
8 people				

Name _____

Adding Sums of 10

Holiday Cookies

Jack Rabbit and his sister made holiday cookies. Some were carrot cookies. Some were sugar
cookies. There were 10 cookies in all. How many cookies could they have made of
each kind? Write your answers in equations.

_____ carrot + _____ sugar = 10 cookies   _____ carrot + _____ sugar = 10 cookies

_____ carrot + _____ sugar = 10 cookies   _____ carrot + _____ sugar = 10 cookies

Keep going! Write more equations on the back.

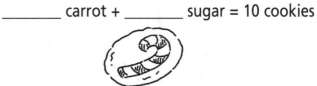

Snowflakes on Mittens

Estimate how many snowflakes are on each mitten. _____   _____

For the first mitten, skip count by 2s
to find out. (You can circle groups of 2.) _____

For the second mitten, skip count by 5s
to check your answer. (You can circle groups of 5.) _____

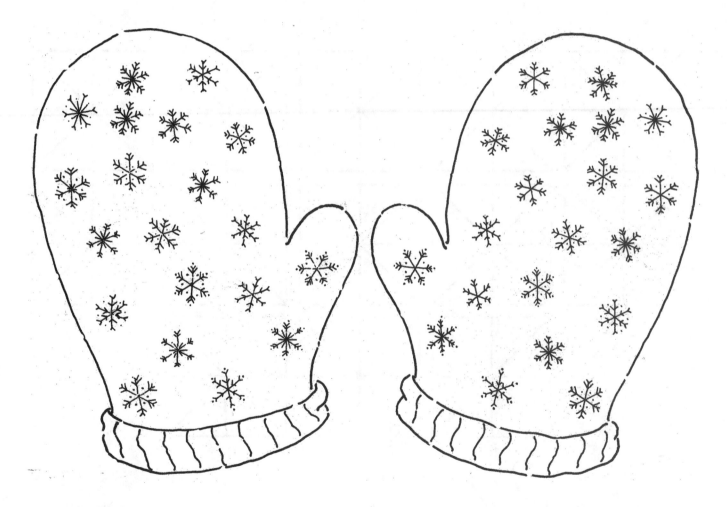

Extra

Would snowflakes really wait for you to count? _____

Explain your answer: _____

Name _____

Quilt Colors

Grandpa Squirrel wants to make Baby Squirrel a warm winter quilt. Here is the quilt pattern he's using:

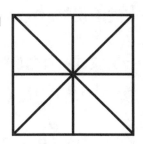

He'll be using 4 red triangles and 4 blue triangles. Find different ways to make the quilt.   Color the triangles below.

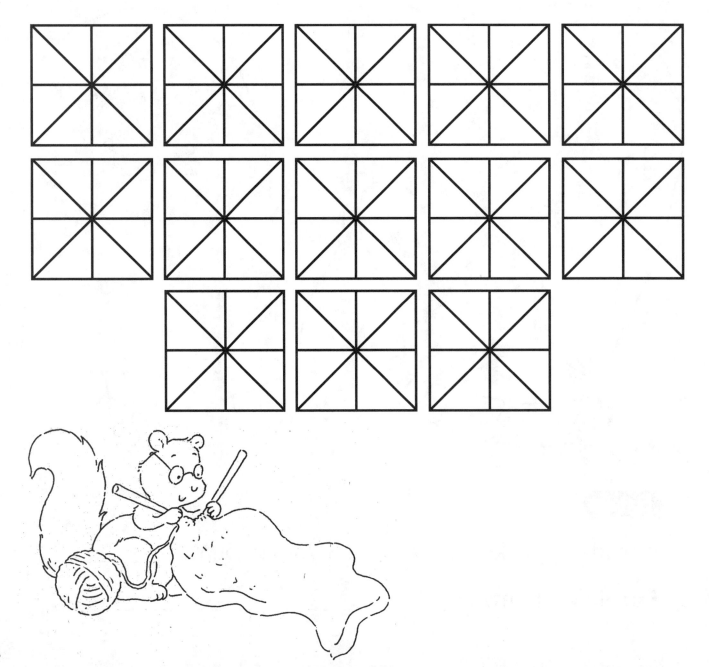

Cabin in the Snow

Fill in the blanks in the poem. Look at the pictures to help you.

Little Cabin in the Snow

_____ – sided snowflakes, soft and cold.

_____ – sided cabin, warm and bright.

_____ – sided doorway, where Grandma stands

with steamy, round pancakes that taste just right.

Extra

Now name the shapes you see in the picture.

_____

_____

_____

December Weather

In December, Mrs. Monroe's class drew the weather on a calendar. Each kind of weather has a picture:

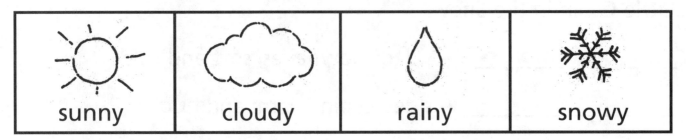

| sunny | cloudy | rainy | snowy |

Look at the calendar. Answer the questions below.

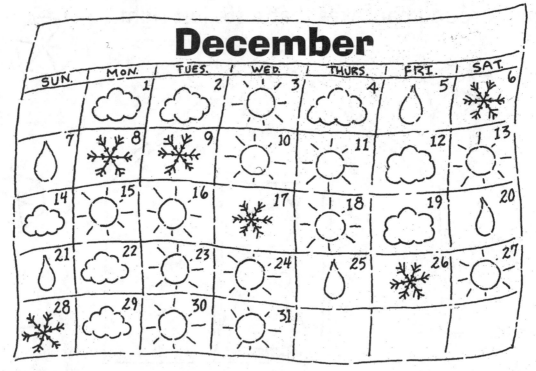

How many sunny days did they have?_____

How many cloudy days did they have?_____

How many rainy days did they have?_____

How many snowy days did they have?_____

Which kind of weather did they have the most?_____

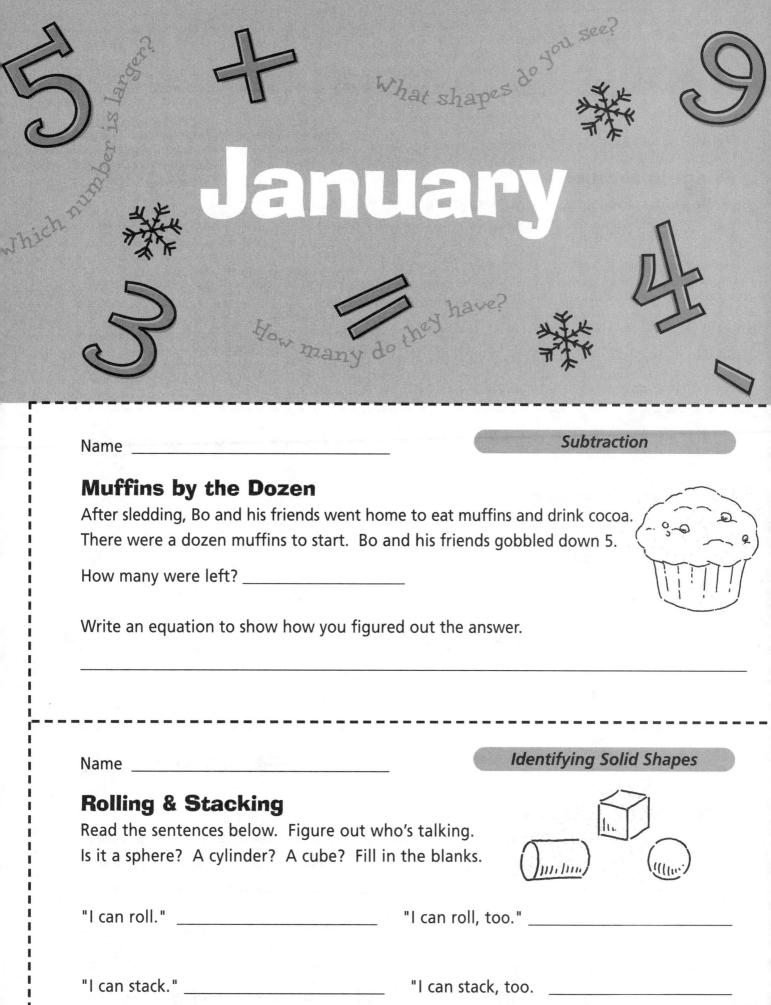

January

Name _____

Subtraction

Muffins by the Dozen

After sledding, Bo and his friends went home to eat muffins and drink cocoa. There were a dozen muffins to start. Bo and his friends gobbled down 5.

How many were left? _____

Write an equation to show how you figured out the answer.

_____

Name _____

Identifying Solid Shapes

Rolling & Stacking

Read the sentences below. Figure out who's talking.
Is it a sphere? A cylinder? A cube? Fill in the blanks.

"I can roll." _____   "I can roll, too." _____

"I can stack." _____   "I can stack, too. _____

47

January

How many in each group? What patterns do you see?

Name _____

Penguin School

In the winter, the Penguin School is not open on weekends.
Polly Penguin learns one new thing every day of school.

How many new things does she learn in 1 week? _____

Explain your answer: _____

Extra: What if Polly learns one new thing each day of school for 2 weeks?

How many new things would she learn then? _____

Name _____

Guess My Number

Gordo Gecko said, "Guess my number.   It is between 32 and 37."

Which number could it be?

_____

His number was 33. Did Gordo give a good enough hint? _____

What other hints could he have given? _____

Name _____

Hibernation Breaks

In winter, chipmunks hibernate. At times they might wake up. Every time Chad Chipmunk wakes up, his mother asks him a math problem. Help Chad answer these math questions so he can go back to sleep.

Which has more flat sides—a cylinder or a cube?_____

How many more? _____

Hint: Compare a cube and a cylinder to solve the problem.

Name _____

Danny Duck's Dinner

Danny Duck went to buy some food for dinner.   He had 10¢.

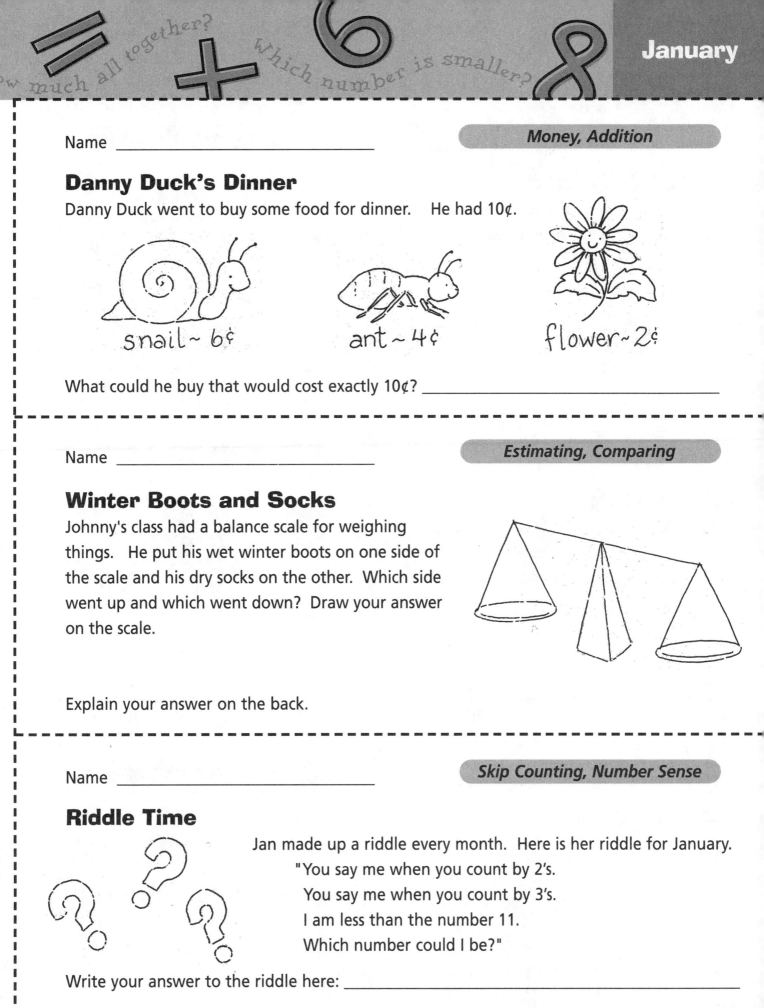

snail ~ 6¢   ant ~ 4¢   flower ~ 2¢

What could he buy that would cost exactly 10¢? _____

Name _____

Winter Boots and Socks

Johnny's class had a balance scale for weighing things.   He put his wet winter boots on one side of the scale and his dry socks on the other. Which side went up and which went down? Draw your answer on the scale.

Explain your answer on the back.

Name _____

Riddle Time

Jan made up a riddle every month. Here is her riddle for January.

"You say me when you count by 2's.
You say me when you count by 3's.
I am less than the number 11.
Which number could I be?"

Write your answer to the riddle here: _____

How many in each group?   What patterns do you see?

Name _____

MLK Jr.'s Birthday

Martin Luther King, Jr.'s actual birthday falls in January between the numbers 14 and 19.   Figure out which day it is with these clues.

It's an odd number.
It's lower than 16.
Which day is it?   _____

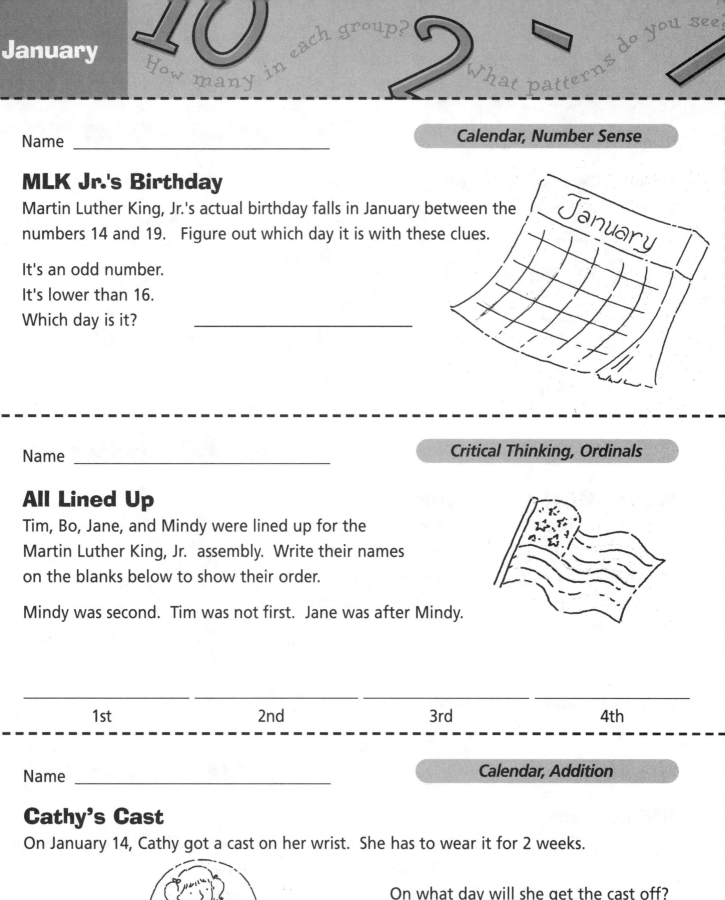

Name _____

All Lined Up

Tim, Bo, Jane, and Mindy were lined up for the Martin Luther King, Jr. assembly. Write their names on the blanks below to show their order.

Mindy was second. Tim was not first. Jane was after Mindy.

_____   _____   _____   _____
        1st   2nd   3rd   4th

Name _____

Cathy's Cast

On January 14, Cathy got a cast on her wrist. She has to wear it for 2 weeks.

On what day will she get the cast off?

_____

Hint: Look at a calendar to help you.

Name _____

Cool Calculations

Penny Pig's favorite numbers were 3 and 4. She tried to make different numbers appear
on her calculator by pressing the 3, the 4, the plus sign, and the equal sign in different orders.

How did she get to 16? Write the equation here.

_____

How did she get to 11? Write the equation here.

_____

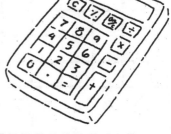

Name _____

Bear Family Quilts

Baby Bear's quilt looks like this:

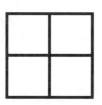

Mama Bear's quilt is bigger and looks like this:

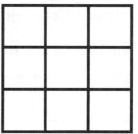

Papa Bear's quilt is the biggest. On another sheet, draw what Papa Bear's quilt would look like.
Extra: Use color tiles to make all the quilts.

Name _____

Temperature Matcheroo

Every morning, Jimmy looked at a thermometer outside his window. The thermometer
measured the temperature. Draw a line to match these temperatures with the seasons.

90°	fall
70°	summer
50°	winter
30°	spring

Hint: Remember which seasons are usually warmest and coolest

Name _____

Favorite Number Graph

Favorite Numbers

1 2 3 4 5 6 7 8 9 10

Ask your classmates to pick their favorite numbers between 1 and 10. On another sheet of paper make a bar graph, like the one here, to record their answer. Draw one X in the column for each choice.

What did you learn from the graph? Did more people pick even numbers or odd numbers? Write what you learned on the back.

Name _____

Place Value, Addition

Squirrel Math

Sally Squirrel had 25 acorns. She made 3 piles. She made 2 piles with 10 acorns each and 1 pile with 5 acorns.   Sally said, "10 + 10 + 5 = 25."

Sidney Squirrel had 36 acorns. He brought them to Sally. Sally made 4 piles. How many acorns were in each pile?

Pile #1 _____ Pile #2 _____ Pile # 3 _____ Pile #4 _____

What do you think Sally said? _____

Name _____

Subtraction

Pie Fight

To celebrate National Pie Day, the circus clowns made 26 cream pies. They threw 11 at each other in a pie fight. They ate the rest.

How many pies did they eat? _____

Write an equation to show how you got your answer.

_____

Name _____

National Popcorn Day

National Popcorn Day is at the end of January. It is the same day as Super Bowl Sunday. Bring in some wrapped popcorn kernels. Fill a tablespoon with popcorn kernels. Estimate how many kernels are on the spoon.

Write your estimate here: _____

Now count them. Write the exact number here: _____

Show the two numbers you wrote in a greater than/less than equation. _____

Name _____

Coin Puzzler

January 29 is National Puzzle Day. Solve this riddle to celebrate.

<u>3</u> shiny coins inside the piggy bank
are worth <u>16</u> cents. Clank, clank, clank.

What coins are in the bank? _____ _____ _____

<u>Extra:</u> Now substitute <u>4</u> and <u>26</u> for the numbers in the poem. Write your answer on the back.

Scarf Patterns

Marla's grandmother is knitting three scarves. Help her finish each scarf by continuing each pattern.

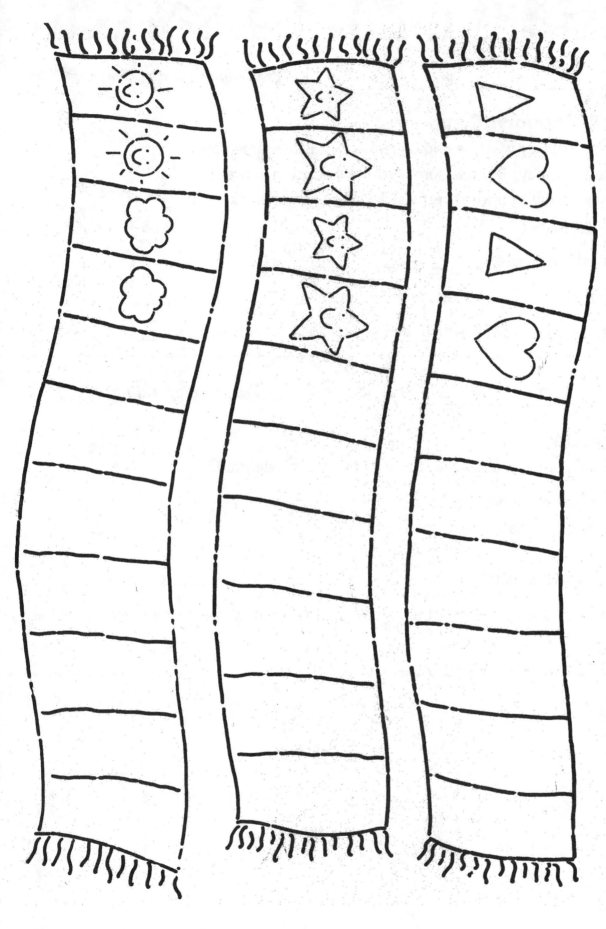

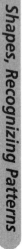

54

What to Wear?

Tina had 2 pairs of pants. One was black. One was white. She had 3
sweaters. They were red, yellow, and blue. Color in the clothes below.
Cut them out. Make as many different outfits as you can.

How many did you make? _____

Do you think Tina would be late for
school if she tried on all your outfits? _____

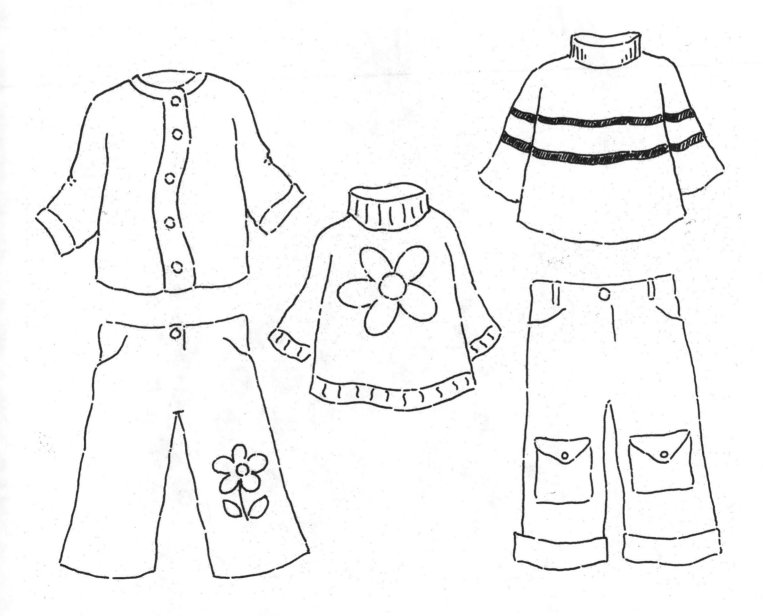

Dalmatian Spots

Dana's Dalmatian has lots of spots.
How many do you think it has?_____

Check your estimate by skip counting by fives.
(Circle groups of five.)

How many spots does it have?_____

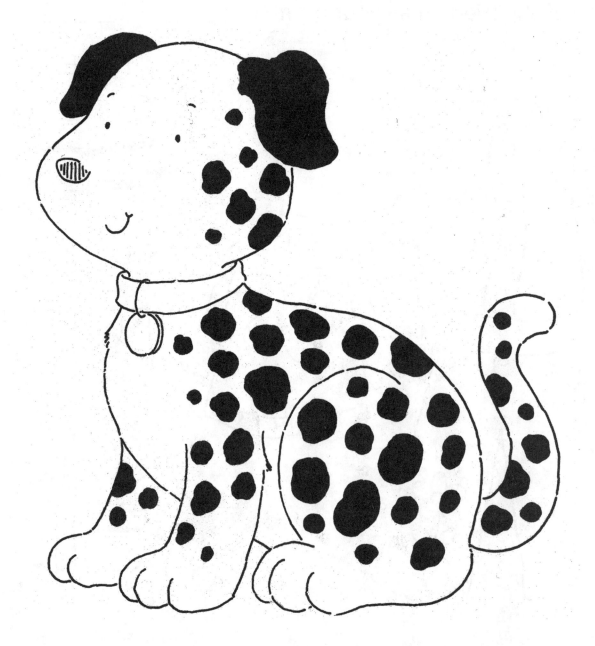

February

Name _____

Money, Addition

Chinese New Year

For Chinese New Year, some children receive money in red envelopes.
Which would you rather have in your envelope—3 quarters or 7 dimes?

I would rather have _____

Explain your answer. _____

_____

Name _____

Time

Ground Hog Day

The ground hog woke up at 10:00. Two hours later,
he popped his head out of his hole to look at his shadow.

What time did the ground hog check his shadow?

_____

57

How many in each group? What patterns do you see?

Name _____

Black History Month

George has 39 stamps in his stamp collection. He bought 3 new stamps that show "Black Heroes in History." George said, "Now I have 43 stamps in all."

Was George correct? Circle Yes or No.   **YES**   **NO**

Explain your answer. _____

_____

Name _____

Estimating Weight and Length

Pennies and Paper Clips

On the 100th day of school, Joan's class weighed 100 pennies and 100 paper clips.

Which do you think was heavier? _____

Then they put the 100 pennies in one line and the 100 paper clips in another.

Which line do you think was longer? _____

Hint: Get a few pennies and a few paper clips. Experiment to figure out the answers.

Name _____

Skip Counting, Patterns

100th Day of School

Read this math riddle:

To celebrate the 100th day, count to 100 by 10s.
If you say all the numbers out loud, estimate how many will you say?

Write the numbers you used to count to 100 by 10s. _____

How many numbers did you write? _____

Talk with a classmate about the patterns you see.

58

Name _____

Thirsty, Anyone?

A cup of hot cocoa is perfect on a cold winter day. But lemonade hits the spot in the summer, . What is your favorite drink? What drinks do your classmates like? On another sheet of paper, make a bar graph to record their choices.

Which drink is the most popular? _____

How can you tell? _____

Name _____

Bear Riddles

Solve these riddles about bears. Write the bear name on the lines.

My fur is white. I live in the Arctic.
The first letter of my name is the 16th letter of the alphabet.
What kind of bear am I? _____ _____ _____ _____ _____ bear

My fur is brown. I am one of the biggest bears in the world.
The first letter of my name is the 7th letter of the alphabet.
What kind of bear am I? _____ _____ _____ _____ _____ _____ _____ bear

---

Name _____

Pictures of Presidents

Solve this math riddle.

I have 2 bills that show President Lincoln's head.
I have 3 bills with Washington on them instead.

How much money do I have? _____

Write an equation to show how you know.

How many in each group? What patterns do you see?

Name _____

Who Is Older?

Josh and Ashley turned 7 years old this year. Ashley's birthday is in January on Martin Luther King, Jr. Day. Josh's birthday is in February on Valentine's Day.

Who is older? _____

Explain your answer. _____

_____

Name _____

Sloppy Winter Boots

Solve this math riddle.

12 sloppy winter boots
are sitting by the door.
How many children are
sipping cocoa on the floor? _____

Hint: Use manipulatives to help solve the riddle.

Extra: Now 16 boots are by the door. How many children are there? _____

Name _____

Odd + Odd

Jerry added two odd numbers and came up with 8.

What numbers did Jerry use? Write 2 equations to show your ideas.

_____   _____

Jerry tried adding two odd numbers to come up with an odd number. Explain why it didn't work.

_____

Name _____

Multiplication

So Many Stamps!

Sandy is sending a very large Valentine's Day
card to a friend. To mail it, she needs 12 stamps.
She is arranging the stamps in rows. Each row
has the same number of stamps. How many
different arrangements can she make? Try it!
On the back, or on another sheet of paper, draw
a picture to show the ways you could arrange
the stamps in equal rows.

Name _____

Addition, Multiplication

Valentine Count

Mario received 6 valentines. Barb received 6 valentines. Maria received 6 valentines, too.

How many valentines did they get in all? _____

Explain how you figured out the answer. _____

_____

Name _____

Number Sense, Calendar

Special Birthday

Justin's brother was 20 years old on the day after February 19 in the year 2000.
Why was this birthday special? These questions will help you.

Which month is February? (1st, 2nd, 3rd, ...?) _____ Which day is his birthday? __

How old was he?_____ In which year was he this age?_____

What do the numbers have in common?_____

Extra: What would be a special birthday in the year 1999? Write your idea on the back.

Measuring His Shadow

When the ground hog came out to check his shadow, the inchworm said the shadow was 10 inchworms long. The frog said the shadow was 5 frogs long. Cut out the inchworms, the frogs, and the shadow to find out.

How many inchworms equal the shadow? _____

How many frogs equal the length of the shadow? _____

Who was right? _____

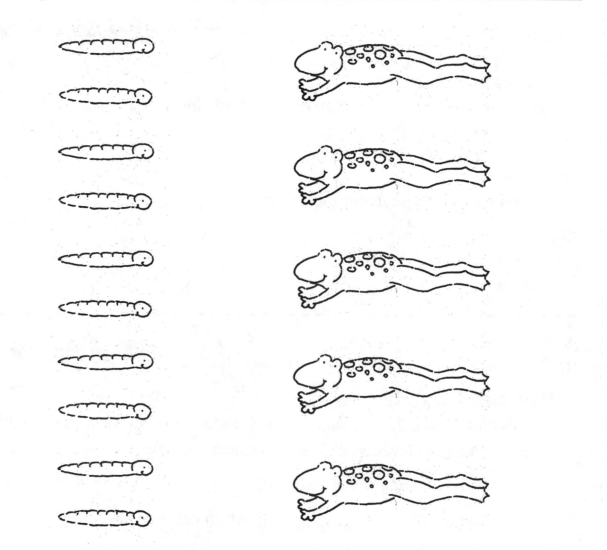

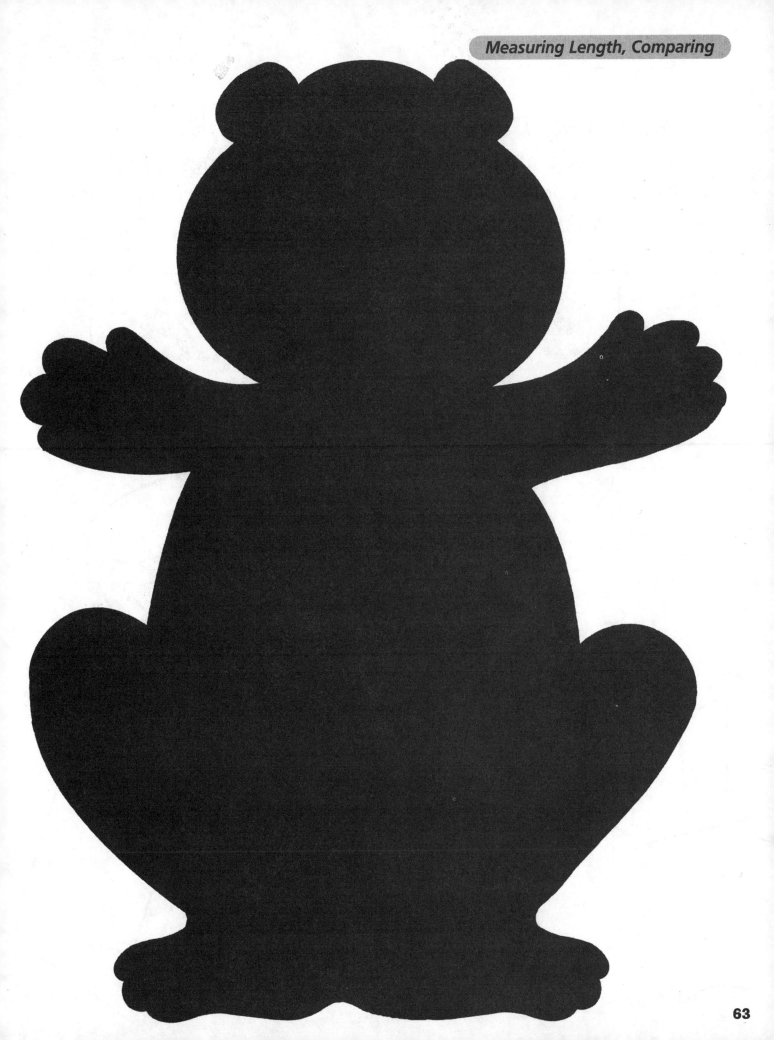

Snow-Print Detective

Sally dropped a big box in the snow. Lots of things fell out.
Look at each object. Below it, write which kind of print it would
make in the snow. Use the shape words in the box.

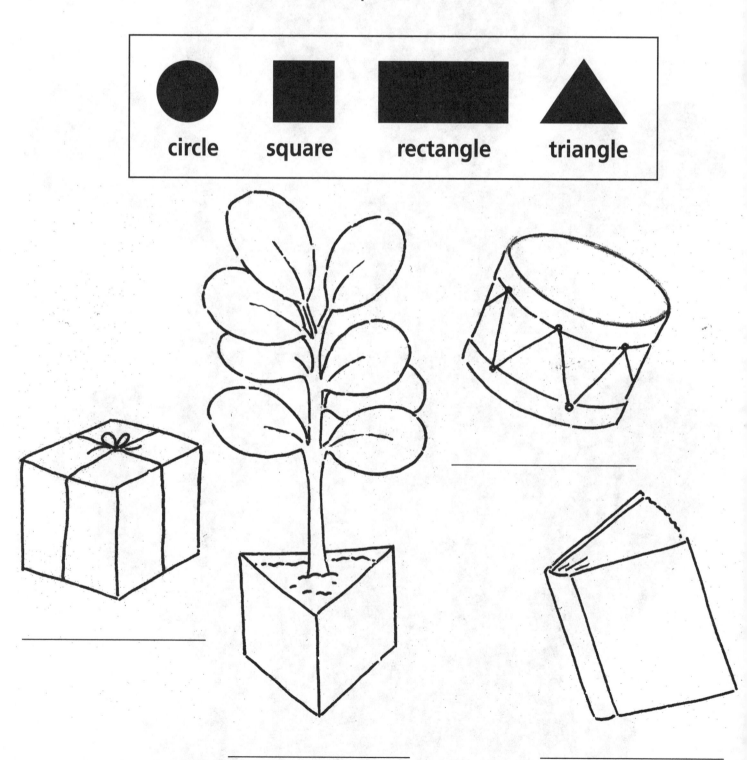

circle　　square　　rectangle　　triangle

Valentine Symmetry

Janis folded all her valentines in half. Some were symmetrical.
That means, one half matches the other half. Some valentines
were not symmetrical.

Cut out the valentine shapes below. Fold them in half
so you make a crease that runs from top to bottom.
Which ones are symmetrical?

_____   _____

_____   _____

Fold the symmetrical shapes in half so that
you make a crease running from left to right.

Which shape is symmetrical this way? _____

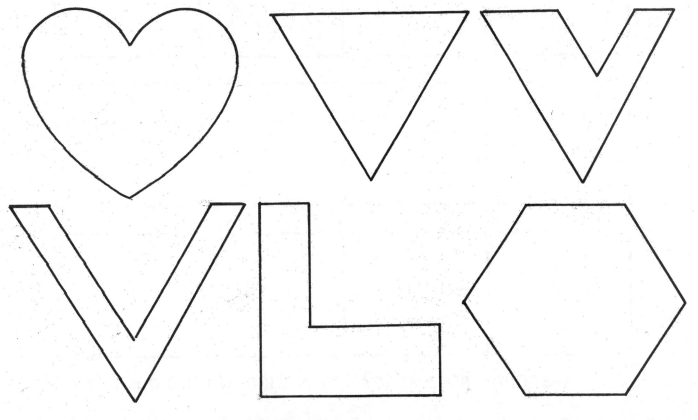

Valentine Stickeroo

Martha Mule made a valentine for Max Mule. She had 4 stickers in 2 different colors. How many ways could she arrange the stickers on the card?

Here are the stickers:

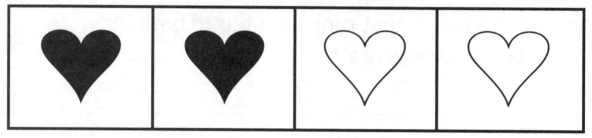

Here are some blank cards:
Draw stickers in the squares of the cards to
show how Marla could arrange them.

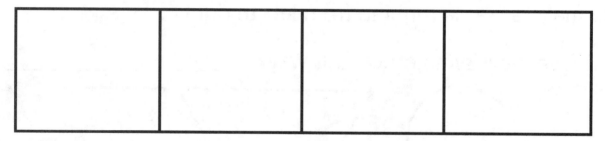

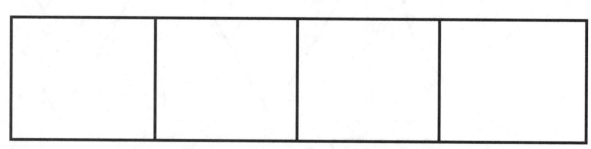

Are there more ways? Draw them on the back.

Picking Out Patterns

On the 100th day of school, everyone in Pat's class picked out patterns on the 100 Chart. Look at the chart below.

1	2	3	4	5	6	7	8	9	10
11	12	13	14	15	16	17	18	19	20
21	22	23	24	25	26	27	28	29	30
31	32	33	34	35	36	37	38	39	40
41	42	43	44	45	46	47	48	49	50
51	52	53	54	55	56	57	58	59	60
61	62	63	64	65	66	67	68	69	70
71	72	73	74	75	76	77	78	79	80
81	82	83	84	85	86	87	88	89	90
91	92	93	94	95	96	97	98	99	100

Find and finish the pattern starting with 2, 12, 22,...

_____

Find and finish the pattern starting with 100, 90, 80,...

_____

Find and finish the pattern starting with 97, 87, 77,...

_____

Find and finish the pattern starting with 11, 22, 33,...

_____

Presidents' Day Problem

The first 18 Presidents of the United States are listed below.
They are shown in order.

1. George Washington (1789–1797)
2. John Adams (1797–1801)
3. Thomas Jefferson (1801–1809)
4. James Madison (1809–1817)
5. James Monroe (1817–1825)
6. John Quincy Adams (1825–1829)
7. Andrew Jackson (1829–1837)
8. Martin Van Buren (1837–1841)
9. William Henry Harrison (1841)
10. John Tyler (1841–1845)
11. James Knox Polk (1845–1849)
12. Zachary Taylor (1849–1850)
13. Millard Fillmore (1850–1853)
14. Franklin Pierce (1853–1857)
15. James Buchanan (1857–1861)
16. Abraham Lincoln (1861–1865)
17. Andrew Johnson (1865–1869)
18. Ulysses S. Grant (1869–1877)

1. Which President was Washington? _____ **The 1st** _____

2. Which President was Lincoln? _____

3. Which President came before Lincoln? _____

4. Which President came after Lincoln? _____

5. How many Presidents were there
   <u>between</u> Washington and Lincoln? _____

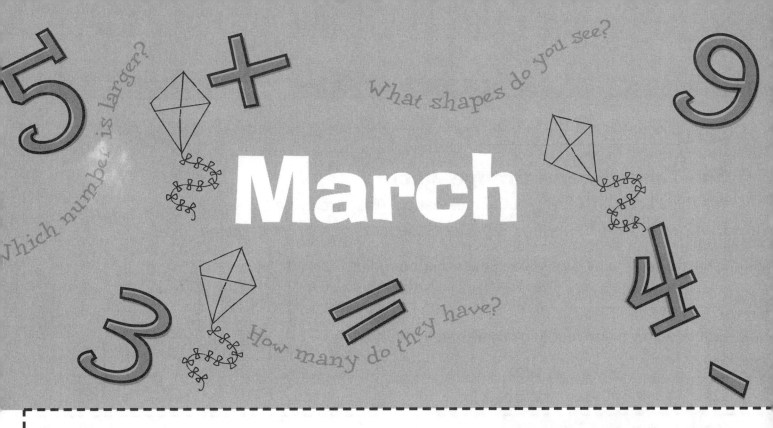

March

Name _____

Colorful Kites

It was a windy March day. Some kids in the park were flying kites.

• The yellow kite was the highest.

• The red kite was between the yellow kite and the blue kite.

• The green kite was the lowest.

On another sheet of paper, draw a picture and color it to show the positions of the kites.

Name _____

What's for Breakfast?

The first week of March is National School Breakfast Week. Take a survey of your class to find out each classmate's favorite breakfast. Show the results on a graph. Model your graph after the one shown here .

Which breakfast was the most popular? _____

How could you tell? _____

Cereal			
Pancakes			
Eggs			
Oatmeal			
French Toast			

69

How many in each group? What patterns do you see?

Name _____

The Three Bears' Orange Juice

The three bears are coming out of hibernation. They are going for a walk.
Look at the thermoses below. Papa Bear's thermos holds 8 cups of orange juice.

Estimate how many cups Mama Bear's thermos holds.

_____ cups

Estimate how many cups Baby Bear's thermos holds.

_____ cups

Explain your estimates on the back.

8 cups

Name _____

Money Riddle

A second-grade class is having a spring taco sale to raise money. Tim has 10¢
to spend on tacos. Jen has 5¢ more than Tim. How much money does Jen have? _____

Write an equation to show how you figured out the answer.

_____

Ralph has 2¢ more than Jen. How much money does Ralph have? _____

Write another equation to show the answer. _____

Name _____

The Shrinking Teddy Bear

Pat's teddy bear is shrinking! On Monday, the bear's waist measured 20 inches around.
On Tuesday, it measured 18 inches. On Wednesday, it measured 16 inches.

At this rate, what would it measure on Thursday? _____

What would it measure on Friday? _____

What would it measure on Saturday? _____

Why do you think the bear was shrinking? _____

Name _____

Finding Gold

March 17 is St. Patrick's Day. Leprechauns are in Irish folklore. A leprechaun found 7 gold coins under a bush. He found 8 more at the end of a rainbow. He spent 3 of the coins on a tiny hammer.

How many coins does he have left to spend? _____

Write 2 number sentences to show how you figured out the answer.

_____

_____

Name _____

Leprechaun Gold

Larry Leprechaun put his gold coins on the right side of the balance scale. Lizzy Leprechaun put hers on the left side. Here is how the balance scale looked.

Count Larry's gold coins. Write the number here: _____

Now draw in the number of gold coins Lizzy might have had.

Write a greater than/less than equation to show your ideas: _____ > _____

Name _____

Leprechaun Steps

On another sheet of paper, draw what you imagine a leprechaun footprint might look like. Cut it out. How many leprechaun footprints would it be from your desk to the door?

Write your estimate here: _____
Now use your cutout to measure the distance.

Write how many footprints it really is from your desk to the door. _____

How many in each group? What patterns do you see?

Name _____

Who Won?

Jane's team played Kira's team in basketball. Jane's team had a score of 6 tens and 4 ones.

What was their score? _____

Kira's team had a score of 4 tens and 6 ones.

What was their score? _____

Write the numbers in this greater than/less than equation: _____ > _____

Which team won? _____

Name _____

Dog Calculations

Sara pressed 5 + on her calculator. Her dog started thumping his paw on the + key. He pressed it 4 more times. Fill in the blanks below to show the numbers that came up on the calculator.

5, _____ , _____ , _____ , _____

You will need to use calculator. Press 5 +.
Press the + key again and again.

Name _____

Lost-and-Found Mystery

Daniel counted clothes at the school Lost and Found. In the winter, he counted 26 items. In the spring, there were only 4 items. How many more items were in Lost and Found in the winter than in the spring?

Write an equation to show your answer. _____

Extra: Why do you think there were more items in the Lost and Found in the winter? Explain your idea on the back.

Name _____

Kite Store

Fred the Flying Squirrel had 5 boxes in his kite store. Each box had 10 kites.

How many kites did he have?

_____

Write an equation to show your answer:

_____

Hint: The number is more than 40 and less than 60.

Name _____

The Year of the Dragon

The year 2000 was the Year of the Dragon.
Sheila was 10 years old that year.
In 12 more years it will be the Year of the Dragon again.

How old will Sheila be then? _____

Write an equation to show how you figured out the answer.

_____

Name _____

Johnny Appleseed Math

Johnny Appleseed was planting seeds in a field. He said,

"10 seeds here, 10 seeds there,
10 seeds in each handful, I plant them with care."
Johnny ended up planting 8 handfuls of seeds. He also planted 6 extra seeds.

How many seeds did he plant in all? _____

How many in each group? What patterns do you see?

Name _____

Paul's Peanut Machine

Go Nuts Over Peanuts Week is the third week of March. To celebrate, Paul made a peanut machine.

When he put 2 peanuts in the machine, 12 came out.

When he put 5 peanuts in the machine, 15 came out.

When he put 6 peanuts in the machine, 16 came out.

What would happen if he puts in 7, 8, or 10 peanuts? _____

What is the machine doing? _____

Name _____

Mark's Baby Sister

Mark's baby sister Krista is 1 year old. Mark is 8 years old. Write the answers on the lines below.

When Krista is 1, Mark is 8.   When Krista is 2, Mark is _____.

When Krista is 3, Mark is _____.   When Krista is 4, Mark is _____

When Krista is 5, Mark is _____.   When Krista is 6, Mark is _____

When Krista is 7, Mark is _____.   When Krista is 8, Mark is _____

Circle the one where Mark's age is double his sister's age.

Name _____

Amusement Park Math

The amusement park opened on the first day of spring. 12 people were in line for the "Over the Falls" ride. 4 people fit in each boat. All the people got into their boats.

How many boats were filled? _____

Explain how you figured out the answer.

Name _____

Peter Piper's Pickled Peppers

In the fall, Peter Piper stored 26 jars of pickled peppers.
During the winter, he ate 7 jars of pickled peppers. Now it is spring.

How many jars does Peter have left? _____.

Write an equation to show your answer.

_____

Name _____

Would You Rather Have . . . ?

When Carrie put away her winter clothes, she found 5 dimes in her coat pocket. Her brother said he would trade her his 46 pennies for her 5 dimes.   Should she trade?

Circle Yes or No   **YES**   **NO**

Explain your answer. _____

_____

Classroom Garage Sale

Tolu's class did some spring cleaning. Then they had a garage sale. They sorted the things they were selling. Sort these objects into like groups. Draw the items of each group on one of the tables below.

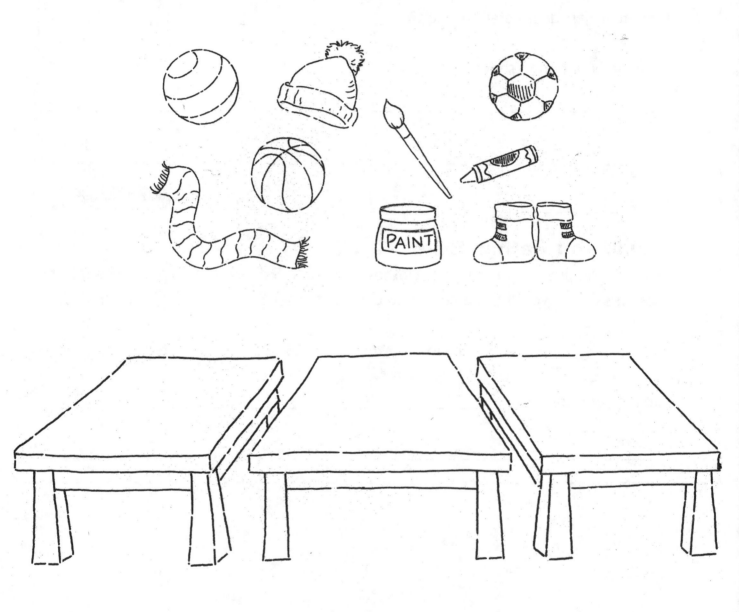

_____   _____   _____

Below each table, write a label for the group.

Name _____

Patterns for the Mail Carrier

Meimei the mail carrier is delivering letters. Give her some help.
Fill in the missing addresses on the houses below.

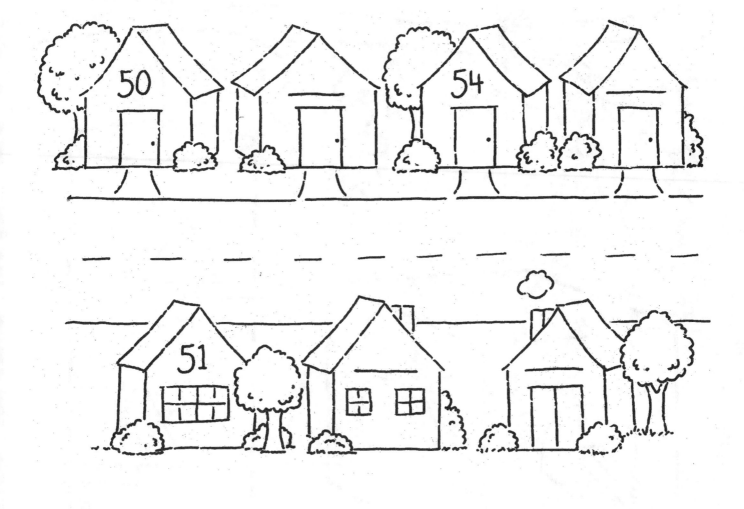

Extra

What pattern do you see in the house numbers? _____

_____

_____

Bird Feeder Geometry

It's spring! The birds are coming back. Kwaku and his mother made two bird feeders. What shapes can you find on their feeders? Write your ideas on the lines.

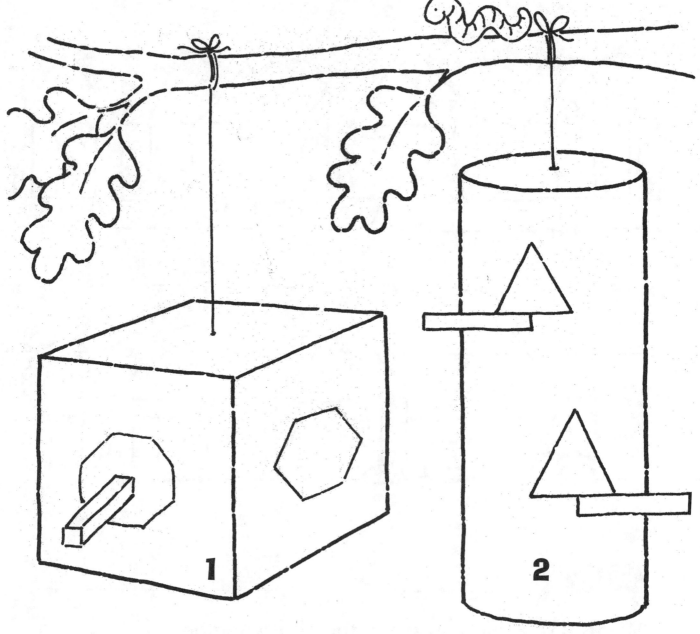

_____   _____

_____   _____

_____   _____

April

Which number is larger?

What shapes do you see?

How many do they have?

Name _____

April Fool's?

On April Fool's Day, Jeff said to his mom, "I'd rather have 2 dimes and 13 pennies than 3 dimes and 2 pennies." Do you think this was an April Fool's Day joke?

Circle Yes or No.   **YES**   **NO**

Explain your answer: _____

_____

Name _____

Party Balloons

At the end of the April Fool's Party, Li divided the balloons. He had 15 balloons for 3 children. "The balloons don't divide evenly!" said Li. Is he right?

Circle Yes or No.   **YES**   **NO**

Explain your answer: _____

How many balloons does each child get? _____

April

How many in each group? What patterns do you see?

Name _____

Ricky Recycles

Every Friday, Ricky takes the recycling bin to the curb.

Look at a calendar. How many times will Ricky take out the recycling bin in April? _____

How many times in May? _____ How many times in June? _____

How many times altogether in April, May, and June? _____

Write an equation to show your last answer. _____

Name _____

Baseball Shapes

Baseball season starts in April. A baseball field is made up of many shapes.
Look at this baseball field. What shapes do you see?

_____ _____

_____ _____

Draw the baseball field on a bigger sheet of paper. Label the shapes.

Name _____

Donuts in a Bag

Davey bought some donuts for his class. 6 donuts were in the bag.
4 were sugar donuts. 2 were glazed donuts.

If you reached in the bag without looking,
what kind of donut would you probably get? _____

Explain your answer. _____

Extra: Try this activity with colored tiles.

Name _____

Addition

Benny's One-Man Band

Benny Bunny is a one-man band. He needs to take a boat to the Spring Parade. The boat holds 27 pounds.

6 lbs   5 lbs   2 lbs   4 lbs   8 lbs

How much does Benny and his instruments weigh? _____

Can the boat hold Benny and all his instruments? _____

Name _____

Time

A Tricky Way to Tell Time

Jack doesn't use numbers to tell the time. Instead, he describes how the clock hands look. Try Jack's method. Tell what time it is:

1. The hands are shaped like the letter L. _____

2. The hands are shaped like a backwards L. _____

3. The hands are straight up and down. They are on top of each other. _____

4. The hands are straight up and down. They are not on top of each other. _____

Name _____

Multiplication

Barnyard Patterns

At the farm, it was time to shoe the horses. Jayson was counting the horses' hooves. Give him a hand.

How many total hooves for 2 horses? _____   How many total hooves for 3 horses? _____

How many total hooves for 4 horses? _____   How many total hooves for 5 horses? _____

How many total hooves for 6 horses? _____

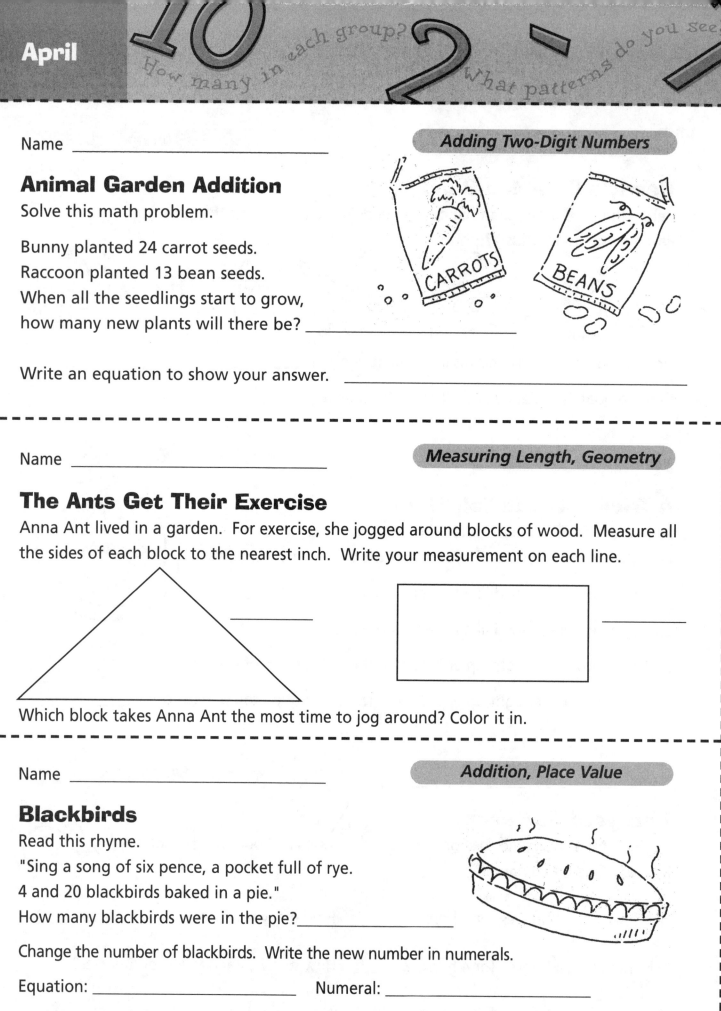

Name _____

Animal Garden Addition
Solve this math problem.

Bunny planted 24 carrot seeds.
Raccoon planted 13 bean seeds.
When all the seedlings start to grow,
how many new plants will there be? _____

Write an equation to show your answer. _____

Name _____

Measuring Length, Geometry

The Ants Get Their Exercise
Anna Ant lived in a garden. For exercise, she jogged around blocks of wood. Measure all the sides of each block to the nearest inch. Write your measurement on each line.

Which block takes Anna Ant the most time to jog around? Color it in.

Name _____

Addition, Place Value

Blackbirds
Read this rhyme.
"Sing a song of six pence, a pocket full of rye.
4 and 20 blackbirds baked in a pie."
How many blackbirds were in the pie?_____

Change the number of blackbirds. Write the new number in numerals.

Equation: _____   Numeral: _____

Name _____

A Prickly Problem

Mrs. Porcupine was sorting shapes.
This is what she did:

Where do these shapes go?

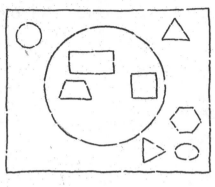

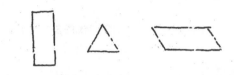

Draw the shapes in the correct place.

Name _____

The Biggest Number

It was time for the Math Olympics. The Ladybug Team
had the numbers 2, 3, 4, and 5 on their backs. Their
challenge was to make the largest sum they could using
the numbers on their backs. Write the numbers in the
boxes to make the largest sum.

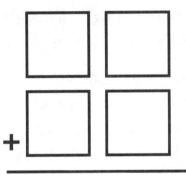

Name _____

Planting Beans

Tom planted 23 jellybeans and 16 string beans.
How many "beans" did he plant in all?
Place the numbers in these boxes to add and find out.

Extra: Which "beans" do you think really grew?
Write your answer on the back.

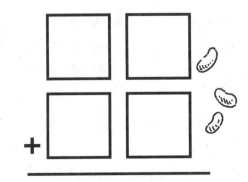

How many in each group? What patterns do you see?

Name _____

Mr. McGregor's Garden

Peter Rabbit went into Mr. McGregor's garden to eat the carrots. He counted 30 carrots. He nibbled on 10 before he heard Mr. McGregor's footsteps.

How many carrots did he leave alone? _____

Explain how you figured out the answer. _____

_____

Name _____

Farm Animals Weigh In

Jody helped her mom weigh the baby animals on the farm.

The baby goat weighed 12 pounds.
The chick weighed 2 pounds.
The lamb weighed 7 pounds.
The piglet weighed 19 pounds.

_____   _____

_____

Then she put 2 animals on one side of a large balance scale and 1 animal on the other side. The scale balanced! Which animals did she put on each side? Write their names on the line.

Name _____

Groups of Geese

In April, when the weather is warm, geese fly north. They fly in the shape of an upside down V. 37 geese are flying north. Each V has 10 geese.

How many groups of 10 are there? _____

How many geese are left over? _____

Name _____

National Coin Week

The fourth week of April is National Coin Week. Joan and John found 3 dimes and 4 nickels. How can they divide the money so each gets the same amount?

Joan could get _____ dime(s) and _____ nickel(s).

John could get _____ dime(s) and _____ nickel(s).

Name _____

Billy Goat's Raisins

The billy goat needed to cross the bridge. A troll stopped him.
"Give me your raisins," said the troll.
"I'll share them with you," said the billy goat. "I have 24 raisins. You can have half. Tell me how many you should get."
While the troll was figuring out the problem, the billy goat went right on by, keeping all his raisins.

What answer should the troll have come up with? _____

Hint: Use manipulatives to figure out the answer.

Creature Categories

Nick's class took a field trip to the beach. When they looked in the tide pools, they saw a lot of animals. Group the animals they saw. Color the animals in each group the same color.

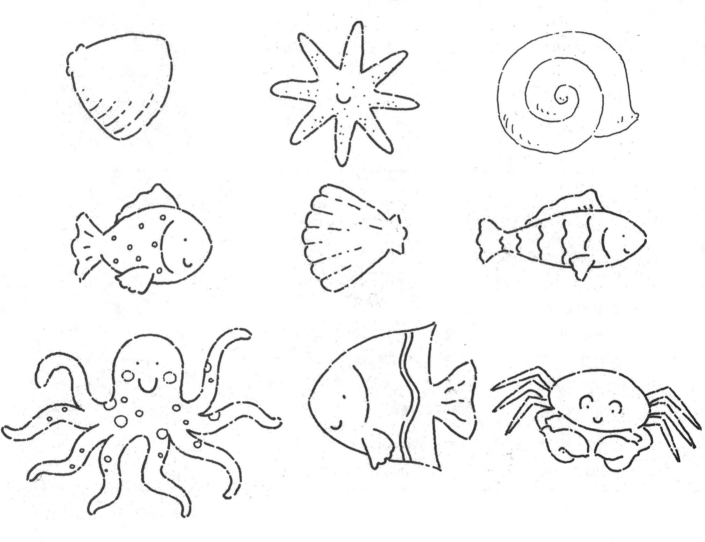

Write a word or phrase that explains how you grouped them.

Group #1_____

Group #2_____

Group #3_____

Name _____

Time to Get Up!

Twenty animals were hibernating near Sleepy Pond.
5 of them woke up. Color 5 animals below.

How many are still sleeping? _____

A week later, 7 more woke up.   Color 7 other animals.

How many are still sleeping? _____

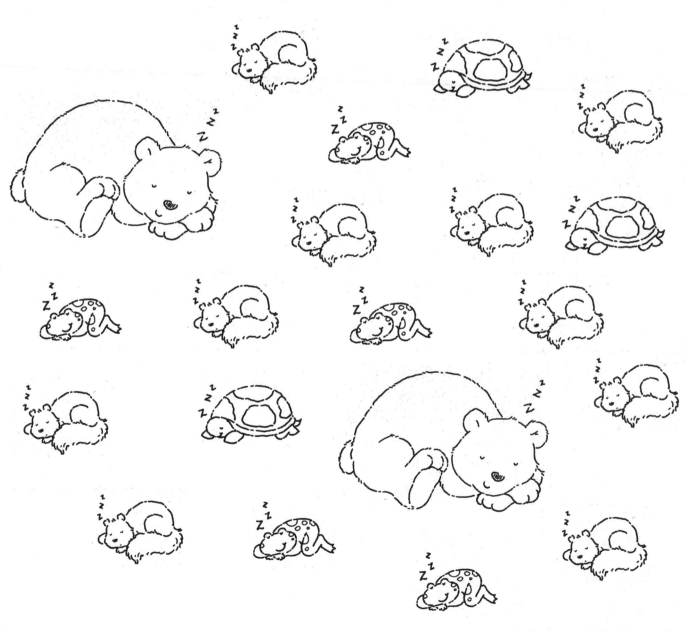

Jack's Beanstalk

Jack's class was growing bean plants.   After 1 week, Jack's was the tallest.

Measure Jack's plant below.   Record its height: _____

After 2 weeks, Jack's plant had doubled in height.

How tall was it now? _____

Draw a picture to show how tall the plant grew.
Measure your drawing to make sure it is the correct height.

2 weeks.

After 3 weeks, Jack's plant was still growing!

How tall would it be now? _____

Explain your answer. _____

May

Which number is larger? What shapes do you see? How many do they have?

Name _____

Diagramming

Ice-Cream Favorites

Take a class survey. First, copy the Venn diagram below on a sheet of paper. Make it as big as possible. Then ask your classmates which they like more—chocolate ice cream or strawberry ice cream. Write their names in the correct circle. If they like both flavors equally, write their names in the center circle. If they don't like either one, write their names outside the circle.

How many like chocolate?_____

How many like strawberry?_____

How many like both? _____

Name _____

Identifying Solid Shapes

Shape Riddles

Solve these shape riddles. Try to picture the shapes in your mind.

I have 6 sides, and all of them are square.
I'm number cubes, I'm blocks. I'm everywhere.

What solid shape am I? _____

I'm orange at a construction site, and ice cream sits on top of me.
You sometimes run around me when you're playing in P. E.

What solid shape am I? _____

How many in each group?   What patterns do you see?

Name _____

Getting Ready

It took Dina's grandmother 1 1/2 hours to braid Dina's hair.   She started at 11:00 in the morning.

At what time did she finish? _____

The party was at 1:00.
Did Dina's grandmother finish braiding Dina's hair in time for her to go to the party?

Circle Yes or No.   **YES**   **NO**

Extra: How much extra time did they have? _____

Name _____

Using a Calculator, Multiplication

Snoozing in May

May is "Better Sleep Month." Using a calculator, Kezia taught Jamal how to figure out how many hours a week he sleeps. This is what she did. She pushed **8+** on the calculator. Then she pushed the + key 6 more times. Try it! Write the number on the calculator each time you push the keys.

Day 1: + _____   Day 2: + _____

Day 3: + _____   Day 4: + _____

Day 5: + _____   Day 6: + _____

Day 7: + _____

Name _____

Patterns

Cluck, Neigh, Moo

Figure out the pattern of the barnyard symphony below. Fill in the missing sounds.

Cluck, neigh, meow,   Oink, _____, _____,

Cluck, neigh, moo.   Oink, _____, _____,

Woof, neigh, meow,   Cock-a-doodle, doodle, doo.

Woof, _____, _____.

Name _____

Birthdays in May

Sam and Danielle both have birthdays in May. Sam's birthday is 3 weeks away.
Danielle's birthday is 18 days away.

Whose birthday comes first? _____

Explain your answer. _____

_____

Name _____

Spider Survey

In May many spiders make their webs. Do you like spiders? Do your classmates?
Take a class survey.   Draw a tally mark next to each.

Do Like Spiders _____   **Do Not Like Spiders** _____

How many of your classmates like spiders? _____

How many classmates do not like them? _____

Write the numbers in a greater than/less than equation: _____ > _____

Name _____

Mother's Day Decisions

Sera went to the store with 30¢ to buy a gift for Mother's Day.
She bought 2 things. Circle 2 gifts she could buy with 30¢.

10¢   12¢

How much money did Sera spend? _____

How much did she have left? _____

15¢   5¢

91

How many in each group?   What patterns do you see?

Name _____

Spring Shelter

The wildlife shelter received two new animals. The new raccoon has 5 toes on each foot.
The new parrot has 4 toes on each foot.

Total number of raccoon toes: _____

Total number of parrot toes: _____

The raccoon has _____ more toes than the parrot.

Name _____

Heads and Feet

Solve this math riddle.

Chickens are clucking in the hen house. Horses are neighing in the barn.
There are 12 legs and 4 heads altogether, making a racket on Grandma's farm.

How many horses are on the farm? _____

How many chickens are on the farm? _____

Hint: Draw a picture on the back to find the answer.

Name _____

International Pickle Week

The third week of May is International Pickle Week.
Jeffrey's class had a pickle picnic. They had 35 dill pickles and 32 sweet pickles.

How many pickles in total were at the pickle picnic? _____
On the back, show how you figured out the answer.

Name _____

"Bee" a Mathematician

Kathy watches a beehive from her window.
She notices that no bee works in a cell that touches
another cell. Draw bees in the cells to show
what Kathy sees. One bee is drawn in for you.

How many bees are working in this beehive?

_____

Name _____

Parade Hats

For the May Day parade, 27 children and 7 adults were playing in the marching band.
The band ordered 35 fancy hats with feathers.

Did everyone get a hat?

Circle Yes or No.   **YES**   **NO**

Write an equation to explain your answer _____

Name _____

Cricket Jumps

A cricket jumped along a number line. He took equal jumps to the number 12.
He could do this in 4 ways.
Circle the numbers he jumped on. (Hint: He didn't start on 1.)

Jump #1: 1 2 3 4 5 6 7 8 9 10 11 12   Jump #3: 1 2 3 4 5 6 7 8 9 10 11 12

Jump #2: 1 2 3 4 5 6 7 8 9 10 11 12   Jump #4: 1 2 3 4 5 6 7 8 9 10 11 12

Name _____

Zoo Weigh-In

Zoey's class went to the zoo. They wrote down how much the animals weighed. Cut out the animals below. Arrange them in weight order—from lightest to heaviest.

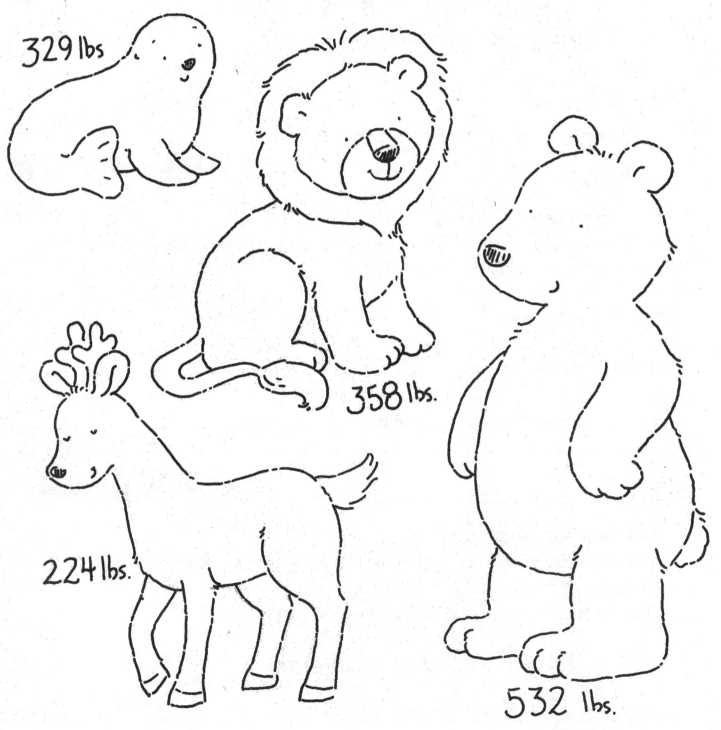

329 lbs

358 lbs.

224 lbs.

532 lbs.

Name _____

Chester's Cakes and Pies

Fill in the blanks. Chester Chipmunk was cutting cakes and pies.
Bobby Bear said, "Some aren't cut in half.

When you cut something in half, there are _____

pieces and both of the pieces are the same _____."

Here is how Chester cut the cakes and pies.
Circle the desserts that are cut in half correctly.

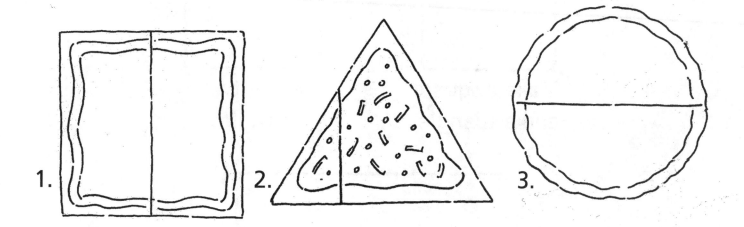

1.   2.   3.

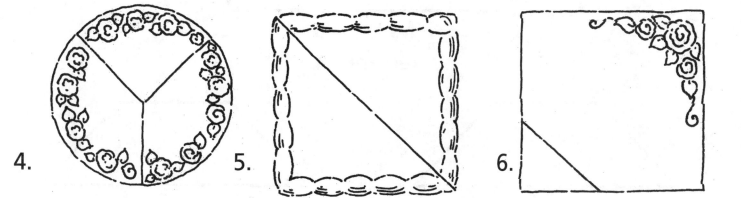

4.   5.   6.

Shape Tricks

Danny's class was learning about shapes. He noticed that you could draw a line across one shape to make two shapes. Draw a line through each shape below to make two new shapes. (Hint: Pattern blocks may help you.)

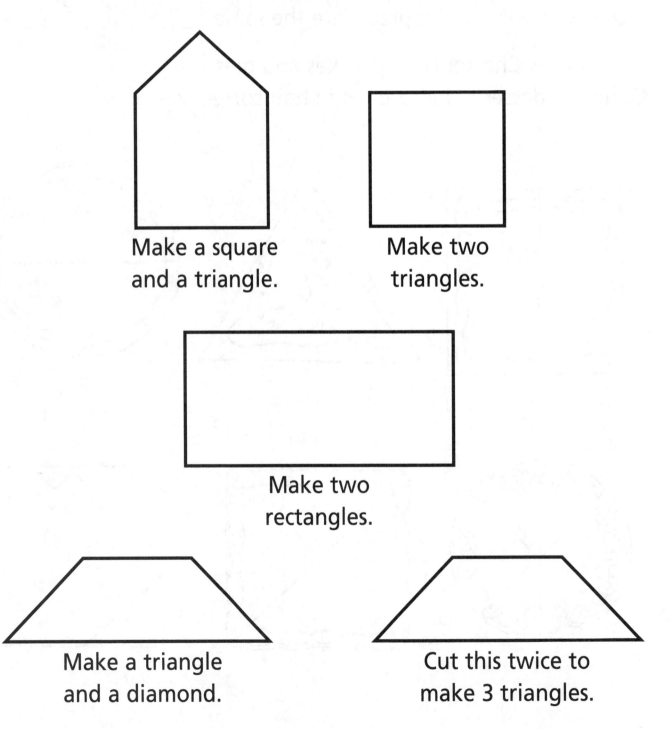

Make a square
and a triangle.

Make two
triangles.

Make two
rectangles.

Make a triangle
and a diamond.

Cut this twice to
make 3 triangles.

Candy Boxes

Steve works in a candy store. He puts candy into boxes. Each box has 10 spaces. Steve has 32 candies. Try to draw 32 candies in the boxes below. Write the number of candies in each box on the line. Write the number of any leftover candy at the bottom of the page.

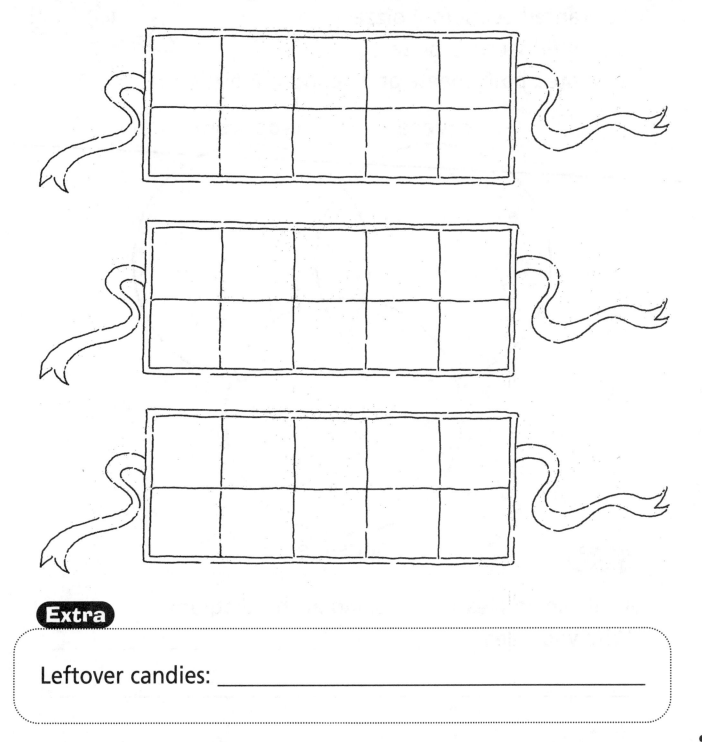

Extra

Leftover candies: _____

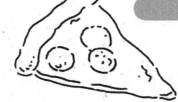

Pizza Party

Garth's class is having a pizza party. They made a diagram to show which pizzas they would like. Draw an X in each circle to show how many classmates wanted each kind of pizza.

- 5 wanted cheese pizza.
- 10 wanted pepperoni pizza.
- 3 wanted sausage pizza.
- 2 wanted both cheese and pepperoni pizza.

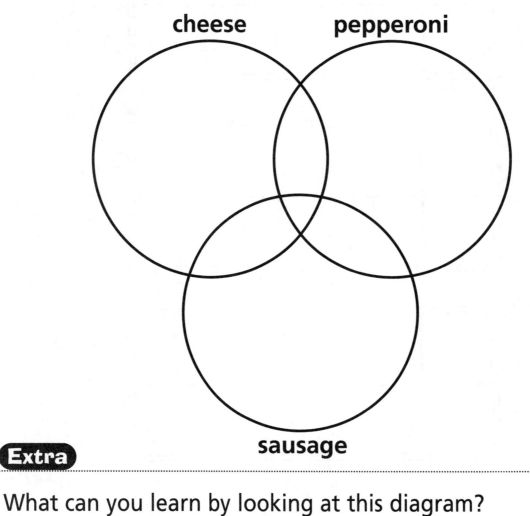

Extra

What can you learn by looking at this diagram?

Write your ideas: _____

_____

June

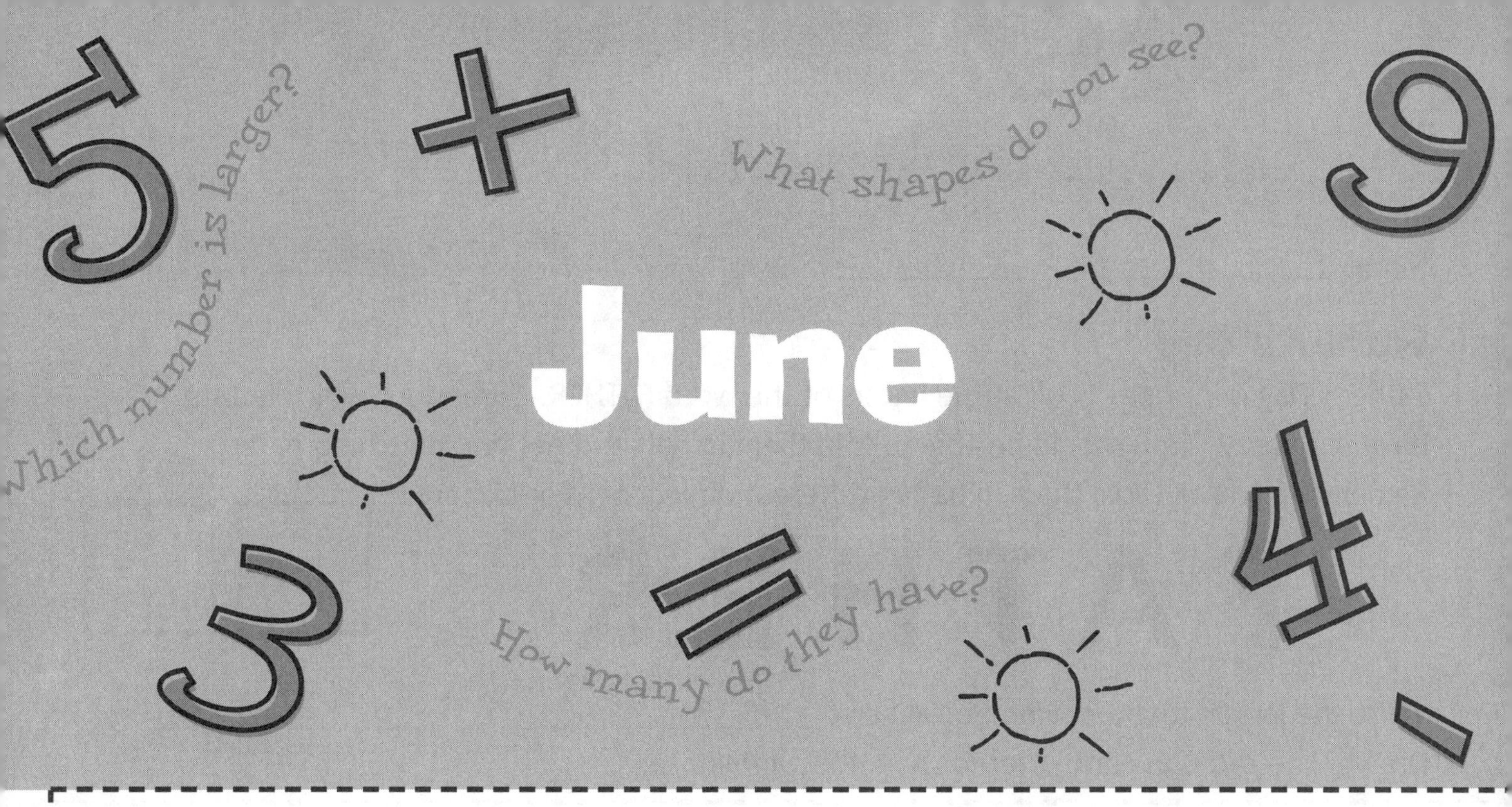

Which number is larger?
What shapes do you see?
How many do they have?

Name ______________________________

Recognizing Patterns, Addition

Picnic Patterns

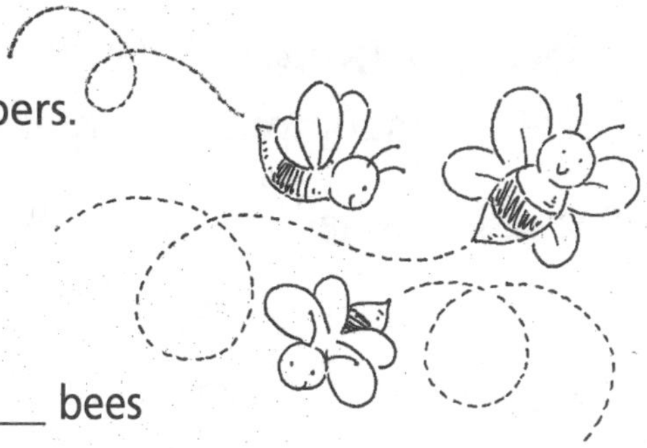

Figure out the pattern below by filling in the correct numbers.

5 flies, 8 chickadees

11 gnats, ____________________ fleas

____________________ ants, and ____________________ bees

Are all at the picnic with you and me.

What pattern do the numbers have? ____

Name ______________________________

Graphing, Comparing

Favorite Ball Games

Which ball games do your classmates like to play?
Record their answers on a bar graph, like the one below

Soccer								
Baseball								

Look at your graph. Complete this sentence with information you learn from the graph.

More children like______________________ than______________________ .

How many in each group?

What patterns do you see?

Name _____

Name _____

Name _____

Symmetry

Father's Day

Father's Day is in June. Look at the letters of the word FATHER. Figure out which letters have symmetry. (You should be able to fold them in half and get two matching parts.) Remember, you can fold them in half in different directions. For example:

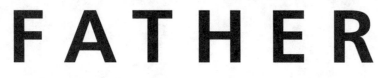

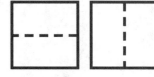

Write the letters that are symmetrical here: _____
Draw a line through each letter to show the symmetry.

Money, Multiplication

She Sells Seashells

Solve this math tongue-twister riddle.

She sells seashells by the seashore.

If each seashell sells for 3¢,
how much do 6 seashells cost? _____

Addition, Greater Than/Less Than

Baseball Scores

Jesse's team was playing baseball with Harry's team. Look at the scoreboard below. Add the numbers.

| Jesse | 1 | 4 | 0 | 2 | 0 | 1 | 0 | 0 | 2 | Total _____ |
| Harry | 2 | 2 | 0 | 3 | 1 | 2 | 0 | 0 | 1 | Total _____ |

Who won? Show the winner in a greater than/less than equation _____ > _____

Winner _____

Name _____

Flag Day Patterns

Look at the flag of the United States.
Color in the flag here so it looks like the
flag in your classroom.

What patterns do you see on the flag? On the
back of this paper, or on another sheet, list all
the patterns. Then describe the patterns, or
draw them. Hint: How many stars in each row?

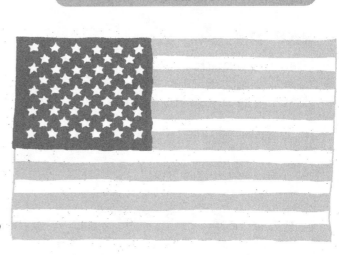

Name _____

Probability, Fractions

Spinners for the School Fair

Joey was making spinners for a game booth at
the school fair. Each spinner had a red section
and a white section. Look at the spinners below.
Which spinners are fair?
(Hint: A fair spinner has the same chance of landing on
a red section as a white section.) Circle the fair spinners.

Extra: On the back, explain why one spinner is not fair.

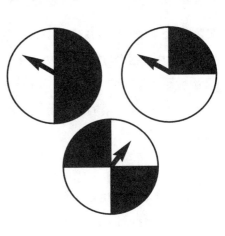

Name _____

Fractions

Quilt Squares

Lenny's class is making a class quilt for the
end of the year. Each child can use two colors.
On the back, or on another sheet of paper,
draw quilt squares with two colors. Each color
must cover 1/2 of the square.

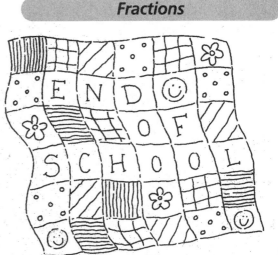

How many in each group?
What patterns do you see?

Name _____

365 Days to Go

Shauna's birthday was today. Her next birthday will be in 365 days. That's one whole year.

How many hundreds is that? _____

How many tens is that? _____

How many ones is that? _____

Extra: A leap year has 366 days. How many hundreds, tens, and ones are in a leap year?

Name _____

Pizza Party Puzzler

The porcupines had a pizza party on the last day of school. Peter Porcupine was very hungry. Should he have 1/4 of a pizza or 1/3 of a pizza?

_____

Look at these pizzas. Circle the correct one to show which fraction is more.

Name _____

All Sorts of Animals

Milo's class learned about all sorts of animals. Look at the
animals below. Cut them out. Sort them into groups that
show how some animals are alike. Then share your
groups with a friend. Did you sort them in the same way?

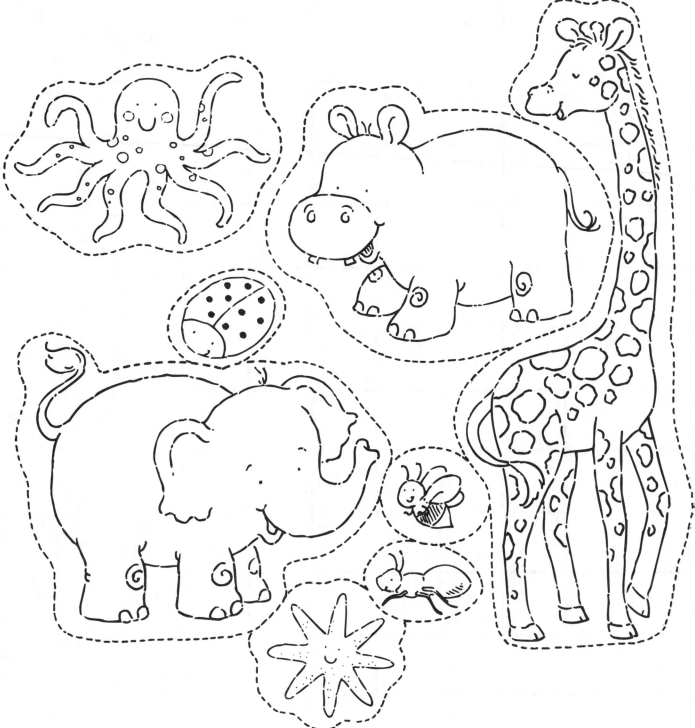

Favorite Class Subject

Which subjects do you and your classmates like the most?
Ask them to find out. Read each subject in the bar graph on
this page. Color in the square's to show each vote.

Math												
Science												
Reading												
Geography												
Social Studies												
Art												
P. E.												
Music												

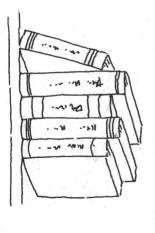

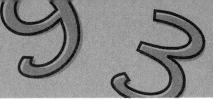

September

The Name Game, p. 7
Answers will vary but should reflect
the correct number of letters in each name.

Name Sort, p. 7
Answers will vary, but should accurately reflect the number of students in class. Other sorting ideas include: names that start with vowels, names that start with consonants; names with 1 syllable, 2 syllables, and so on; names with same beginning letters, names with same ending letters.

Off to School, p. 8
Answers will vary.

One Friend a day, p. 8
7, 7 Extra: 14

More Than 10, Less Than 10, p. 8
Answers will vary, depending on the group you set up.

Hide-and-Seek Countdown, p. 9
8 . . .5, 4 . . .2 Extra: 19 . . . 16 . . . 13, 12

Apple Colors, p. 9
Answers will vary.

Adding in Code, p. 9
EE, OU, E . . . E (THREE, FOUR, SEVEN)

Pencil Puzzler, p. 10
6 - 4 = 2, 2 + 2 = 4
Katie now has 4 pencils.

One Bee in Our Classroom, p. 10
7, 9

Apple Problems, p. 10
4, 4, Extra: 5, 5; 6, 6; 7, 7; 8, 8; 9, 9

Shapes All Around, p. 11
Answers will vary, but should reflect actual classroom objects and correct shape names.

Red, Black, Snap, Clap, p. 11
Black, black, red; ABBABBABBA
Extra: snap, clap, clap, snap, clap, clap snap

The Last Leaves, p. 11
The maple tree has 8 leaves. 5 + 3 = 8

Falling Leaves, p. 12
7 Extra: Answers will vary.

Classroom Zoo, p. 12
Groups: mice (3), turtles (3), fish (3)

Who Needs Glasses?, p. 12
14; 2, 4, 6, 8, 10, 12, 14

Frog School, p. 13
Extra: 2

Big Foot, p. 14
Estimates will vary. Actual length is 5".

Mary Had a Little Puppy, p. 15
followed, above, under, in, up

Fall Leaf Patterns, p. 16
Leaf patterns will vary.

October

Coin Detective, p. 17
The dime is smaller than the nickel, but it's worth more.

Finger-Adding Game, p. 17
Answers will vary.

Finding Favorite Colors, p. 18
Answers will vary, but should reflect the rows of color tiles students set up.

Falling Pumpkins, p. 18
7

Waiting in Line, p. 18
6, 10

One and Only One, p. 19
5 - 4 = 1   3 - 2 = 1   4 - 3 = 1   2 - 1 = 1

Shape Hunters, p. 19
1. cylinder   2. sphere   3. cone   4. cube   5. rectangular or cube

Poodles and Beagles, p. 19
2 poodles + 6 beagles = 8 dogs in all   3 poodles + 5 beagles = 8 dogs in all
4 poodles + 4 beagles = 8 dogs in all   5 poodles + 3 beagles = 8 dogs in all
6 poodles + 2 beagles = 8 dogs in all   7 poodles + 1 beagles = 8 dogs in all

Big Bad Wolf Math, p. 20
1. handspan   2. giant step   3. giant step   4. handspan

National Cookie Month, p. 20
3 Extra: 4

Disappearing Counting Cubes, p. 20
Answers will vary.

Nan's Number Cubes, p. 21

Jack-o'-Lantern Designer, p. 21
Answers will vary.

Three Halloween Kittens, p. 21
4 + 1 + 5 = 10   4 + 2 + 4 = 10   4 + 5 + 1 = 10   4 + 4 + 2 = 10   4 + 3 + 3 = 10

Trick or Treat?, p. 22
yes; 3 + 2 = 5; 2 + 3 = 5

Comparing Costumes, p. 22
3; 11 - 8 = 3

What's Your Costume?, p. 22
Answers will vary. Graph should be set up as a bar graph.
Answers should reflect information from the graph.

A Friendly Scarecrow, p. 23
4, 2 + 2 = 4
Extra: 6, 8, The numbers are double.

Sign Shape, p. 24
Yield sign: triangle, 3   Caution sign: diamond, 4
Speed-limit sign: rectangle, 4   Stop sign: octagon, 8

Ladybug Dots, p. 25
4 + 4 = 8   5 + 5 = 10   6 + 6 = 12   7 + 7 = 14   8 + 8 = 16
Extra: 6, 8, 10, 12, 14, 16   Pattern: Count by 2s, even numbers, doubling

Sorting Treats, p. 26
Great than: 10: 12 chocolate bars, 11 pennies, 15 pieces of gum, 13 candied apples.
Less than: 10: 7 boxes of raisins, 8 lollipops, 4 oranges, 1 cookie

November

Piggy Bank Puzzle, p. 27
dimes; nickels

Favorite Pet Tally, p. 27
Answers will vary. The favorite pet is the animal with the most tallies.

Playing in the Snow, p. 28
6 + 6 + 12,   6 + 7 = 13

ABC Sort, p. 28
Possible categories: vowels and consonants; letter will all curved lines, all straight lines, and both curved and straight lines; letters with and without symmetry; the number of strokes it takes to make each letter.

How Many Birthdays?, p. 28
4, 11 - 7 = 4 Extra: 15

Game and Puzzle Week, p. 29
2 + 7 = 9   9 - 2 = 7   7 + 2 = 9   9 - 7 = 2

Birthday Riddle, p. 29
9

Sledding Time, p. 29
Example: How many children in all?   5+3=8
How many more girls than boys?   5-3=2

Wildlife Shelter, p. 30
45 > 39, 45 > 28   28 < 39, 28 < 45   39 > 28, 39 < 45

Mystery Drawing, p. 30
Students should draw a turkey.

Gobbler Riddle, p. 30
1 + 9 = 10   2 + 8 = 10   3 + 7 = 10   4 + 6 = 10
5 + 5 = 10   6 + 4 + 10   7 + 3 = 10
8 + 2 = 10   9+1=10

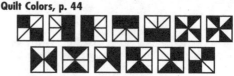
Thanksgiving Puzzler, p. 31
11-3=8
Possible answer: The more you take away from 11, the smaller the answer is.

Mystery Holiday, p. 31
11th month: November   Date: Answers will vary.   Holiday: Thanksgiving

Mashed, Baked, or Fried?, p. 31
Answers will vary.

Scavenger Hunt, p. 32
Answers will vary.

Collecting Food, p. 33
The answer could be a graph with 3 cans of chili, 3 cans of veggies, and 4 cans of soup.

Money Matters, p. 34
Alex's coins: 5¢ + 25¢ + 10¢ = 60 ¢
Billy's coins: 10¢ + 10¢ + 10¢ + 10¢ + 10¢ + 5¢ + 5¢ + 1¢ + 1¢ + 1¢ = 63¢
63¢ > 60¢ Billy has more money.

Penguin Family on Parade, p. 35
3 1/2 inches, 2 inches, 1 1/2 inches, 3 inches. Patty, Peter, Petunia, Paul.

Thanksgiving Play, p. 36
2; Pilgrims, 4; Native Americans, Extra: 6,2

December

One and Off the Bus, p. 37
5; 4 - 2 = 2; 2 + 3 = 5

Magic Tricks, p. 37
Trick 1: 6 - 6 = 0   Trick 2: 0 + 5 = 5

Beehive Hexagons, p. 38

Basketball Time, p. 38
1 minute, 5 minutes, 2 hours

Barn Owl's Mistake, p. 38
Wrong answers: 4 + 5 = 7, 6 + 7 = 11   Correct answers: 4 + 5 = 9, 6 + 7 = 13
Barn owl is doubling and subtracting 1, instead of doubling and adding 1.

Cold Fingers and Toes, p. 39
Children could skip count by fives or tens.
Multiplication: 4 x 20 = 80; or 5 x 16 = 80; or 4 x 10 (fingers) = 40 fingers;
4 x 10 toes = 40 toes; 40 + 40 = 80

Two by Two, p. 39
Answers will vary. If the class has an even number of students, each student will have a partner. If the class has an odd number of students, one student will not have a partner.

The Goldfish Gift, p. 39
Possible answers: 1 quarter; 25 pennies; 2 dimes + 1 nickel; 2 dimes + 5 pennies;
1 dime + 3 nickels; 1 dime + 2 nickels + 5 pennies; 1 dime + 1 nickel + 10 pennies;
5 nickels, 15 pennies + 1 dime; 15 pennies + 2 nickels; 20 pennies + 1 nickel

Exactly in the Middle, p. 40
65

Pie Slices, p. 40
1; 2 Extra: 3

A Nickel a Month, p. 40
60¢; 5 x 12 = 60   5, 10, 15, 20, 25, 30, 35, 40, 45, 50, 55, 60

Thumb Prints and Hand Spans, p. 41
hand span; answers will vary; answers will vary (Note: The total number of hand spans should be less than the total number of thumb prints.)

A Wingful of Books, p. 41
You need to know the total number of books Owl took out.
Answers will vary, but should include the number 7: [student's number] - 7 = _____

Holiday Piggy Bank, p. 41
4 pennies; 5 pennies; 15

Family Time at Holiday Time, p. 42
Answers will vary.

Holiday Cookies, p. 42
1 carrot + 9 sugar = 10 cookies   2 carrot + 8 sugar = 10 cookies
3 carrot + 7 sugar = 10 cookies   4 carrot + 6 sugar = 10 cookies
5 carrot + 5 sugar = 10 cookies   6 carrot + 4 sugar = 10 cookies
7 carrot + 3 sugar = 10 cookies   8 carrot + 2 sugar = 10 cookies
9 carrot + 1 sugar = 10 cookies

Snowflakes on Mittens, p. 43
Estimates will vary. 2, 4, 6, 8, 10, 12, 14, 16, 18, 20, 5, 10, 15, 20
Extra: no; Snowflakes would melt before you could count them.

Quilt Colors, p. 44

Cabin in the Snow, p. 45
6, 5, 4 Extra: hexagon—snowflake, pentagon—cabin, rectangle—doorway, circle—pancake

December Weather, p. 46
Sunny days: 12   Cloudy days: 8   Rainy days: 5   Snowy days: 6

January

Muffins by the Dozen, p. 47
7; 12 - 5 = 7

Rolling and Stacking, p. 47
sphere, cylinder, cube, cylinder

Penguin School, p. 48
5; Without weekends, a week has only 5 days.
Extra: 10

Guess My Number, p. 48
33, 34, 35, 36; no
Possible hints: It is an odd number. Both numerals are the same. You can get there if you skip count by 3's. It's less than 34.

Hibernation Breaks, p. 48
a cube; 4 (A cylinder has 2 flat sides. A cube has 6.)

Danny Duck's Dinner, p. 49
snail, ant.

Winter Boots and Socks, p. 49
Students might say that the boots weigh more because they are bigger and because they are wet.

Riddle Time, p. 49
6 (2, 4, 6, 8, 10; 3, 6, 9)

MLK, Jr.'s Birthday, p. 50
January 15

All Lined Up, p. 50
Bo, Mindy, Jane, Tim

Cathy's Cast, p. 50
January 28

Cool Calculations, p. 51
4 + 4 + 4 + 4 = 16; 4 + 4 + 3 = 11

Bear Family Quilts, p. 51

Temperature Matcheroo, p. 51
90°—summer   70°—spring   50°—fall   30°—winter

Favorite Number Graph, p. 52
Answers will vary.

Squirrel Math, p. 52
Pile #1: 10 Pile #2: 10 Pile #3: 10 Pile #4: 6
10 + 10 + 10 + 6 = 36

Pie Fight, p. 52
15; 26—11 = 15

National Popcorn Day, p. 53
Estimates will vary. Answers will vary. Greater than/less than equations will vary.

Coin Puzzler, p. 53
1 dime, 1 nickel, 1 penny
Extra: 2 dimes, 1 nickel, 1 penny

Scarf Patterns, p. 54
Pattern #1: triangle, heart, triangle, heart, triangle, heart
Pattern #2: little star, big star, little star, big star, little star, big star
Pattern #3: sun, sun, cloud, cloud, sun, sun, cloud

What to Wear?, p. 55
Total amount of outfits = 6
Answers to second question will vary.

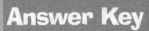

Dalmatian Spots, p. 56
Answers (estimates) will vary. Total amount: 50
Skip count by 5's: 5, 10, 15, 20, 25, 30, 35, 40, 45, 50

February

Chinese New York, p. 57
3 quarters; 3 quarters is 75¢, which is more than 7 dimes, which is only 70¢.

Ground Hog Day, p. 57
12:00

Black History Month, p. 58
no; 39 + 3 = 42, not 43

Pennies and Paper Clips, p. 58
Answers will vary. When experimenting, students should discover that the pennies will be heavier, but the paper clips will be longer.

100th Day of School, p. 58
Estimates will vary. 10, 20, 30, 40, 50, 60, 70, 80, 90, 100; 10

Thirsty, Anyone?, p. 59
Answers will vary.

Bear Riddles, p. 59
polar bear; grizzly bear

President Pictures, p. 59
13 dollars; 5 dollars + 5 dollars = 10 dollars
1 dollar + 1 dollar + 1 dollar = 3 dollars
10 dollars + 3 dollars = 13 dollars

Who Is Older?, p. 60
Ashley; January comes before February, so Ashley is about one month older than Josh.

Slopping Winter Boots, p. 60
6 Extra: 8

Odd + Odd, p. 60
1 + 7 = 8; 3 + 5 = 8
Two odd numbers always add up to an even number. One even number and one odd number always add up to an odd number.

So Many Stamps!, p. 61
2 rows of 6 stamps
3 rows of 4 stamps
4 rows of 3 stamps
6 rows of 2 stamps

Valentine Count, p. 61
18; 6 + 6 + 6 = 18, or 6 x 3 = 18

Special Birthday, p. 61
2; 20; 20; 2000; They all have 2s, or 2s and 0s.
Extra: Turning 9 on September 9, 1999 (9/9/99)

Measuring His Shadow, pp. 62–63
10; 5; They were both right.

Snow-Print Detective, p. 64
stringed box = square
plant pot = triangle
drum = circle
book = rectangle

Valentine Symmetry, p. 65
symmetrical: heart, triangle, even V, hexagon
symmetrical twice: hexagon

Valentine Stickeroo, p. 66

O	O	X	X		X	X	O	O		X	O	X	O
O	X	O	X		X	O	O	X		O	X	X	O

Picking Out Patterns, p. 67
1. 32, 42, 52, 62, 72, 82, 92   2. 70, 60, 50, 40, 30, 20, 10
3. 67, 57, 47, 37, 27, 17, 7   4. 44, 55, 66, 77, 88, 99

Presidents' Day Problem, p. 68
1. the 1st   2. the 16th   3. James Buchanan   4. Andrew Johnson   5. 14

March

Colorful Kites, p. 69
Students' pictures should look like this:

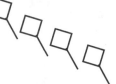

What's for Breakfast?, p. 69
Answers will vary.

The Three Bears' Orange Juice, p. 70
Possible estimates: 6 cups, 4 cups. Explanation: Baby Bear's thermos is about half the size of Papa Bear's thermos, or 4 cups. Mama Bear's thermos is about in between in size, or 6 cups.

Money Riddle, p. 70
15¢; 10 + 5 = 15
17¢; 15 + 2 = 17

The Shrinking Teddy Bear, p. 70
Thursday: 14 inches   Friday: 12 inches   Saturday: 10 inches
The bear could be shrinking because it has a hole and is losing stuffing.

Finding Gold, p. 71
12; 7 + 8 = 15; 15 - 3 = 12

Leprechaun Gold, p. 71
5; 6 or more; [student's answer] > 5

Leprechaun Steps, p. 71
Estimates will vary. Number of steps will vary.

Who Won?, p. 72
64; 46; 64 > 46; Jane's team won.

Dog Calculations, p. 72
10, 15, 20, 25

Lost-and-Found Mystery, p. 72
22; 26 - 4 = 22
Extra: Possible answer: Children wear jackets and sweatshirts in the wnter.

Kite Store, p. 73
50; 10 x 5 = 50 or 10+10+10+10+10=50

The Year of the Dragon, p. 73
22; 10 + 12 = 22

Johnny Appleseed Math, p. 73
86

Paul's Peanut Machine, p. 74
17, 18, 20; The machine is adding 10 more peanuts to the original amount put in the machine.

Mark's Baby Sister, p. 74
When Krista is 1, Mark is 8.   When Krista is 2, Mark is 9.
When Krista is 3, Mark is 10.   When Krista is 4, Mark is 11.
When Krista is 5, Mark is 12.   When Krista is 6, Mark is 13.
When Krista is 7, Mark is 14.   When Krista is 8, Mark is 15.
Double: When Krista is 7, Mark is 14.

Amusement Park Math, p. 74
3; 12 ÷ 4 = 3

Peter Piper's Pickled Peppers, p. 75
19; 26 - 7 = 19

Would You Rather Have . . .?, p. 75
no; 5 dimes = 50¢, which is more money than 46¢

Classroom Garage Sale, p. 76
Possible groups: Balls: soccer ball, basketball, rubber ball
Winter clothes: scarf, hat, boots   Art supplies: paint, paint brush, crayon

Patterns for the Mail Carrier, p. 77
Top side of the street: 50, 52, 54, 56   Bottom side of the street: 51, 53, 55
Extra: The even numbers are on one side of the street. The odd numbers are on the other side of the street.

Bird Feeder Geometry, p. 78
1. cube, octagon, hexagon, rectangle, square, rectangle solid
2. cyclinder, triangle, circle, rectangle

April

April Fools?, p. 79
no; 2 dimes + 13 pennies = 33¢;
This is more money than 3 dimes + 2 pennies, which is 32¢.

Party Balloons, p. 79
no; 15 ÷ 3 = 5 or three divides evenly into 15

Ricky Recycles, p. 80
Answers will vary, depending on current year's calendar. There will be 4–5 Fridays for each month. Number sentences will vary, but show all 3 numbers being added, for example, 4 + 5 + 4 = 13

Baseball Shapes, p. 80
bases = squares   home plate = pentagon
infield = diamond   pitcher's mound = circle and square

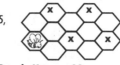

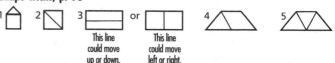

Donuts in a Bag, p. 80
sugar donut; There are more sugar donuts than glazed donuts.

Benny's One-Man Band, p. 81
25 pounds; yes

A Tricky Way to Tell Time, p. 81
1. 3:00, or 12:15   2. 9:00, or 11:45   3. 12:00   4. 6:00

Barnyard Patterns, p. 81
8 (2 x 4)   12 (3 x 4)   16 (4 x 4)   20 (5 x 4)   24 (6 x 4)

Animal Garden Addition, p. 82
37; 24 + 13 = 37

The Ants Get Their Exercise, p. 82
triangle: 7 inches
rectangle: 7 inches

Blackbirds, p. 82
24; students' new number sentences and numerals will vary. Make sure they
follow the same pattern as the rhyme, with the ones coming before the tens.

A Prickly Problem, p. 83
The rectangle and the parallelogram go inside the circle because all shapes here have
four sides. The triangle goes outside the circle because it does not have four sides.

The Biggest Number, p. 83
53 + 42 = 95

Planting Beans, p. 83
23 + 16 = 39
Extra: The string beans grew. Jelly beans are not real beans, but candy.

Mr. McGregor's Garden, p. 84
20; 30 - 10 = 20

Farm Animals Weigh In, p. 84
lamb and baby goat on one side; piglet on the other side

Groups of Geese, p. 84
3 groups of 10; 7 geese are left over

National Coin Week, p. 85
One child gets: 2 dimes + 1 nickel (25¢)   One child gets: 1 dime + 3 nickels (25¢)

Billy Goat's Raisins, p. 85
12

Creature Categories, p. 86
3 groups: fish, shells, animals with multiple legs/arms

Time to Get Up!, p. 87
15; 8

Jack's Beanstalk, p. 88
2 inches; 4 inches
Two possible answers:
6 inches, because it grew 2 inches each week; or
8 inches, because it doubled in height each week

May

Ice-Cream Favorites, p. 89
Answers will vary.

Shape Riddles, p. 89
cube; cone

Getting Ready, p. 90
12:30; yes; Extra: 1/2 hour or 30 minutes

Snoozing in May, p. 90
Day 1: 8   Day 2: 16   Day 3: 24   Day 4: 32   Day 5: 40   Day 6: 48   Day 7: 56

Cluck, Neigh, Moo, p. 90
Woof, neigh, moo; Oink, neigh, meow, neigh, moo

Birthdays in May, p. 91
Danielle; 3 weeks is 21 days, which is longer than 18 days.

Spider Survey, p. 91
Answers will vary.

Mother's Day Decisions, p. 91
Answers will vary.

Spring Shelter, p. 92
raccoon toes: 20   parrot toes: 8
12

Heads and Feet, p. 92
2 horses, 2 chickens

International Pickle Week, p. 92
67

"Bee" a Mathematician, p. 93
5,

Parade Hats, p. 93
yes; 27 + 7 = 34

Cricket Jumps, p. 93
Jump # 1: 2, 4, 6, 8, 10, 12   Jump #2: 3, 6, 9, 12   Jump #3: 4, 8, 12   Jump #4: 6, 12

Zoo Weigh-In, p. 94
deer (224 pounds), seal (329 pounds), lion (358 pounds), bear (532 pounds)

Chester's Cakes and Pies, p. 95
2, size; Correct pies: 1, 3, 5

Shape Tricks, p. 96
1   2   3   This line could move up or down.   or   This line could move left or right.   4   5

Candy Boxes, p. 97
10, 10, 10 Extra: 2

Pizza Party, p. 98
Extra: Answers will vary. Possible: Pepperoni is the most popular topping.
Cheese is the next favorite topping. Sausage is the least favorite topping.

June

Picnic Patterns, p. 99
14 fleas; 17 ants 20 bees
Pattern: Each number is the previous number plus 3.

Favorite Ball Games, p. 99
Answers will vary.

Father's Day, p. 100
A, T, H, E

She Sells Seashells, p. 100
18¢

Baseball Scores, p. 100
Jesse's total: 10   Harry's total: 11   11 > 10   winner: Harry

Flag Day Patterns, p. 101
red strip, white stripe, red stripe, white stripe;
horizontally, stars are in rows of 6, 5, 6, 5;
vertically, stars are in columns of 5, 4, 5, 4;
every other row of stars is indented

Spinners for the School Fair, p. 101
1. fair; the red and white sides are the same size.
2. not fair; the spinner would probably land on white because the white section
   is larger than the red section.
3. fair; both colors have two sections that are the same size.

Quilt Squares, p. 101
Possible answers:

365 Days to Go, p. 102
3 hundreds, 6 tens, 5 ones
Extra: 3 hundreds, 6 tens, 6 ones

Pizza Party Puzzler, p. 102
1/3, the pie with 3 pieces should be circled.

All Sorts of Animals, p. 103
Answers will vary. Possible ways to sort:
insects/fish/mammals; number of legs; live in air vs. water

Favorite Class Subject, p. 104
Answers will vary.

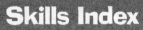